T0212301

Ethics and Error in Medicine

This book is a collection of original, interdisciplinary chapters on the topic of medical error. Given the complexities of understanding, preventing, and responding to medical error in ethically responsible ways, the scope of the book is fairly broad. The contributors include top scholars and practitioners working in bioethics, communication, law, medicine, and philosophy. Their contributions examine preventable causes of medical error, disproportionate impacts of errors on vulnerable populations, disclosure and apology after discovering medical errors, and ethical issues arising in specific medical contexts, such as radiation oncology, psychopathy, and palliative care. They also offer practical recommendations for respecting autonomy, distributing burdens and benefits justly, and minimizing injury to patients and other stakeholders. *Ethics and Error in Medicine* will be of interest to a wide range of researchers, students, and practitioners in bioethics, philosophy, communication studies, law, and medicine who are interested in the ethics of medical error.

Fritz Allhoff is Professor in the Department of Philosophy at Western Michigan University. He has had fellowships in the Institute for Ethics of the American Medical Association and in the Center for Law and the Biosciences at Stanford Law School. His books have been published by Oxford University Press, University of Chicago Press, among others.

Sandra L. Borden is Professor in the School of Communication and Director of the Center for the Study of Ethics in Society at Western Michigan University. Her books include the award-winning *Journalism as Practice: MacIntyre, Virtue Ethics and the Press* (Ashgate 2007; Routledge 2009).

Routledge Research in Applied Ethics

The Capability Approach in Practice
A New Ethics for Setting Development Agendas
Morten Fibieger Byskov

The Ethics of Counterterrorism
Isaac Taylor

Disability with Dignity
Justice, Human Rights and Equal Status
Linda Barclay

Media Ethics, Free Speech, and the Requirements of Democracy
Edited by Carl Fox and Joe Saunders

Ethics and Chronic Illness
Tom Walker

The Future of Work, Technology, and Basic Income
Edited by Michael Chobli and Michael Weber

The Ethics of Eating Animals
Usually Bad, Sometimes Wrong, Often Permissible
Bob Fischer

Self-Defense, Necessity, and Punishment
A Philosophical Analysis
Uwe Steinhoff

Ethics and Error in Medicine
Edited by Fritz Allhoff and Sandra L. Borden

Ethics and Error in Medicine

Edited by
Fritz Allhoff
Sandra L. Borden

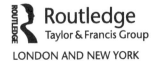

Routledge
Taylor & Francis Group

LONDON AND NEW YORK

First published 2020 by Routledge

2 Park Square, Milton Park, Abingdon, Oxon OX14 4RN
605 Third Avenue, New York, NY 10017

Routledge is an imprint of the Taylor & Francis Group, an informa business

First issued in paperback 2021

Library of Congress Cataloging-in-Publication Data
A catalog record for this book has been requested

ISBN: 978-0-367-21791-4 (hbk)
ISBN: 978-1-03-217682-6 (pbk)
DOI: 10.4324/9780429266119

Typeset in Sabon
Apex CoVantage, LLC

In Memory of Shirley Bach

Contents

Figures

Foreword

This book is a fitting tribute to the life and career of Dr. Shirley Bach, who specialized in the field of biomedical ethics. Sadly, she passed away on February 13, 2018, at age 86, before she would have had an opportunity to enjoy reading the contents of this edited volume on ethics and medical error. As one of her longtime friends and colleagues, I would like to write a few words about this very special person.

Shirley and her husband, Michael, received their doctorates in chemistry from the University of Wisconsin-Madison in the late 1950s. They came to Kalamazoo, Michigan, shortly after that, as Michael began working as a researcher at the Upjohn Pharmaceutical Company. Shirley began teaching part time in Western Michigan University's (WMU) Department of Chemistry in 1961, and she served as a research associate from 1964 to 1971. In 1971, Shirley became a full-time assistant professor of Natural Science in the College of General Studies. It was shortly after this that she developed her popular and highly acclaimed course in biomedical ethics. Before doing so, however, she consulted with the Department of Philosophy to see if anyone there was interested in collaborating with her in examining this rapidly developing area of academic and societal interest. The answer at that time was that there was not. But this did not dissuade her from proceeding in creating the course. Largely due to her persistent desire to talk with philosophers about ethical issues in the biomedical world, members of the Department of Philosophy began to shed their initial indifference.

By 1985, it was evident that quite a number of faculty from a variety of departments at WMU had developed serious academic interests in major ethical issues of the day—issues in medicine, medical research, nursing, business, communication, criminal justice, engineering, political science, research ethics, social work, sociology, and so on. Shirley had a keen interest in all of them. So, in the fall of 1985, she, James Jaksa (from the Department of Communication Arts and Science), and I launched WMU's Center for the Study of Ethics in Society. The Center was sponsored by the Graduate College, rather than locating itself in any particular academic department. An advisory board for the center was organized that had representatives from every college in the University.

Shirley remained in the College of General Studies until it was dissolved in 1989. By then a full professor and well-entrenched in the field of bioethics, she was eagerly welcomed into the Department of Philosophy, her choice of a department in which to relocate. Although she retired from WMU in 1997, she stayed active in the Center for the Study of Ethics in Society as Associate Director up until the time of her passing.

Shirley was an outstanding teacher, receiving WMU's top teaching award—the Alumni Award for Teaching Excellence—as well as the Honors Convocation Award of the Association of Governing Boards of State Universities. I was fortunate to have the opportunity to team-teach with her a couple of times. So, I know firsthand how deserving of those awards she was.

Shortly after the issuance of the Belmont Report in 1978, Shirley led the way in establishing WMU's Institutional Review Board (IRB), serving as its first chair. From the outset, under Shirley's strong leadership, WMU's IRB secured a reach beyond the natural science areas, covering the social sciences as well. This required both determination and courage, as this was met with strong resistance by some research faculty in the social sciences. But Shirley was more than up to the task.

During her long and distinguished career, Shirley established strong ties with Michigan State University's Center for Ethics and Humanities; the Karolinska Institute in Stockholm, Sweden; Bronson and Borgess Hospitals' Biomedical Ethics Committees in Kalamazoo; and the Western Michigan University Homer Stryker M.D. School of Medicine. She also served on the Michigan Medical Ethics Resource Network. She was well known and highly regarded as a presenter, consultant, and committee member throughout the Kalamazoo area, the State of Michigan, and elsewhere—including the Hastings Center in New York. Among the topics of her many presentations locally, statewide, and nationally were cloning, genetic screening, end-of-life decisions, organ transplants, and health care and research errors.

The topic of medical error was of special interest to Shirley. Tragically, her husband, Michael, died as a result of medical error at a renowned hospital. The hospital refused to offer her an apology for its mistakes. This, she said, was all that she wanted from the hospital. However, given this refusal, she reluctantly decided to file a lawsuit charging the hospital with gross negligence. She did this, not to obtain money, but to force into the open the issue of the importance of acknowledging and apologizing for medical mistakes. She won the lawsuit and used its proceeds to establish the Michael K. and Shirley R. Bach Endowment for the Center for the Study of Ethics in Society. This endowment has been used to sponsor public programs on medical ethics, especially ones that address the topic of medical error.

Shirley was an extraordinary person, much loved and admired by all who had the privilege of knowing her. She very much exemplified the spirit of the sort of collaborative inquiry that serious reflection on issues in practical ethics requires. This is especially so in regard to the importance of taking constructive steps to minimize the occurrence of medical errors and of acknowledging them when they occur. She would have been very pleased to have lived to be able to see this edited volume come to fruition.

Michael S. Pritchard
Professor of Philosophy, Emeritus
Western Michigan University
Kalamazoo, MI 49001

Acknowledgments

Most importantly, we acknowledge Dr. Shirley Bach, whose life's work and vision were the principal catalysts for this project.

Several of these chapters were first presented at a mini-conference organized by Western Michigan University's Center for the Study of Ethics in Society in partnership with the Association for Practical and Professional Ethics and the Western Michigan University Homer Stryker M.D. School of Medicine (Chicago, 2018). Several more were presented at a mini-conference at the Western Michigan University Medical Humanities Conference (Kalamazoo, 2018). We thank the presenters, audiences, and hosts for these fora, which contributed to the strength of the chapters.

For manuscript preparation, we received a grant from the Office for the Vice President of Research at Western Michigan University. We received additional funding and administrative assistance from the university's Center for the Study of Ethics in Society. We thank both these sources for their support.

Our research assistant, Luke Golemon, provided invaluable help in terms of author correspondence, copy-editing, formatting, and indexing. We are very grateful to him for his efforts. At Routledge, we thank Andrew Weckenmann for commissioning the project and for his support throughout the process. We also thank Allie Simmons, his editorial assistant. We also thank Umamaheswari Chelladurai for [her] help in the publication process, including copy-editing and typesetting.

We thank Michael S. Pritchard for his eloquent foreword. We also thank our authors for their chapters. They worked tirelessly through myriad rounds of editing and were gracious in their responses to feedback and ultimately produced excellent chapters. Finally, we thank you, the readers, for your interest in this topic; we hope that this book advances your understanding of and interest in ethics and medical error.

1 Introduction

Medicine, Mistakes, and Moral Evaluation

Sandra L. Borden

So often it is the little things.

A sophisticated computer-based system to match organ donors with organ recipients. A world-class tertiary medical facility. A team of expert surgeons. A rare heart–lungs combo that fit the cavity of a 17-year-old girl. Speedy transportation of the donated organs synchronized with the removal of the teenager's failing ones. Perfectly executed implantation of the donated organs.

The transplant surgeon, Dr. James Jaggers, takes the patient off bypass, ready to close the incision. Everything looks set for the medical miracle that drove Jésica Santillán's family to smuggle her over the border from Mexico and got her school and community in North Carolina to rally around her. And then the blood bank at Duke University Hospital informs the operating room that the organs are the wrong blood type (Diflo 2006, 73).

After urgent treatments to prevent hyperacute rejection of the donor's type-A organs, Dr. Jaggers immediately went to Jésica's family and personally informed them of the mistake; he also informed the United Network for Organ Sharing (UNOS). Duke, however, did not make a public statement about the error for several more days. Nearly two weeks after the first surgery and a TV plea by Jésica's mother, a new, blood-compatible heart and lungs became available for Jésica, who was now near death. Dr. Jaggers obtained the family's consent for a second surgery with the help of a family friend because the Santilláns did not speak English (Kopp 2003).

Fewer than 24 hours after the second transplant, Jésica suffered from bleeding and swelling in her brain, and, soon after, her brain stopped functioning. She was taken off life support and pronounced dead at 1:25 p.m. on February 22, 2003 (Kopp 2003).

A number of individuals at Duke, UNOS, the Boston hospital where the donor was treated, or the local organ procurement organization could have checked to make sure the donated organs matched Jésica's type O-positive blood type before the surgery. But no one did. Carolina Donor Services did not ask for Jésica's blood type before releasing the organs, as required by UNOS policy. Dr. Jaggers did not ask the donor's blood type as is standard practice. The cooler prepared for the donated organs was not labeled with the donor's blood type as required under transplantation protocols. Even if it had, the procuring surgeon did not know what Jésica's blood type was (Kopp 2003; Diflo 2006).

Everyone was focused on the amazing high-wire act of organ transplantation. Meanwhile, no one made sure there was a net on the ground before the act got started.

Attention to Patient Safety

Just four years before Jésica's transplant, the U.S. Institute of Medicine (IOM) issued the landmark report *To Err is Human: Building a Safer Health System.* The IOM report marked the unofficial beginning of the patient safety movement. Among other impacts, the report has been associated with a significant increase in the number of research articles published about patient safety, as well as in the number of federal grants awarded on the same topic (Stelfox et al. 2006). Hospitals and healthcare professionals have instituted a number of interventions to improve patient safety, such as the 2003 Michigan Keystone project for reducing IV line infections and other common ICU complications. Such checklists, along with information technology and other safety measures targeting systemic weak spots, have also been institutionalized since the report (for a summary of reforms, see Chapters 3 and 9). Nevertheless, the incidence of medical error continues to be alarmingly high.

Error is defined in the IOM report as "Failure of a planned action to be completed as intended or use of a wrong plan to achieve an aim" (Kohn, Corrigan, and Donaldson 2000, 210). Although this definition does not hinge on the occurrence of patient injury, or "adverse events," nevertheless patient safety advocates are quick to point out the toll medical error has on patients.[1] According to a 2016 analysis by Johns Hopkins experts, nearly 10 percent of all deaths in the United States are estimated to be the result of medical errors; the number of deaths attributable to medical error is exceeded only by heart disease and cancer. And that is not accounting for the fact that conventions used for billing codes and death certificates may be systematically undercounting medical error deaths (Makary and Daniel 2016).

Those dedicated to the IMO report's systems approach for preventing and catching medical errors (discussed in more detail later in the chapter) are hampered by a number of factors. These include misguided efforts to blame and punish individuals, the decentralized way in which health care is delivered and purchased in the United States, and the perverse incentives that exist in health-care organizations to take shortcuts, underreport errors and circumscribe systemic improvements in view of pragmatic considerations (Bosk 2006; Kohn, Corrigan, and Donaldson

2000). In addition, another major recommendation of the IMO report—toughening laws and regulations to exert external pressure on health-care organizations to improve their performance—has not gotten much traction beyond the passage of a patchwork of state laws requiring reporting of hospital-acquired infections and other selected medical errors (Editorial Board 2009).[2]

Ethical Principles in Medicine

Given that the incidence of medical error continues to be high, it is somewhat surprising that medical error has received relatively little scholarly attention in the last decade. Even less has been written about the ethical issues raised by medical error. The purpose of this volume is to bring much-needed attention to this context.

Beauchamp and Childress's (2012) *Principles of Biomedical Ethics*, now in its seventh edition, is the most widely used ethical framework in medical ethics. The framework proposes four general principles reflecting multiple theoretical approaches: respect for autonomy, non-maleficence, beneficence, and justice. All except justice are focused primarily on the patient. Respect for autonomy concerns the patient's freedom to choose for oneself without interference from others or under conditions that limit meaningful choice. Non-maleficence concerns providers' obligation to refrain from intentionally injuring patients. Beneficence requires helping patients by promoting good or preventing or removing harm. Justice concerns the fair and equitable treatment of all members of a society or system based on what they are due, as well as the fair distribution of benefits and burdens within that society or system.

These broad norms can be further specified into moral rules reflecting the particulars of the medical context. For example, Beauchamp and Childress (2012) propose moral rules for autonomy concerning informed consent for medical treatment. The general principles may conflict in practice; if they cannot be balanced, one must determine which obligation is overriding in that specific situation. Here, Beauchamp and Childress model their approach after W.D. Ross's distinction between a prima facie obligation—one that is binding all things being equal—and an actual obligation—one that is binding all things considered; that is, in view of the relative weight of all the relevant obligations in the particular circumstances.

The framework relates the four principles and their moral rules to virtues in biomedical ethics, as well as professional–client relationships and various ethical theories. In sum, it aims to provide a comprehensive account of applied ethics in medicine (and research). As such, Beauchamp and Childress (2012) have adjusted the framework over the years in response to criticism, and scholars have been interested in testing the framework empirically (see, e.g., Ebbesen, Andersen, and Pedersen 2012 on the principles' cross-cultural applicability). Because of its wide-ranging influence and its aspirations to provide a comprehensive approach to biomedical ethics, it is not surprising that a number of the contributors to this volume use Beauchamp and Childress's framework to consider a number of broad ethical questions pertaining to medical error, including:

- Who count as stakeholders with interests that need to be considered when preventing or responding to medical error based on the principles of autonomy, non-maleficence, beneficence and justice?
- When responding to medical error, is it just to blame or punish those responsible for "human error" in complex systems characterized by flaws attributable to no one in particular?
- How do we go about fulfilling beneficence and non-maleficence when it comes to medical error, given the inevitable tradeoffs?
- To what degree does the context for moral action constrain moral choice, and thus limit the autonomy of those who might be held responsible for medical errors? And if individuals are not fully responsible for those errors, then who is?

Responsibility for Medical Error

When we hear about medical errors, it is those rare, catastrophic cases, such as Jésica's, that explode into public consciousness precisely because they are rare and catastrophic. Nevertheless, her case is useful for illustrating a number of important ethical considerations concerning medical error. Among these is the importance of personal responsibility as well as its limits. Although experts agree that medical mistakes, as a rule, cannot be simply attributed to careless, incompetent or malicious providers, medical error may nevertheless feel like a betrayal of trust. Patients in pain and fear literally put themselves in the hands of highly trained health-care providers with the confidence that they can rely on their expertise and experience. Providers' professional training emphasizes their fiduciary relationship with patients given this asymmetry; hence, the obligation to always prioritize the patient and to act in her best interest (Bosk 2006).

In an interview with CBS correspondent Ed Bradley (Kopp 2003) on *60 Minutes*, Dr. Jaggers recalled with remorse that decisive moment when he accepted the first organ donation:

> I'm ultimately responsible for this because I'm Jésica's doctor and I'm arranging all this. But honestly, I look back, and yeah, if I'd made one more phone call or if I had told somebody else to make a phone call or done something different, maybe it would have turned out differently. But you know, those are all 20/20 hindsight.
>
> (Kopp 2003, paragraph 19, sic)

As tempting as it is in individualistic cultures to look for specific persons to blame, however, subsequent analyses of what went wrong concluded that the medical error was the result of breakdowns in both local and national systems. Analysts identified a number of contributing factors, including wrong assumptions, failure to follow protocol, communication lapses, poor coordination across institutions and providers, and time and resource constraints. Add to that list the sheer difficulty of minding all the details involved in such a complex procedure as an organ transplant, let alone one that is performed as infrequently as a heart–lungs transplant. Transplant surgeon Thomas Diflo wrote of the case years later:

> Transplantation in the United States, particularly deceased-donor transplantation, has become an exquisitely choreographed dance between the listed patients, their transplant physicians and surgeons, the OPOS, the hospitals where the donors have been treated, and the donor families. The logistics are staggering, and I am frequently amazed that the system works at all.
>
> (Diflo 2006, 72)

And, so, little things—unnoticed, unexamined, innocuous on their own, but of outsized importance when combined—undercut the best efforts of the most professional and dedicated providers and health-care facilities. Root-cause analyses of medical errors, such as those in Jésica's case, almost always converge on systemic explanations: "The attribution of the accident to 'human error' comes from the linking together of complex systems failure and hindsight bias during post-accident review" (Cook 2006, 46,). Implicit bias and other known sources of medical error may be baked into the very technologies, protocols, discourses, and role expectations that characterize health-care delivery no matter where a patient receives treatment. Therefore, it is not enough to examine the individual decisions medical providers make. We also need to pay attention, as Jésica's case illustrates, to professional and institutional structures.

Silke Schicktanz and Mark Schweda (2012) argue that Beauchamp and Childress (2012) do not systematically conceptualize "responsibility" even though it seems basic to their account. Schicktanz and Schweda propose multiple "responsibilities" in bioethics based on a relational model of moral agency. These include a collective model of responsibility that may be relevant here:

> If we have good reasons to believe that an action was based on the condition of a joint commitment or a system effect that goes beyond the impact of single actors, we can identify a collective as agent and therefore also claim collective responsibility. This is even more so if collectives possess economical, structural, or political power.
>
> (135)

The IOM report, in fact, warned that patient safety could only be improved using a systems approach: "The problem is not bad people; the problem is that the system needs to be made safer" (Kohn, Corrigan, and Donaldson 2000, 49). In Jésica's case, there was a geographically dispersed organ transplant system, its computer-based matching system, and the systems within the donor hospital and the recipient hospital, including the equipment, the operating rooms and other physical spaces, the providers, the communication among them, and policies within all these structures. In accidents—or harmful system failures—a number of things go wrong and combine in ways that were not (and rarely could have been) anticipated. These things gone wrong are errors. Multiple errors build up into serious events that would not have occurred absent that particular combination of factors. Examples of accidents mentioned in the report include the Three Mile Island nuclear accident and the explosion of the Challenger space shuttle.

Because of the unique combination of factors that result in accidents, the report noted that system adjustments to correct for "active errors" in medicine—such as accepting an organ bloc for transplant that was incompatible with the recipient's blood type—are unlikely to prevent similar accidents in the future. Rather, system interventions are more likely to nip in the bud "latent errors" inherent in organizational design, staff scheduling, and other aspects of the system itself. This is important, though, because latent errors can lead to active errors. To quote from the report again, "The active error is that the pilot crashed the plane. The latent error is that a previously undiscovered design malfunction caused the plane to roll unexpectedly in a way the pilot could not control and the plane crashed" (55). In Jésica's case, latent errors included lack of redundancy in the processes requiring blood type matching between organ donors and recipients and work-flow routines that had normalized leaving off the blood-type label from coolers storing donated organs (Bosk 2006). If it had not been Dr. Jaggers and Jésica's other providers, it could well have been other operators in the system, given these flaws.

Ethical Précis

Aside from the complexities involved in conceptualizing and assigning moral responsibility, Jésica's case illustrates a number of other important ethical considerations concerning medical error. These include:

- **The possibility for error from preventive treatment and diagnosis to treatment and follow-up care** (Kohn, Corrigan, and Donaldson 2000, 4). The scenario in which a team of surgeons gives a patient organs that are incompatible with her blood type is precisely the kind of scenario we imagine when thinking about medical error. But, as we saw in this case, medical error may happen well before treatment—while diagnosing symptoms, obtaining informed consent for medical procedures or making notes in a patient's chart. Medical error can happen after treatment as well, as reflected in the high maternal mortality rate in the United States compared to similar countries (Sawyer and McDermott 2019). Vigilance is key at every stage of the patient's journey through the system.

- **Harm caused by medical errors; i.e., "adverse events."** A tendency toward error, or committing a fundamental error of the sort that Dr. Jaggers did, are morally problematic aside from any resulting consequences. This is because they indicate deficiencies in standards of excellence to which health-care providers have committed themselves and given the rest of us reasonable grounds to count on. However, errors that do result in harm, especially harm to the very persons who are supposed to be cared for by health-care providers, seem especially egregious.

- **The range of stakeholders implicated and considerations for treating all with fairness and respect.** Medical ethics rightly centers patients as stakeholders in health-care decisions, as they are the most vulnerable in this setting, dependent on the judgment and goodwill of health-care providers. However, Jésica's case illustrates the range of others implicated in medical errors: colleagues, institutions, the patient's family and other advocates, health-care professions, the media and their audiences, providers themselves, other patients (such as those who might have benefited from the organs implanted in Jésica), and society as whole.

- **The causal role of communication problems.** As we saw in Jésica's case, communication (or lack thereof) can play an outsized role in both contributing to, and preventing, medical error. Furthermore, the very insidiousness of medical error means that providers need to think about how to communicate risks ethically to patients whose diminished health and lack of expert knowledge make them vulnerable to injury (e.g., physical and otherwise). Such communication is even more challenging in a case such as Jésica's, in which an (untrained) community advocate acted as an intermediary between her Spanish-speaking family and her English-speaking providers.

- **The vulnerability of patients generally and of disadvantaged populations in particular.** Not only was Jésica dying due to unhealthy organs, she was a minor, a Mexican national of LatinX ethnicity subject to deportation due to her undocumented status in the United States. Being situated at the intersection of these various identities made her even more vulnerable to error, as the possibility entered for paternalism and implicit bias to negatively affect her care. Indeed, much of the media coverage of her case focused on how she was not entitled to the transplant surgery in the first place and how ungrateful her family was not to donate any of her organs after she died (Wailoo, Livingston, and Guarnaccia 2006).

- **Responsibility for disclosure, apology and reparation for error.** After providers discover an error, they should consider how to report it in a way that is honest, helpful and fair. They also should consider how—and whether—to attribute blame and offer reparation. In Jésica's case we can see how what was said about the medical error, to whom, how, and when all constituted decision points regarding the best way to ethically disclose what had happened and why. Although Duke accepted public responsibility eventually for the error, spokespeople continued to point the finger at Dr. Jaggers, undermining the hospital's systemic account of why Jésica received the wrong organs (and, since Duke's was not the only system involved, it is not accurate to discuss this error as if it were only Duke's [Bosk 2006]). The family eventually sued, and the defendants settled out of court ("Duke, Santillan Family Reach Settlement" 2004).

- **Media publicity and framing of medical error.** Jésica's case received substantial press coverage between the two surgeries and after Jésica's death. However, such accounts are often inaccurate, or at least incomplete, due to the confidentiality of much of the data collected in investigations of medical error and cultural scripts used by the media to frame news stories. This means they do not always provide useful guides for future action; they also can act as disincentives to disclosure (Bosk 2006).

- **The efficacy of investigations and reforms to prevent similar errors in the future.** Institutions react to cases such as Jésica's by putting into place processes that can reduce the chance for error (at least the same kind of error). This happened at Duke after Jésica's death prompted a federal investigation that found Duke's transplant procedures lacking in several areas.[3] But for every sensational case of medical error such as Jésica's, there are thousands of cases that never make the headlines. And, whether we like it or not, there is no way to practice medicine without some risk of medical error.

Organization and Scope of Volume

This volume engages these ethical considerations with contributions from leading and emerging scholars and practitioners working in communication, law, medicine, and philosophy. Given the complexities of understanding, preventing, and responding to medical error in ethically acceptable ways, the scope of this project is fairly broad. Contributors examine preventable causes of medical error, disproportionate impacts of errors on vulnerable populations, disclosure and apology after discovering medical errors, and ethical issues arising in specific medical contexts, such as radiation oncology, psychopathy, and palliative care.

The contributions in this volume offer practical recommendations for respecting autonomy, distributing burdens and benefits justly in health-care systems, and minimizing injury to patients and other stakeholders. The chapters have been grouped into the following units: "Questions of Justice," "Communication and Risk," "Vulnerable Populations," and "Learning from Error." Medical professionals, hospital ethics commit-tees, health communication scholars, bioethicists, and patient advocates should benefit from the thorough analyses presented here of ethical issues to be considered when guarding against error, communicating risk, and making amends for preventable errors.

The chapters in Part I, "Questions of Justice," address the kinds of fair-ness issues raised earlier when it comes to deciding what counts as medi-cal error and how one should react to error's aftermath. As Beauchamp and Childress (2012) note, there are a number of different conceptions of justice, and these have not always been used consistently in biomedical ethics. What the various versions agree on is that justice has to do with giving people what they are due—according to standards such as equality, merit or need—and distributing benefits and burdens fairly based on justi-fied norms. In his chapter, "Medical Error and Moral Luck," philosopher Fritz Allhoff examines conceptual and normative questions associated with the IOM's definition of medical error, in particular with reference to patient injury and tying medical error to moral luck. Bioethicists Jeremy Garrett and Leslie McNolty pick up on the normative significance of adverse events and moral luck in their chapter, "Toward a Restorative Just-Culture Approach to Medical Error." In arguing for just cultures in health-care facilities, they propose that it is unfair to assign, and ulti-mately ineffective, to blame individual providers for systemic problems largely out of their control. They contrast a restorative justice approach, emphasizing collective responses to medical error and the restoration of all the parties affected, with a retributive justice approach focused on punishment. Philosopher Samuel Reis-Dennis, for his part, critiques the just-culture approach in his chapter, "Rehabilitating Blame." Although some observers blame lawsuits for the unwillingness of providers and hospitals to apologize for medical error, Reis-Dennis argues that blaming attitudes can be morally appropriate in such situations as expressions of righteous anger and as prods for the two parties to move toward each other in mutually respectful moral dialogue.

Communication problems in medical practice persist despite the wide use of electronic medical records and other strategies meant to standard-ize vital information and expand providers' access to it. A physician may neglect to draw attention to a serious underlying condition when making a referral, or a nurse may be reluctant to flag a problem with a treatment plan for fear of contradicting someone higher up in the chain of com-mand. Especially fraught are patient handoffs—when one tired, over-worked shift of providers turns over care of patients to the next shift, or a patient is transferred from one facility to another. Handoffs are estimated to be a contributing factor in 24–28 percent of medical errors; communication problems have been consistently found to play a major role in handoff errors, as well as in medical errors more generally. Communication problems are a factor in up to 31 percent of malpractice claims in the United States (Riesenberg et al. 2009).[4]

In fact, communication enters into the ethics of medical error in lots of other ways as well. As we saw in Jésica's case, it is important for providers and health-care facilities to communicate honestly, completely and quickly about mistakes so that they can be addressed responsibly and so that patients can make informed choices about their care and their options when injured. Promises of confidentiality are legally codified around the world in privacy laws and licensing requirements that limit disclosure of medical records, personnel actions, and patient–physician communication. Such guarantees are seen as vital to patient well-being and trust in the health-care professions. However, such guarantees also hide out of sight information that could help patients make more informed choices about their providers and health-care facilities; they also hamper our ability to address latent errors in health-care systems (Bosk 2006). And that does not even touch on micro-aggressions and omissions that issue from implicit bias or hierarchical pressures, potentially affecting intake and diagnosis at the very beginning of the medical-care chain. Neither does it account for the difficult issue of whether, when, and how to acknowledge responsibility for error or apologize for it at the very end of that chain. Communication affects the quality of medical care at virtually every juncture, as it calibrates the relationships between providers and patients, within medical teams, between administration and medical staff, between health-care facilities, even between computers.

Part II, "Communication and Risk," examines the importance of interaction on patient safety and how it is conditioned by medical hierarchies, roles, specialization, and the prestige and respect each of these commands. As much as systems interventions tend to emphasize the "hard" side of things (procedures, physical layouts, etc.), the authors in this section make the case that providers who care about their patients need to cultivate "soft" skills. Health communication scholar Leah Omilion-Hodges identifies tensions between competing medical models on transdisciplinary care teams as a possible source of medical error in her chapter, "A Communication-Based Approach to Safeguarding Against Medical Errors: The Case of Palliative Care." Based on her research with palliative-care units, she recommends storytelling and other intentional communication strategies to defend against organizational flaws that can lead to mistakes. In their chapter, "Communicating about Technical Failures in Assisted Reproductive Technology," physicians Rashmi Kudesia and Robert Rebar take a look at the unique risks involved in assisted reproductive technologies. These include equipment maintenance failures and other errors that can lead to adverse events with impacts that cross generations. Specifically, they examine the implications of catastrophic errors, such as the recent laboratory failures in Ohio and California that resulted in the loss of thousands of patients' gametes and embryos. Here the authors focus on communicating risk ahead of procedures, but also how to communicate ethically about such catastrophic errors after the fact with transparency and integrity. The final chapter in this section is "Respecting Patient Autonomy in Radiation Oncology and Beyond" by medical physicist Megan Hyun and philosopher Alexander Hyun. They argue that the potential for error in the field of radiation oncology obligates health-care facilities to change their communication practices to better respect the autonomy of patients throughout radiation treatment for cancer. Enter the medical physicist: someone already in the system with the training and experience needed to fill in the education gap so that patients are better informed about the risks of radiation treatment and the safety measures in place to minimize them. The authors make suggestions for applying some of their recommendations to patient health literacy more generally.

Patients are by definition vulnerable in medical settings, not only dependent on medical expertise, but often scared, hurting and in distress, sometimes to the point of their very lives being on the line. As we have seen, health-care providers thus assume a fiduciary duty toward patients as those with the most power in the patient–provider relationship. But many patients enter the medical setting further disadvantaged by histories of marginalization and injustice that make them skeptical of providers' commitment to act in their best interest. Providers, for their part, may be prone to medical error when dealing with these populations because of implicit bias that compromises their professional judgment from the get-go. And health-care systems continue to be marked by structural racism, sexism, ableism, and other forms of oppression that contribute to large health disparities for racial minorities and other historically disadvantaged populations. Despite the high maternal mortality rate in the United States, to go back to an earlier example, childbirth is understudied, and there is too little in the way of data collection to understand why mothers die while giving birth or shortly thereafter. For black women, the danger is compounded: in a system that already underserves women, they are roughly three times more likely to die giving birth than their white counterparts (Kozhimannil 2018).

The first chapter in Part IV, "Vulnerable Populations," defends a counterintuitive approach to mitigating such race-based disparities in health care. In "Medical Overtesting and Racial Mistrust," philosopher Luke Golemon documents the history of racism in U.S. medicine, then argues that health-care providers should over-test racial minorities as a counterbalance to under-testing motivated by racist medical mythology. At least until race-based disparities can be reduced in medicine, Golemon suggests racial minorities may suffer less harm from medical error in such a regime—and may have their trust in the health-care system shored up besides. In the next chapter, "The Epistemology of Medical Error in an Intersectional World," philosopher Devora Shapiro argues that the very concept of medical error is marked by power relations among social identities with different health expectations in settings shaped by particular legal, political, economic, and cultural features. In short, how medical error is defined depends on whose interests are at stake and how these are construed; the same goes for its close cousin, "standard of care." Shapiro demonstrates how dominant definitions of medical error may perpetuate disparities in access to quality health care by serving interests that do not coincide with those of marginalized individuals and groups and how these are multiplied for those at the intersection of several disadvantaged social positions.

The next chapter, "The Harm of Ableism: Medical Error and Epistemic Injustice," argues that disabled patients face a higher prospect of harm from medical error than non-disabled patients because of ableism. Philosophers Joel Michael Reynolds and David Peña-Guzmán conceive of ableism as an epistemic schema and show how this schema distorts communication between patients and providers, thus contributing to "schematic error." They also employ the concept of "contributory injustice" to argue that providers operating from a position of privilege are obligated to learn about non-dominant bodies of knowledge (for example, how disability communities themselves understand the meaning of disability). This can help providers challenge their own limited epistemic schemas and integrate alternative models of disability into the medical establishment.

Philosopher Kelsey Gipe closes out the "Vulnerable Populations" section with her chapter, "Errors and Determinations of Decision-Making Capacity in Mentally Ill Patients." She argues that we need to more closely examine the occurrence of medical error at the point at which providers determine a patient's capacity to give informed consent. She is particularly concerned about the difficulties in doing this when mentally ill patients request medical aid in dying in the absence of terminal illness or imminent death. After considering the complexities in these sorts of situations, Gipe recommends a blanket assumption of incapacity with room for exceptions.

The collection closes with a section on "Learning from Error" that examines the potential of various sensitizing and education strategies to help medical students and practitioners to learn from medical error; namely how to avoid error and limit its damage when it occurs. In "Medical Error as a Collaborative Learning Tool," Jordan Joseph Wadden, a philosopher, suggests that reporting medical error should be encouraged as a way to remind providers that they cannot possibly know everything there is to know about the practice of medicine. Besides learning with each other so that they can reduce the incidence of medical error, providers who contribute to such a culture of openness can cultivate a healthy capacity for epistemic humility.

In "Inference to the Best Explanation and Avoiding Diagnostic Error," philosopher David Kyle Johnson argues that diagnostic reasoning has been mistakenly reduced to running tests and probabilities—the "Dr. House syndrome." In fact, diagnostic reasoning is more like the kind of reasoning that is at the heart of the scientific method: comparing multiple hypotheses using theoretically informed observation and choosing the best explanation. We could make progress on reducing diagnostic error if we incorporated this understanding of diagnostic reasoning into medical textbooks and other aspects of medical education. Rasmus Rosenberg Larsen, another philosopher, looks at flawed historical evidence as the basis for ongoing error in the case of psychopathy assessments. He argues in "Psychopathy Treatment and the Stigma of Yesterday's Research" that years of conventional wisdom based largely on flawed studies has led psychiatrists to mistakenly surmise that psychopathy is not amenable to treatment. This error is especially consequential in the legal and correctional settings where forensic psychiatry is practiced, as it may influence patients' chances of entering rehabilitation and treatment programs.

For the last chapter in this collection, "Reducing Medical Error through Simulation: An Ethical Alternative for Training Medical Practitioners," philosopher T.J. Broy teams up with physicians Maureen Hirthler, Robin Rockhold, and Ralph Didlake to examine the ethical costs and benefits of using various simulation options to give medical students experience practicing techniques and teamwork without any chance of their errors hurting actual patients. Using Beauchamp and Childress's (2012) four principles, the authors lay out the ethical rationale for using simulation in medical education. However, a closer look at factors beyond efficiency and risk reduction reveals costs that must be considered for a full ethical assessment of this teaching strategy. These costs mirror the concerns that have cropped up in the ethics of robotics literature, such as the possible inhibition of empathy. The authors provide reasons to think that simulation, if done well, could overcome such reservations. Nevertheless, they urge that development of simulation in medical education proceed carefully to ensure that its benefits outweigh any costs in the long run.

Although these chapters account for many of the ethical issues surrounding medical error, we do not claim to have covered all of them. The issues our contributors have identified, moreover—though analytically distinct—are in practice related to each other in complicated ways. Therefore, it is productive to read these chapters as being in conversation with one another, reflecting multiple (sometimes conflicting) perspectives relevant to a fuller understanding of ethics and medical error. We hope this collection will inspire additional voices to join the conversation.

Notes

1. Fritz Allhoff explores the implications of this and other wrinkles in the IOM's conception of medical error in his chapter.
2. *The National Medical Error Disclosure and Compensation Act,* introduced in 2005 by then-Sen. Hillary Rodham Clinton, never got out of the Senate's Committee on Health, Education, Labor, and Pensions (www.Congress.gov).
3. For a summary of changes Duke made after this case, see Diflo (2006, 78–79).
4. Medical error linked to an adverse event rises to the level of (legally actionable) malpractice when it can be proven that the error was caused by negligence and the injury directly resulted from the error. See Kapp (1997) for further discussion.

Works Cited

Beauchamp, Tom L., and James F. Childress. 2012. *Principles of Biomedical Ethics, 7th Edition.* New York: Oxford University Press.

Bosk, Charles I. 2006. "All Things Twice, First Tragedy Then Farce: Lessons from a Transplant Error." In Peter Joseph Guarnaccia, Julie Livingston and Keith Wailoo (eds.), *A Death Retold: Jesica Santillan, the Bungled Transplant, and Paradoxes of Medical Citizenship.* Durham, NC: The University of North Carolina Press: 97–116.

Cook, Richard I. 2006. "Hobson's Choices: Matching and Mismatching in Transplantation Work Processes." In Peter Joseph Guarnaccia, Julie Livingston and Keith Wailoo (eds.), *A Death Retold: Jesica Santillan, the Bungled Transplant, and Paradoxes of Medical Citizenship.* Durham, NC: The University of North Carolina Press: 46–69.

Diflo, Thomas. 2006. "The Transplant Surgeon's Perspective on the Bungled Transplant." In Peter Joseph Guarnaccia, Julie Livingston and Keith Wailoo (eds.), *A Death Retold: Jesica Santillan, the Bungled Transplant, and Paradoxes of Medical Citizenship.* Durham, NC: The University of North Carolina Press: 70–81.

Ebbesen, Mette, Svend Andersen, and Birthe D. Pedersen. 2012. "Further Development of Beauchamp and Childress' Theory Based on Empirical Ethics." *Journal of Clinical Research & Bioethics* S6: e001.

Editorial Board. 2009. "A National Survey of Medical Reporting Laws." *Yale Journal of Health Policy, Law, and Ethics* 9 (1): 4.

Kapp, Marshall B. 1997. "Medical Error Versus Malpractice." *DePaul Journal of Health Care Law* 1 (4): 751–772. Retrieved from https://via.library.depaul.edu/jhcl/vol1/iss4/4

Kohn, Linda, Janet Corrigan, and Molla Donaldson. 2000. *To Err Is Human: Building a Safer Health System.* Washington, DC: National Academies Press.

Kopp, Carol. 2003, March 16. "Anatomy of a Mistake: The Tragic Death of Jesica Santillan." *60 Minutes. CBS News.* Retrieved from www.cbsnews.com/news/anatomy-of-a-mistake-16-03-2003/.

Kozhimannil, Katy. 2018. "Reversing the Rise in Maternal Mortality." *Health Affairs* 37 (11): Patient Safety.

Makary, Martin, and Michael Daniel. 2016. "Medical Error—The Third Leading Cause of Death in the US." *British Medical Journal* 353.

Riesenberg, Lee Ann, Jessica Leitzsch, Jaime Massucci, Joseph Jaeger, Joel Rosenfeld, Carl Patow, Jamie Padmore, Kelly Karpovich. 2009. "Residents' and Attending Physicians' Handoffs: A Systematic Review of the Literature." *Academic Medicine* 84 (12): 1775–1787.

Sawyer, Bradley, and Daniel McDermott. 2019. "How Do Mortality Rates in the U.S. Compare to Other Countries?" *Peterson-Kaiser Health System Tracker Chart Collections.* Retrieved from www.healthsystemtracker.org/chart-collection/mortality-rates-u-s-compare-countries/#item-healthcare-access-quality-1990–2016.

Schicktanz, Silke, and Mark Schweda. 2012. "The Diversity of Responsibility: The Value of Explication and Pluralization." *Medicine Studies* 3: 131–145.

Henry Thomas Stelfox, Stelfox Palmisani, Michael C. Scurlock, E. John Orav, and David W. Bates. 2006. "The '*To Err is Human*' Report and the Patient Safety Literature." *Quality and Safety in Health Care* 15 (3): 174–178.

Wailoo, Keith, Julie Livingston, and Peter Guarnaccia. 2006. "Introduction: Chronicles of an Accidental Death." In Peter Joseph Guarnaccia, Julie Livingston and Keith Wailoo (eds.), *A Death Retold: Jesica Santillan, the Bungled Transplant, and Paradoxes of Medical Citizenship.* Durham, NC: The University of North Carolina Press: 1–16.

WARAL.com. 2004, June 26. "Duke, Santillan Family Reach Settlement." Retrieved from www.wral.com/news/local/story/111895/

Part I
Questions of Justice

2 Medical Error and Moral Luck[1]

Fritz Allhoff[2]

Medical Error

In 1999, the Institute of Medicine released a report, *To Err Is Human: Building a Safer Health System* (Kohn, Corrifan, and Donaldson 1999).[3] The report noted that at least 44,000 (American Hospital Association 1999, 1; Institute of Medicine 2000, 1)—and perhaps as many as 98,000 (American Hospital Association 1999, 1; Institute of Medicine 2000, 1)—Americans died each year as a result of medical errors (Institute of Medicine 2000, 1). At the time, this would have been the eighth-leading cause of death, comprising more deaths than other high-visibility causes, such as motor vehicle accidents (43,000), breast cancer (42,000), or AIDS (17,000) (Institute of Medicine 2000, 1; Centers for Disease Control and Prevention 1999, 6). In the intervening years, medical error has moved up the charts, now comprising the third leading cause of deaths in the United States (Makary and Daniel 2016; Allen and Pierce 2016). The overall number of deaths from medical error in 2016 was more than 250,000, which was 9.7 percent of deaths nationwide (Makary and Daniel 2016), over double what had been reported in 1999 (Centers for Disease Control and Prevention 2001, 1).[4]

But what is lost in these statistics is how medical error is *defined*; obviously the numbers have to be predicated on some antecedent definition, lest it be unclear what actually counts as a death due to medical error. The Institute of Medicine defined error "as the failure of a planned action to be complete as intended or the use of a wrong plan to achieve an aim" (Institute of Medicine 2000, 4). The report went on to note that "errors depend on two kinds of failures: either the correct action does not proceed as intended (an error of execution) or the original intended action is not correct (an error of planning)" (Institute of Medicine 2000, 4). It further emphasized that error "can happen in all stages of the process of care, from diagnosis, to treatment, to preventive care" (Institute of Medicine 2000, 4).

The report then went on to build a taxonomy of medical error that tracks these three categories. Diagnostic error includes: error or delay in diagnosis, failure to employ indicated tests, use of outmoded tests or therapy, and failure to act on results of monitoring or testing. Treatment error includes: error in the performance of an operation, procedure, or test; error in administering the treatment; error in the dose or method of using a drug; avoidable delay in treatment or in responding to an abnormal test; and inappropriate (not indicated) care. Preventive error includes failure to provide prophylactic treatment and inadequate monitoring or follow-up of treatment. A fourth catchall category, "other," includes failure of communication, equipment failure, and other system failure (Institute of Medicine 2000, 36).

The next section will problematize these categories, but let me make some further comments on the Institute of Medicine's approach in the remainder of this section. First, the report acknowledges that not all errors result in actual harm (Institute of Medicine 2000, 2). This is an important observation, and one worth lingering on. Say, for example, a health-care provider[5] prescribes penicillin to a patient with a known penicillin allergy, but the patient never takes the penicillin. Maybe she never fills the prescription, maybe she loses it after having it filled, maybe she feels better by the time she gets home and elects to not use it at all, or whatever. The analysis here is that the provider *erred*, but that error did not eventuate in harm to the patient. We can easily contrast that patient—and indeed we will—to another who both received the errant prescription *and* took it, suffering anaphylaxis. What contrasts these patients is not the error, but whether there was an "adverse event" (i.e., bad outcome) after the error (Institute of Medicine 2000, 4).[6] And what ultimately matters is adverse events, not errors per se. Or, to put it another way, the principal reason that we care about errors is that they tend to lead to adverse events. But if a provider committed an isolated error that did not lead to such an adverse event—and setting aside any propensity for future recurrence—it just seems like something closer to good luck than to pernicious error.

Second, one of the major contributions of the report was to pivot from blaming *individuals* to blaming *institutions*. In its words:

> The common initial reaction when an error occurs is to find and blame someone. However, even apparently single events or errors are due most often to the convergence of multiple contributing factors. Blaming an individual does not change these factors and the same error is likely to recur. Preventing errors and improving safety for patients require a systems approach in order to modify the conditions that contribute to errors. People working in health care are among the most educated and dedicated workforce in any industry. The problem is not bad people; the problem is that the system needs to be made safer.
>
> (Institute of Medicine 2000, 36)

And this is important. We can think of some archetypical medical error, such as when a surgeon amputates the wrong leg. It should probably be the case that no surgeon, independently, exercises sole judgment over which appendage to amputate. So if the wrong leg does get amputated, it would not just be the surgeon who is implicated: the medical records could be incorrect, thus implicating any number of providers; the records could have been verified, thus implicating hospital oversight; the patient's family could have noticed the wrong markings while the patient was being prepped for surgery; or, frankly, a huge range of other possibilities could have contributed to the error.

Even think of some particularly nefarious errors, like those effected by a drunk surgeon. Here it is perfectly reasonable to blame that surgeon, but, even in cases like this, there is plenty of blame to go around. How was the *hospital* configured such that a drunk surgeon got access to an operating room? Think of some fairly simple remediation, like putting a breathalyzer on the operating rooms' doors: would that be a good idea? Did the surgeon have to sign a form, declaring lack of compromised abilities? If not, would the implementation of such a form promote better outcomes? These are just examples, but the simple point is that, even in the limited number of cases in which we might attribute blame to "bad apples," there are a range of institutional safeguards that could be in play. And thinking through error invites us to countenance all of these—some of whose costs could exceed the associated benefits—at myriad institutional levels. In fact, this sort of "systems-based thinking" is a manifest strength of the report, particularly insofar as it broadens the conversation beyond individual practitioners.[7]

Finally, it goes beyond present purposes to indicate, specifically, how we should deal with medical error. But, in recognition that this discussion does not take place in a vacuum, let me indicate broad thinking on how to mitigate error. The Institute of Medicine proposes a four-tiered approach that can be usefully summarized. First, it proposes a national focus to create leadership, research, tools, and protocols to enhance the knowledge base about safety.[8] Second, it recommends identifying and learning from errors by developing a nationwide public mandatory reporting system and by encouraging health-care organizations and practitioners to develop and participate in voluntary reporting systems.[9] Third, it aims to raise performance standards and expectations for improvements in safety through the actions of oversight organizations, professional groups, and group purchasers of health care.[10] Fourth, it suggests implementing safety systems in health-care organizations to ensure safe practices at the delivery level.[11]

Asymmetric Errors

In order to motivate the discussion of medical error and moral luck that will come in subsequent sections, it is worth teeing up how the Institute of Medicine's conception of error is, in some key regards, asymmetric. In that regard, let me start with an example, use that example to motivate a contrast with fairly standard thinking in moral philosophy, and then return to the issue more directly. As the example, consider the diagnostic error described as "failure to employ indicated tests" (Institute of Medicine 2000, 36). Suppose a health-care provider were looking at potentially cancerous tissue and that biopsy would be the indicated procedure. Further suppose that, for whatever reason, the provider fails to order the biopsy. Per above, we are going to call this an error whether or not it leads to an adverse event (i.e., patient harm)—simply because the test should have been ordered. If the failure to order it leads to the development of melanoma, that would be both an error and an adverse event. But even if the tissue were benign—but could have been malignant— there would have been a harm-free error.

On the other hand, though, suppose the provider orders the biopsy even when it was not indicated. Here we can imagine a patient coming to the clinic, fearing skin cancer. The patient has a mole on her forearm, but it is shallow, small in circumference, lacks irregular edges, there is no family history, and so on. So, after a visual exam, the provider deems skin cancer to be a low risk and the biopsy not to be medically indicated. Suppose, though, that the patient presses, persistently asking for the biopsy. Despite the procedure not being medically indicated, we can imagine the provider relenting for any number of reasons. Maybe the provider dislikes conflict. Maybe the patient is particularly strident or annoying. Maybe the provider's husband died of skin cancer last year. Maybe the provider gets to bill for the extra procedure, as well as follow-up care. It is not to say that any of these are good reasons, but it would hardly be surprising for any of them to drive clinical care.

And so the provider does order the biopsy. Here is the important question, though: is that a medical error? Or can over-testing in general comprise error? On the Institute of Medicine's report, the answer is pretty clearly no. The reason is that the types of error that it countenances in this regard trade on "*failure* to employ indicated tests": there simply is no prong on their analysis for "ordering non-indicated tests." There are two ways we could go on this. The first is to draw a distinction between "error" and something else, like "mistake." On this approach "error" is a term of art, as defined by the report. And if we say over-testing is not—or *cannot*—be error, we are just tracking that definition. "Mistake" would just pick out when providers get something wrong, whereas "error" would be a subset of "mistake," and would be circumscribed by the list in the report. So, to continue this example, over-testing and under-testing would, *ex hypothesi*, both be instances of "mistake," but only *under-testing* would be an instance of "error."

There is nothing incoherent about this, but it seems curious. Specifically, it introduces a distinction between "error" and "mistake" that just does not track our ordinary usage of the terms—rather, we treat them as co-extensive. For example, the Oxford English Dictionary defines "error" as "[s]omething incorrectly done through ignorance or inadvertence; a *mistake*, e.g., in calculation, [judgment], speech, writing, action, etc." (OED Online 2019, emphasis added). Conversely, it defines "mistake" as "misapprehension, misunderstanding; *error*, misjudgment" (OED Online 2019, emphasis added).[12] So it seems fair to say that the report is, at best, being idiosyncratic. The second way to go, though, would just be to say that the report's conception is implausible: both over-testing and under-testing are forms of error (i.e., not just mistake), and we are being supplied with an analysis that is not just idiosyncratic, but instead downright silly. Is this just terminological, or is there anything that hangs on it, theoretically?

The biggest thing that hangs on it is the numbers. If we expand "error" beyond the report's more limited definition, there would obviously be more error, probably a lot more.[13] In other words, to stay with our example, we would have to figure out all the instances of over-testing, then add those back into the number of errors—whereas we have previously been excluding those. Suffice it to say that there's a lot of over-testing,[14] so the data is going to be affected by the definitions. There might even be optics problems as well: raising the number of things that count as "error" could affect the public's perception of the profession, which could have effects on those seeking treatment. That said, this limited definition should not necessarily be seen as a self-serving metric; maybe there are other theoretical virtues that count in favor of it.

Top among prospective candidates is the idea that over-testing and under-testing are differentially situated with regards to adverse events. So let us suppose that over-testing would rarely lead to an adverse event. We can suppose that needless x-rays, for example, would lead to increased exposure to radiation, and that additional quantum of radiation could be the difference-maker between whether the patient develops cancer or not (Harvard Women's Health Watch 2018). Or we could suppose that needless blood draws could lead to injuries from the phlebotomist, such as nerve damage (Owen and Johnson 2017). But it is probably safe to assume that these interventions are *less* likely to eventuate in patient harms than, for example, failure to order an indicated biopsy for skin cancer. To be sure, there are all sorts of problems with over-testing, but they probably have more to do with health-care economics than with adverse events (Golemon, this volume).

However, even if this is true—and it probably is—why not talk in terms of "adverse events caused by error" instead of redefining "error" to track propensity for adverse events? Remember from the outset that the IoM report *already* draws a distinction between error and adverse event: not all error (even on its own circumscribed definition) eventuates in adverse events. In other words, we have at least the following categories from the Institute of Medicine taxonomy:

1.   Error that leads to adverse events.
2.   Error that does not lead to adverse events.
3.   Non-error that leads to adverse events.
4.   Non-error that does not lead to adverse events.

Set aside (4), which is not so interesting. If a health-care provider fails to order an indicated biopsy and the patient dies of skin cancer; that is (1). If a provider fails to order an indicated biopsy and, the patient does *not* die of skin cancer; that is (2). Suppose, for example, the patient *actually had* skin cancer, but inadvertently lost the affected arm in a chainsaw accident, before the cancer spread. Or suppose that, given the presentation of the skin defect, the patient would *usually* have skin cancer, but just happened not to in this case. Again, (2). But if a provider ordered a non-indicated x-ray, and the patient developed cancer because of radiation exposure (cf., (3)), that would not be error under the Institute of Medicine's definition.

This just does not make much sense. What we ultimately care about is whether health-care providers make errors—in the ordinary usage of the word—that eventuate in adverse events. *Those* are the things we should be counting, if we want to measure the significance of medical error. In this regard, over-testing is just as bad as under-testing (an Institute of Medicine error), at least conceptually; the only difference is that over-testing would be *less likely* to lead to adverse events than under-testing, as discussed above. But we need not sort that out just by defining "error" to exclude over-testing altogether. Rather, we would just say something more straightforward, like that, in general, over-testing is not as bad as under-testing. Not because it is not error, but just because less tends to hang on it.

But note that we also want (2) cognized as medical error—which the Institute of Medicine report does. Conceptually, whether an error leads to an adverse event or not has nothing to do with whether it is an *error* in the first place. Of course, errors that lead to adverse events are *worse* than errors that do not lead to adverse events, but, again, nothing hangs on that for our conception of "error." Rather, we just say that some errors are worse than others, either in isolation or as statistical classes. And we would still care about specific errors that did not lead to adverse events because, statistically, they might tend to. So, again, consider the provider who failed to order an indicated biopsy, yet the patient lost the affected arm to a chainsaw accident. The provider is not vindicated simply because skin cancer never developed. And part of the explanation there would be that, if this error were committed multiple times, skin cancer *would* develop in a bunch of them;

there are not so many chainsaw accidents, for example, such that the provider is usually off the hook.

In summary, the central point is that the Institute of Medicine approach rules out certain sorts of error that, at least intuitively, it should not. Rather, the Institute of Medicine enumerates several classes of error—if a putative error does not fall within one of those delineated classes, it is not an error, at least by its lights. And this is problematic because the list is under-inclusive, or at least it is under-inclusive as against common-sense definitions of "error." Second, the Institute of Medicine definition problematizes error in the sense that it separates "error" from "adverse event." And, insofar as that then makes it conceptually possible to have errors that do not lead to adverse events, it is not immediately clear that we are counting the things we should be counting. Instead, we most proximately care about errors that *do* lead to adverse events—or at least that *tend* to. This is not a conceptual mistake, though, but, rather, just admits of more errors than we necessarily care about. That can be remedied, though, just by focusing on the relevant subset (e.g., errors with adverse events, rather than all errors). By contrast, the conceptual mistake that bars certain errors from counting as errors at all is more problematic. It is not clear what this has going for it—nor does the report wrestle with the implications—and it ignores a relevant source of error. Moving forward, I shall, therefore, revert to the more common usage of "error," under which an error is any sort of mistake that health-care providers make. Those errors are not constrained to an enumerative list, but, rather, could be virtually anything. I will also assume that "error" does not require an "adverse event"—in this regard agreeing with the Institute of Medicine—and will now pivot from this conceptual interrogation into its normative underpinnings.

Moral Luck

In this undertaking, it will be useful to review the doctrine of moral luck. Much has been written on this topic,[15] which originates with Immanuel Kant:

> A good will is not good because of what it effects of accomplishes, because of its fitness to attain some proposed end, but only because of its volition, that is, it is good in itself. . . . Even if, by a special disfavor of fortune or by [mother nature], this will should wholly lack the capacity to carry out its purpose—if with its greatest efforts it should yet achieve nothing and only the good will were left . . . then, like a jewel, it would still shine by itself, as something that has its full worth in itself. Usefulness or fruitlessness can neither add anything to this worth nor take anything away from it.
>
> (Kant 1998, 50)[16]

The contemporary conversation owes to Thomas Nagel (1979, 26) and Bernard Williams (1981), though Nagel is more accessible.[17] Specifically, he notes that "[w]here a significant aspect of what someone does depends on factors beyond his control, yet we continue to treat him as an object of moral judgment, it can be called moral luck" (Nagel 1979, 32).

One reason this becomes a compelling problem in moral philosophy is that we typically "seem to be committed to the general principle that we are morally assessable only to the extent that what we are assessed for depends on factors under our control" (Nelkin 2013). Nevertheless, we routinely assess moral agents *despite* the existence of factors outside their control. For example, consider this thought experiment by Jeremy Waldron:

> Two drivers, named Fate and Fortune, were on a city street one morning in their automobiles. Both were driving at or near the speed limit, Fortune a little ahead of Fate. As they passed through a shopping district, each took his eyes off the road, turning his head for a moment to look at the bargains advertised in a storefront window. (The last day of a sale was proclaimed, with 25 percent off a pair of men's shoes.)
>
> (Waldron 1995, 387)

From a moral perspective, it seems that Fate and Fortune are similarly situated. But further suppose:

> In Fortune's case, this momentary distraction passed without event. The road was straight, the traffic in front of him was proceeding smoothly . . . and he completed his journey without incident. Fate, however, was not so fortunate. Distracted by the bargain advertised in the shoe store, he failed to notice that the traffic ahead of him had slowed down. His car ploughed into a motorcycle ridden by . . . Hurt. Hurt was flung from his motorcycle and gravely injured.
>
> (Waldron 1995, 387)

And now it suddenly looks as if they are differently situated, specifically with regards to the injury Fate causes to Hurt. The issue, though, is that injury has nothing to do with anything under the control of Fortune or Fate. Rather, what sets them apart is simply whether there was a slowed motorcycle in front of only one of them, which is something completely outside of their control.[18]

So the problem is that we either have to give up on the control principle—thus morally assessing people for features outside their control—or else we have to retreat to moral parity between Fortune and Fate. The latter may sound more initially plausible, but it quickly runs aground. Specifically—and this is why I chose Waldron's formulation—consider tort law. If the purpose of tort law is to promote something like rectifi-catory justice (i.e., restoration of the *status quo ante*), then what?[19] In Fortune's case, there is no injury, and so no rectification needed. In Fate's, there is, and it hardly makes any sense to foist the burden of that injury onto Hurt. In one case, we need to collect damages to ensure that Hurt does not bear the costs of Fate's negligence. In the other, there's nothing for Fortune to pay for. And so parity—for example, between carelessness and damages—is asymmetrical. Waldron proposes to resolve this in a creative way; namely charging a tax to *all drivers*, sort of like a national-ized insurance scheme (Waldron 1995, 389).[20] That would equalize tort liability across both drivers, but the moral intuition lingers that Fortune is differently situated in virtue of *causing harm* that Fate did not cause. To credit that intuition, though, is to relent on the control principle that we otherwise take to be morally perspicuous.

But let us now pivot and approach all this through the lens of medi-cal error. Specifically, we can readily acknowledge that our moral assess-ments of error can be colored by exogenous environmental factors (e.g., the presence of motorcycles)—as opposed to endogenous agential factors (e.g., the driver's negligence)—owing to moral luck. To use the language developed in previous sections, suppose that a health-care provider errs, but further suppose that whether that error results in an adverse event is wholly predicated on luck. Return to the case where the provider should have ordered a biopsy, but failed to. Because this is an instance of under-testing, it is properly regarded as medical error (i.e., under the Insti-tute of Medicine classification). But whether we "care" about the error ultimately depends on non-agential features of the case, such as if the patient has an errant chainsaw accident, rendering the failure to resect the cancer—which would only have been revealed through the neglected biopsy—medically irrelevant.

Again, I only mean irrelevant in the instant case. If a health-care pro-vider systematically fails to order indicated tests, at least some of those omissions will eventuate in adverse events. Therefore, we can identify a critical locus of moral evaluation; namely whether actions (or omissions), when common, *tend to* lead to adverse events. Or even suppose "tend to" is too strong: maybe the testing practices of some provider increase the incidence of some particular adverse event from 1 to 2 percent. Here it might not be accurate to say that anything "tends to" happen (i.e., since 2 percent is still something you would rationally bet against). But it would be accurate to say something else, such as the probability of some adverse event is higher given non-testing than it would have been given over-testing. And this fact alone gives us moral purchase on the failure to order the test.[21]

Of course we can say the same thing in the Fate/Fortune case: we do not morally exculpate Fate simply because no motorcycle was in front of him. Rather, we say that he "got lucky," that there easily *could have been* a motorcycle, and that, if he is routinely negligent, he will eventually hit a motorcycle—or something else, like a pedestrian. The associated probabilities between negligence causing a traffic accident and an unordered biopsy failing to prevent a death by melanoma could obviously be different. But, structurally, the cases are isomorphic. Or at least seem to be: the potential difference-maker is that we might be inclined to categorize the Fate/Fortune case as trading on actions (e.g., hitting motorcyclists), whereas the unordered biopsy looks closer to an omission. But without wading too deeply into the act/omission literature, we can make a few ready observations.[22] Chief among them is that this is probably a mischaracterization of Fate/Fortune. The principal problem with Fate here is that he *failed to exercise due care*, and that failure *caused* the injury.

To the extent that it seems odd to talk about omissions being causal, it is not. For example, suppose "Barry promises to water Alice's plant, doesn't water it, and that the plant then dries up and dies. Barry's not watering the plant—his omitting to water the plant—caused its death" (McGrath 2005, 125). The principle is also widely endorsed in tort law.[23] Regardless, the point is simply that moral luck can attach to both acts and omissions; it would be an impoverished account if it only attached to the former. All that moral luck need be committed to is that we seem to morally assess agents, at least in part, on factors beyond their control. That basic claim does not differentiate between acts and omissions, nor need it. Insofar as some of our primary examples (e.g., under-testing) are necessarily omissions, this is an important result.

And so, whether we are considering acts or omissions, our ascriptions of medical error will likely be imbued with moral luck. If a provider errs in a way that does not eventuate in an adverse event, that could just be an instance of the provider getting lucky. This is not necessarily the same as the *patient* getting lucky because various unrelated adverse events to the patient's health might screen off the provider's error: the chainsaw accident superseding the melanoma would be such an example. But other more quotidian examples would make the same point, such as the provider failing to diagnose prostate cancer—where prostate cancer generally afflicts older men who might well die of something else before the prostate cancer becomes lethal. Because the other affliction precludes the provider's error from eventuating in an adverse event, that error remains—or at least could remain—hidden. And yet it still seems as if we would want to say that an oncologist who systematically under-diagnoses prostate cancer is a *bad* oncologist, even if nothing ever seems to hang on it. Or, to put it another way, it seems fraught to say that she is a bad oncologist *only if* her underdiagnoses ultimately kill the patient.

We have yet to explore another way in which moral luck maps onto medical error. Suppose that the provider orders an unindicated test which, by sheer luck, happens to reveal a lethal pathology. For example, suppose the provider should not have ordered an MRI, but that the MRI ultimately reveals an unindicated, but malignant, tumor. Again, under the Institute of Medicine approach, ordering unindicated tests cannot be error at all, but set that aside for reasons previously discussed. Rather, supposing that it was an errant order, it would equally seem odd to praise the provider for discovering the tumor. The errant order is a straight-forward cause of the discovery, but not all causes are morally laudable. If I get in a bar fight and punch out someone's infected tooth, it hardly seems I deserve any moral credit, despite the fact that the punch might have made the recipient better off. Instead, I am morally blameworthy for getting into a fight, regardless of the upshot. In the same regard, the provider who misorders a test is also blameworthy, for failing to fol-low evidence-based practices. There is nothing problematic with saying that, sometimes, bad decisions eventuate in good outcomes; any of us can probably imagine myriad cases of practical deliberation in which we have erred, yet gotten lucky. The point is simply that we should not conflate the conceptual analysis with the moral one (2015).[24]

* * *

The literature on medical error—particularly the ethical dimensions—has been largely underdeveloped, a shortcoming this volume aims to reme-diate. This chapter diagnoses the extent of medical error and updates the conversation in light of the two decades that have passed since the Institute of Medicine report (Kohn, Corrifan, and Donaldson 1999). The chapter also explores conceptual issues relating to the definition of "error," particularly as relates to: (1) the relationship between errors and adverse events; (2) asymmetries in how certain sorts of error—for exam-ple, under- and over-testing—are commonly conceived; and (3) argues for a broader conception of error than is usually proffered (e.g., by allow-ing that over-testing can still comprise error). The last section then con-siders ways in which moral luck bears on our assessments of error, noting that our moral categorization of error—or lack thereof—often trades on features beyond practitioners' control. Insofar as this is true, it raises problems for commonsense conceptions of morality.

Notes

1. Allhoff, Fritz. (2019). "Ethics and Error in Medicine." *Kennedy Institute of Ethics Journal* 29 (3). pp. 187–203. © 2019 Johns Hopkins University Press. Adapted and reprinted with permission of Johns Hopkins University Press.
2. Fritz Allhoff, J.D., Ph.D. is a professor in the Department of Philosophy at Western Michigan University. Parts of this chapter were written while he was a Fellow in the Center for Law and the Biosciences at Stanford University and a Fulbright Specialist in the Faculty of Political Science at the University of Iceland; he thanks those institutions for their support. He also thanks Sandra L. Borden and Luke Golemon for helpful comments on earlier drafts.

3. An executive summary recapitulates the key findings. Available at www.nationalacademies.org/hmd/~/media/Files/Report%20Files/1999/To-Err-is-Human/To%20Err%20is%20Human%201999%20%20report%20brief.pdf.

4. Some of the discrepancy might be due to underreporting on the earlier study (Makary and Daniel 2016). So we need not conclude that the actual rates of death due to medical error doubled, though there is at least plausible evidence for an increase. It seems safe to assume that the Institute of Medicine's stated goal of "a 50 percent reduction in errors over five years" (i.e., from 1999 to 2004) was not realized (Institute of Medicine 2000, 4).

5. For the purposes of this chapter, I will use "health-care provider" when there might be myriad functional roles (e.g., physician, physician's assistant, nurse) that could err in relevant ways. If the instance under discussion requires a more narrow functional role (e.g., surgeon, as a subset of physician), then I will be more specific.

   This approach is conceptually motivated, but also is meant to acknowledge the significance of functional roles beyond physicians, and to serve as a corrective against the fact that bioethics, as a discipline, has overemphasized physicians and underemphasized a broader and more diverse (e.g., by gender, by race, etc.) health-care profession.

6. I will follow the literature and use "adverse event," but the less technical—and more colloquial—"bad outcome" can be used interchangeably.

7. See also Garrett and McNolty (this volume).

8. *Id.*, chapter 4.

9. *Id.*, chapter 5.

10. *Id.*, chapter 6.

11. *Id.*, chapter 7.

12. The semicolon makes the parsing interesting, apparently linking misapprehension/misunderstanding and error/misjudgment separately. Other definitions of "mistake" in the OED make it look cognitive (e.g., relating to judgment), as opposed to action-oriented, whereas the entry on "error" seems to conceive of "mistake" more broadly (e.g., by enumerating a list that includes "calculation, speech, writing, *action*, etc." [emphasis added]). For present purposes, nothing hangs on this.

13. Because the statistics on medical error track the report's definition, it would be hard to be more informative about how much more error there would be on a different definition.

14. See, for example, Golemon (this volume), for a useful survey of the literature.

15. For seminal works, see Statman (1993). For an overview, see Nelkin (2013).

16. Quoted in Nelkin (2013).

17. Williams's position is difficult to understand; even he acknowledges that his original article "may have encouraged" some misunderstandings. Williams (1993, 251). Quoted in Nelkin (2013).

18. Nagel uses a similar—if less descriptive—example. See Nagel (1979). Nagel also classifies four different kinds of moral luck: resultant luck, circumstantial luck, constitutive luck, and causal luck. This is an instance of resultant luck. Circumstantial luck trades on the circumstances in which we find ourselves: some Nazis might be blameworthy for atrocities, but had they been differently situated (e.g., born in Argentina, instead of Germany), they might not have participated in those atrocities at all. Constitutive luck recognizes that moral agents differ in their dispositions and traits. For example, some of us are braver or more cowardly than others, and those traits—over which we may have little control—can affect how we are morally evaluated. (Of course

others, like Aristotle, might be more sanguine about the axes of control we can exert in this regard. See Aristotle [2009, 1152a33–1152a35].) Finally, Nagel proposes causal luck as acknowledging that antecedent circumstances may determine who we are; some commentators have proposed that this category is redundant given constitutive and circumstantial luck. See Nelkin (2013). For present purposes, our examples will focus on resultant luck.

19. See, for example, Owen (1995, 1). See also Aristotle (2009, 1130a13–1131a9).
20. Waldron, originally from New Zealand, favorably comments on a similar scheme there.
21. This could be complicated by any number of considerations, but suffices for present purposes. One complicating set of features would just be that ordering any test carries with it some risks; not just from, for example, radiation, but even for more quotidian reasons, like that the patient could suffer an accident (e.g., vehicular, falling) in transit for the test. And so it *could* be the case that adequate testing *increases* the risks of (some) adverse events. To think this through, we would need more empirical data: how many people die a year from, for example, melanoma? How many of those deaths owe to failure to order a biopsy? How many deaths—or other injuries—are incidental to the biopsy itself (e.g., travel to/from the test site)? And so on: we could drill down into a more detailed analysis. But insofar as the investigation here is structural—as opposed to empirical—we can put these complications aside.
22. See, for example, Kagan (1989), Kamm (2007), Quinn (1989), and Rachels (1975).
23. See, for example, Hart and Honoré (1959, 59) and Wright (1985). But see *Osterland v. Hill* (holding that defendant was not civilly liable for failing to rescue a drowning swimmer, even though it would have been easy for defendant to do so). Regardless, it is uncontroversial that omissions can be causes: the issue is simply which omissions comprise breach of a duty. See Huask (1980).
24. The idea might be fruitfully analogous to knowledge and reliability. In the study of knowledge, knowledge is the end goal. Similarly, in moral reasoning, one might say *one* end goal is good consequences. But there is a push in epistemology to evaluate methods based on their reliability rather than just the end result, since this is most conducive to consistently obtaining the desired end. Thus many epistemologists defend the ability to critique those who do have something like knowledge (true belief with purported justification) but whose justifications come through an unreliable method.

    The analogy for moral methods would be similar. We can still condemn the physician for amputating the wrong leg because amputating the wrong leg is evidence of a very unreliable method more likely to cause harm than good. For more on reliabilist epistemology, see Goldman and Beddor (2015) and

Works Cited

Allen, Marshall and Olga Pierce. 2016, May 3. "Medical Errors Are No. 3 Cause of U.S. Deaths, Researchers Say." *National Public Radio*. Retrieved from https://www.npr.org/sections/health-shots/2016/05/03/476636183/death-certificates-undercount-toll-of-medical-errors

Allhoff, Fritz, and Sandra Borden (eds.). Forthcoming. *Ethics and Medical Error*. New York: Routledge.

American Hospital Association. 1999. "Hospital Statistics." Chicago.

Aristotle. 2009. *Nichomachean Ethics*, trans. David Ross. Oxford: Oxford University Press.

Centers for Disease Control and Prevention, National Center for Health Statistics. 1999. "Births and Deaths: Preliminary Data for 1998." *National Vital Statistics Reports* 47 (25).

Centers for Disease Control and Prevention, National Center for Health Statistics. 2001. "Deaths: Final Data for 1999." *National Vital Statistics Reports* 49 (8).

Goldman, Alvin, and Bob Beddor. 2015. "Reliabilist Epistemology." *Stanford Encyclopedia of Philosophy*. Retrieved from https://plato.stanford.edu/entries/reliabilism/

Hart, H. L. A., and Tony Honoré. 1959. *Causation in the Law*. Oxford: Oxford University Press.

Harvard Women's Health Watch. 2018. "Radiation Risk from Medical Imaging." Harvard Health Publishing. Retrieved form https://www.health.harvard.edu/cancer/radiation-risk-from-medical-imaging

Huask, Douglas. 1980. "Omissions, Causation, and Liability." *Philosophical Quarterly* 30 (121): 318–326.

Institute of Medicine. 2000. *To Err Is Human: Building a Safer Health System*. Washington, DC: National Academies Press.

Kagan, Shelly. 1989. *The Limits of Morality*. Oxford: Oxford University Press.

Kamm, Frances. 2007. *Intricate Ethics*. Oxford: Oxford University Press.

Kant, Immanuel. 1998. *Groundwork of the Metaphysics of Morals*, trans. Mary Gregor. Cambridge: Cambridge University Press.

Kohn, Linda, Janet Corrifan, and Molla Donaldson (eds.) 1999. "Committee on Quality of Health Care in America, Institute of Medicine." *To Err Is Human: Building a Safer Health System* National Academy Press. Retrieved from www.nap.edu/download/9728.

Makary, Martin, and Michael Daniel. 2016. "Medical Error—The Third Leading Cause of Death in the U.S." *BMJ* 353.

McGrath, Sarah. 2005. "Causation by Omission: A Dilemma." *Philosophical Studies* 123: 125–148.

Nagel, Thomas. 1979. *Mortal Questions*. New York: Cambridge University Press.

Nelkin, Dana. 2013. "Moral Luck." *Stanford Encyclopedia of Philosophy*. Retrieved from https://plato.stanford.edu/entries/moral-luck/

OED Online. Retrieved March 2019. Oxford University Press.

Osterland v. Hill 160 N.E. 301 (Mass. 1928).

Owen, David. 1995. *Philosophical Foundations of Tort Law*. Oxford: Clarendon Press.

Owen, Steven, and Jason Johnson. 2017. "Radial Nerve Damage After Venipuncture." *Journal of Hand Microsurgery* 9 (1): 43–44.

Quinn, Warren. 1989. "Actions, Intentions, and Consequences: The Doctrine of Doing and Allowing." *Philosophical Review* 98 (3): 355–382.

Rachels, James. 1975. "Active and Passive Euthanasia." *New England Journal of Medicine* 292: 78–86.

Reynolds, Joel, and David Peña-Guzmán. Unpublished. "The Harm of Ableism: Medical Error and Epistemic Injustice."

Statman, Daniel (ed.). 1993. *Moral Luck*. Albany: State University of New York Press.

Waldron. Jeremy, 1995. "Moments of Carelessness and Massive Loss." In David Owen (ed.), *Philosophical Foundations of Tort Law*. Oxford: Oxford University Press: 387–408.

Williams, Bernard. 1981. *Moral Luck*. Cambridge: Cambridge University Press.

Williams, Bernard. 1993. "Postscript." In Statman Daniel (ed.), 1993. *Moral Luck*. Albany: State University of New York Press: 251–258.

Wright, Richard. 1985. "Causation in Tort Law." *California Law Review* 73 (6): 1735–1828.

3 Toward a Restorative Just-Culture Approach to Medical Error

Jeremy R. Garrett and Leslie Ann McNolty

Engaging With Medical Error as a Matter of Justice

Medical error comes in many forms and will occur in all health-care systems and institutions, regardless of design and management. Consider two clinical scenarios:

1. Dr. Gerard is entering his final chart notes after a 24-hour shift. He receives a call—a boy has been brought in following a car accident and requires emergency surgery. Sandra Ortiz, the nurse who will be assisting with the surgery, notices that Dr. Gerard seems exhausted. She asks him how he is feeling and mentions that he seems to be very tired. Dr. Gerard assures her that he will be fine and proceeds to scrub in for duty. At the end of surgery, Dr. Gerard begins closing the surgical wound before the nurse has had a chance to count all of the sponges to ensure nothing has been left inside the patient's body. Nurse Ortiz tells him she has not yet finished counting, but Dr. Gerard finishes suturing and leaves without responding to her.
2. Dr. Petrovich is entering chart notes following rounds. She enters a new prescription for pain medication for Mrs. Norris, a 45-year-old patient recovering from knee surgery. A series of alerts pop up on the screen. As Dr. Petrovich dismisses a series of 12 notifications of minor drug interactions and standard warnings about the appropriate dosage of the narcotic, she inadvertently dismisses a warning that Mrs. Norris is allergic to the drug Dr. Petrovich has prescribed without reading it.

Although both cases involve deviations from ideal medical practice that may result in harm to patients, they differ in morally important ways, including the intentions of the agents involved, the salience of mitigating factors and structural dynamics, the potential consequences for victims, the relative frequency of the deviation type, and so on. As such, these deviations (arguably) should not be understood, categorized, or managed in the same way.

Unfortunately, the medical establishment historically has disregarded this insight. Conceptualizing all such deviations as "medical error" at odds with medicine's self-professed first principle—*first, do no harm*—it has relied upon simplistic individualized assignments of responsibility: identify the professional(s) in closest proximity to deviations and punish the offending behavior or decisions (Kohn, Corrigan, and Donaldson 2000, 49; Sharpe 2004, 7; Liang 2004, 59). This approach is ethically flawed, both in its *implicit assumptions* (e.g., patient safety justifies any burden to professionals) and in its *practical outcomes* (e.g., holding medical professionals—especially those lower in the medical power hierarchy who handle day-to-day direct care—*individually* responsible for errors even when system design virtually guaranteed such errors would occur). Not only is a blanket punitive approach unfair, it also perversely incentivizes people to hide or miscast errors. As a result, the system cannot be improved.

In this chapter, we will outline and defend a fairer approach to medical error, one that acknowledges that obligations of justice extend beyond patients and derive in part from the distribution of benefits and burdens among professionals. Complex, high-technology, multidisciplinary care entails dynamic systems and teams in which numerous professionals contribute within specialized roles. No provider singlehandedly can ensure safe, quality care, and many medical errors would occur regardless of the individual professionals involved. On a "just- culture" approach, systems are designed to standardize error management, avoid both a "punitive" and a "blameless" culture, balance learning and accountability, openly identify and examine its own weaknesses, and reduce anxiety around error reporting. Importantly, there is no single blueprint for what a just-culture approach to patient safety and medical error looks like (Dekker 2016, xv). Every organization and system must start with the culture it has currently in assessing which cultural shifts are possible and most promising. That said, two broader visions of just culture provide alternative directions for such shifts: (1) a *retributive* just culture, focused on "[imposing] deserved and proportional punishment" and (2) a *restorative* just culture, focused on "[repairing] the trust and relationships that were damaged" (Dekker 2016, 1). In this chapter, we are particularly interested in describing and defending the restorative justice approach. This approach to patient safety improves both system management and health outcomes.

After making an initial case for the restorative justice approach to medical error, we will consider two related objections levied against it. The first objection focuses on how the systems-level focus of restorative just culture threatens traditional professional virtues and individual accountability. The second argues that the forward-looking orientation of restorative just culture rejects backward-looking practices of blame and punishment that are indispensable for respecting persons as moral equals and restoring the equilibrium within our moral community that wrongful medical error disrupts. In responding to these objections, we argue that both rest on misunderstandings about the nature of restorative justice and an inflated regard for the virtues of more punitive approaches. Viewed appropriately, a restorative justice approach to patient safety has sufficient resources to mitigate both concerns while offering greater promise for reducing the prevalence of medical error.

The Varieties, Sources, and Prevalence of Medical Error

Medical practitioners have long been centrally concerned with patient safety, *primum non nocere* ("first, do no harm") serving as the proverbial "basic rule of the physician" and "primary principle of the ethics of the medical profession" (Beecher 1970, 94; Jonsen 1977, 27). Although the precise origins of the Latin expression are controversial among historians of medicine (Jonsen 1977, 27; Herranz 2002, 1463), the origins of the modern patient safety movement are nothing if not precise: November 29, 1999, the date when the Institute of Medicine (IOM) released *To Err is Human*, a major report detailing the astoundingly high rates of injury and death resulting from medical error in the United States (Kohn, Corrigan, and Donaldson 2000). The report was the lead story in news outlets around the country, and its impact redounds to this day.

In the 20 years following the release of the IOM report, new approaches to preventing and mitigating the impact of errors have been developed and adopted by health-care organizations. Increasingly, safety is considered a systems-level issue rather than a problem resulting from individual failures. Drawing from other high-reliability industries, such as aviation and nuclear power, new safety protocols such as checklists have been developed to prevent error in areas including surgery and intensive care. Health care's increasing dependence upon information technology has presented both new opportunities and new challenges for safety in hospitals (Bates and Singh 2018). New insights about the way the physical design of the health-care environment impacts safety are being incorporated into the layout of hospitals—from the placement of sinks for hand washing to the elimination of corners to facilitate cleaning (Joseph, Henriksen, and Malone 2018).

More attention and resources have been directed at the problem, and important changes followed the report, including changes in research, hospital programs, and regulations. Nevertheless, "it has become increasingly clear that safety issues are pervasive throughout health care and that patients are frequently injured as a result of the care they receive" (Bates and Singh 2018, 1736). The cost of errors to individual patients and society as a whole is enormous. Preventable medication errors alone are estimated to cost $21 billion annually (Joseph, Henriksen, and Malone

2018, 1886). Estimates of the number of *deaths* attributable to medical error are controversial; nonetheless "many experts believe that the number is probably in the hundreds of thousands annually, while many more patients are injured unnecessarily" (Bates and Singh 2018, 1737).

The sources and types of medical error are diverse. As the patient safety movement closes out its second decade, one in 20 patients will experience a diagnostic error in any given year, most patients will experience it in their lifetimes, and 10 percent of preventable deaths are attributed to diagnostic delay or error (National Academies of Science, Engineering, and Medicine 2015). Fatal medication errors lead to 7,000–9,000 deaths each year in the United States (Bhimji and Scherbak 2018) with children at an increased risk for harm (AAP 2011, 1199–1210) due to their "different physical characteristics, developmental issues, and dependence on parents and other care providers to prevent medical errors" (Ratwani et al. 2018, 1752). Other common sources of error include communication failures between shift changes and service rotations and understaffing on nights and weekends (Sharpe and Faden 1998, 138–139). In addition, medical error may be caused by poorly designed or implemented technological interventions, such as electronic health-record charting and alerts, and electronic prescribing. These can cause errors by interrupting workflow and communication, or producing resistance or refusal of staff. Clearly, significant work remains to develop and implement systemic solutions to improve patient safety.

The Prima Facie Case for a Restorative Just-Culture Approach

Imagine an institutional committee within a hospital that, against this larger backdrop, is tasked with developing new strategies, policies, procedures, and system improvements for protecting patient safety and preventing medical error. In these deliberations, several points are likely to be widely agreed upon:

- Patient safety is a central goal of medical practice.
- Some human error will occur in any complex system.
- Medical error has enormous costs, including physical and psychosocial harm, staff burnout and turnover, financial and opportunity costs, and diminished social-capital resources, such as institutional reputation and stakeholder trust.
- System design is a crucial factor in minimizing the frequency, scope, and severity of error, as it establishes the choice and action architecture in which clinicians make, or refrain from making, decisions related to the care of patients.
- Systems can only be effectively (re)designed if the true frequency, scope, and severity of error is actually well-understood.

- The true frequency, scope, and severity of error can only be well-understood if all participants are adequately equipped, empowered, and protected to identify and report error when it occurs.
- Trade-offs among important values are inevitable in system and policy design, as many potential safeguards (e.g., more staffing, more layers of oversight, improvements in system infrastructure, etc.) may impact morale, job satisfaction, and turnover among staff, as well as demand significant investments of money, time, and focus that ultimately impact other things the hospital can do.

Assuming that these starting points are widely accepted—and they should be—what defining principles and commitments should guide the committee's thinking about specific strategies, policies, procedures, and system improvements to recommend?

A natural assumption might be that, since the committee's goal is patient safety, non-maleficence—i.e., "a norm of avoiding the causation of harm" (Beauchamp and Childress 2009, 13)—should be the guiding principle. But that proposal stalls out of the gate: if we want the system that produces no amount of error and harm, then we will drastically limit the range of services provided, perhaps even closing up shop entirely. Undoubtedly non-maleficence is not typically understood to require the elimination of harm, but, rather, the minimizing of harm. Nonetheless, although non-maleficence is an important principle to consider in making many decisions, it is ill-suited to serve as the *primary* guiding principle in the design or reform of patient safety systems. Again, some error and harm is inevitable in any complex health-care system, and whether it is ethically justified to trade these (and other) unfortunate results for a system that delivers more benefits to more people is not a question that non-maleficence *itself* can address.

Instead, we must consider and weigh the total package and distribution of benefits and burdens, rights and responsibilities, among various system designs. This makes choosing a particular design first and foremost a matter of *justice*. Here we're reminded of the opening passage from John Rawls' *A Theory of Justice*: "Justice is the first virtue of social institutions, as truth is of systems of thought. . . . Laws and institutions no matter how efficient and well-arranged must be reformed or abolished if they are unjust" (John Rawls 1971, 3). Our imagined committee need not be Rawlsians deliberating behind a veil of ignorance to see its task as one centered on the principle of justice: *their recommendations should seek to fairly distribute the benefits and burdens of providing safe patient care among all relevant stakeholders, including clinicians, current patients and families, and future patients and families.*

As it turns out, this insight is shaping the way that many health-care systems and institutions are making design choices through what has come to be known as the "just-culture" approach to patient safety.

Taking a systemic approach to error reduction and patient safety requires that errors, near-misses, and other deviations are disclosed so that weaknesses and gaps in the system can be identified and improved. This shift in approach presents an opportunity to fundamentally reorient our response to error and harm. In recognizing that most errors are caused by system failures, it no longer makes sense to focus on "who" was responsible for the error. Instead a much broader account of "what" happened is required (Kohn, Corrigan, and Donaldson 2000, 49).

Restorative justice confronts harm from medical error with questions such as (Dekker 2016, 1):

- Who has been (potentially) hurt?
- What are their needs?
- Whose obligation is it to meet those needs?
- What role does the community play in learning from the event?

In more punitive cultures, the person identified as the proximate cause of the error usually is held responsible in the form of blame and/or punishment. But problems arise in punitive systems because they promote perverse incentives. A punitive system encourages people to hide or miscast errors. As a result, the system—a system from which everyone benefits—cannot be improved because the extent and underlying cause of errors are hidden. In a just culture, the source of most error is recognized to have significant systemic dimensions. As such, the presumptive response to error is to (1) review and improve the system and (2) counsel or coach, rather than punish, the relevant team or individuals and collaborate with those harmed. This approach fosters propitious incentives: identify and learn from errors, and improve. This is the standard argument for just culture over a punitive approach. But two additional important factors favor a just-culture approach, both of which are brought out by recognizing obligations of justice to clinical colleagues.

First, it's simply wrong to blame individuals for system errors. What is obscured by the standard argument is that patient safety at any cost cannot be justified. Just as other constraints limit the pursuit of beneficence—veracity, rights of others, and so on—justice also imposes a constraint: *the burdens of providing safe patient care must be fairly distributed.* If the safest system for patients required a grossly unfair distribution of blame for medical errors, then we should reject that system. The typical discussion around patient safety simply ignores this obligation of justice.

Second, restorative just culture better attends to power imbalances in the medical workplace. Every clinician must participate in accurate reporting, but many are made much more vulnerable than others in doing so. On the traditional punitive model, those with diminished power and status more frequently experience a heavier share of certain burdens, such as fearing the loss of their job or even more diminished status within their teams. Justice requires us to consider and correct for this fact.

Two Objections to Restorative Just Culture

Traditional medical ethics emphasizes the professional responsibilities of health-care providers and attributes individual moral culpability when they fail to meet those responsibilities. A frequent objection raised against restorative just culture is that it undermines these traditional notions of individual moral and professional accountability, thereby disrespecting clinicians as moral agents and patients as moral equals. Two features of restorative just culture—its systems-level focus and its forward-looking view of accountability—are especially liable to such criticism. One strand of the objection, then, focuses on the perceived loss of *individual* accountability, while the other strand targets the perceived loss of *backward-looking* accountability. We will consider each objection in turn before responding to both in the next section.

The Individual Accountability Objection

For critics concerned with individual accountability, the systems-level focus of restorative just culture seems to dismiss traditional professional obligations and shift all moral responsibility from the provider to the system. But surely, the objection goes, health-care professionals still have individual moral responsibility for the decisions they make even when practicing within complex systems. It is fine and well to seek improvements to the system, but individuals within the system must remain accountable within their domains regardless of how the system is ultimately structured. To do otherwise is to "let wrongdoers off the hook" for their bad decisions and encourage moral complacency and a sense of moral helplessness.

Though he does not directly engage with restorative just culture per se, Edmund Pellegrino provides an excellent example of this strand of objection to systems-level prescriptions for dealing with medical error. To be clear up front, Pellegrino is not opposed to substantial efforts to reform and improve the microsystems and macrosystems in which every clinical-care decision is made; indeed, Pellegrino explicitly affirms that "a properly organized organizational and systemic context is essential to reduce the prevalence of medical error" (Pellegrino 2004, 84). However, he worries that overemphasis on system-level factors can be detrimental to patient safety and individual professional responsibility by undermining the structures that motivate and support professional virtue.

First, a system narrative can become a kind of "salvation theme" that wrongly assumes systemic changes alone can solve the problem of medical error (Pellegrino 2004, 84). Pellegrino argues, "Systems cannot make the professionals within them virtuous, but they can make it possible for virtuous professionals to be virtuous" (Pellegrino 2004, 84). It is, therefore, crucial to appreciate how the "effectiveness and efficient working" of systems depends on "a parallel affirmation of the moral duty and accountability of each health professional in the system . . . to possess the competence and character crucial to the performance of his or her particular function as well as those of the system as a whole" (Pellegrino 2004, 84). Indeed, as he sees it, "the major function of a system is to reinforce and sustain these individual competencies and virtues" (Pellegrino 2004, 84). Failing to appreciate these factors could be disastrous for system outcomes, Pellegrino argues, since the system design creates the choice and action architecture in which clinicians understand and pursue their individual responsibilities.

For Pellegrino, our models of system design and individual professional accountability should both be guided by the same "architectonic 'first' principle fundamental to what medical and health care are all about"—namely, the principle of "the primacy of the good of the patient" (Pellegrino 2004, 85). This first principle unifies the function and justification of efforts to prevent medical error at both the system and individual levels: "Every action of individual professionals and every organizational policy and regulation must be measured by this gold standard of traditional medical morality" (Pellegrino 2004, 85). A systemic commitment to beneficence and non-maleficence will only be effective if it is supported by individual health-care providers who have made the same professional commitment. If systemic efforts are to be adopted and enforced by the individual human beings who actually provide care, then "it will be necessary to reaffirm the moral nature of medical error, and to retain the notions of blame, accountability, and responsibility" (Pellegrino 2004, 85).

Moreover, Pellegrino argues that the improvement of the system, the purported advantage of a systemic approach, requires that a significant "discretionary space" be retained for health-care providers. This space provides the opportunity for "personalized, individualized, and humanized" care (Pellegrino 2004, 88). It also provides the space for health-care providers to "detect the ill-conceived or poorly designed element in a systems approach . . . and prevent the systemic shortcomings of the system itself from injuring the patient" (Pellegrino 2004, 88). If the system is to be improved, there must be room for providers to recognize and circumvent poor design and find better ways of providing care. Without this space, the very goals of the systemic approach—systems that learn and constantly improve—will be subverted. Yet, at the same time, this discretionary space, though necessary, sometimes allows errors to occur. In those cases, "the character of the health professional is the patient's last safeguard" (Pellegrino 2004, 88). Again, a systemic approach must be supported by a robust affirmation of professional duty and accountability.

Pellegrino argues that moral culpability and blame must be part of this robust affirmation of professional duty and accountability and cannot be eliminated even on a thoroughgoing systemic approach to patient safety:

> A preventable adverse action is a moral failure that cannot be exculpated by the "blame-free" approach advocated by proponents of the system-dimensions of error. Whether it is committed by an individual, a team, or an institution, culpable error is a violation of the implicit promise each of these entities makes when it offers itself as an instrument of help and healing.
>
> (Pellegrino 2004, 87)

Importantly, Pellegrino's criticism is of "blame-free" practices—as though refusing to assign blame could actually eliminate moral culpability. He warns, for example, of the "dangers of complacency and dulling of the moral sensibilities of the humans in the system when either a 'blame-free' approach or a 'blame-the-system' approach is adopted" (Pellegrino 2004, 88).

Pellegrino uses the modern organization of medical care into interdisciplinary teams to demonstrate that the assignment of responsibility and blame cannot be eliminated even within systems. Teams work together in a way that makes the work of the team more than the sum of the actions of each individual. Teams decide and act together and, therefore, they bear a shared responsibility for the functioning of the team. Each member is "implicated in team or system error" to various degrees (Pellegrino 2004, 92). The responsibility to recognize and intervene when the team or the system fails "can only be preserved if individual accountability is retained" (Pellegrino 2004, 93).

The Backward-Looking Accountability Objection

A second strand of objection is less concerned with individual accountability than with *backward-looking* accountability. This objection holds that any virtues gained by restorative justice come at a steep price—namely, the loss of any room for backward-looking practices of blame and punishment. Absent these traditional social practices, the objection goes, we undercut our ability to respect persons as moral equals and restore the equilibrium within our moral community that wrongful medical error disrupts.

In a recent article, Samuel Reis-Dennis outlines this strand of objection to forward-looking prescriptions for dealing with medical error (Reis-Dennis 2018, 739–742).[1] His objection centers on a feature of just culture that he, at least implicitly, regards as *essential* to the approach—namely, its purely "forward-looking" orientation to medical error. In his view, backward-looking practices of blame and punishment play an essential role in morally healthy medical systems.[2] Hence, if a just-culture approach to patient safety and medical error requires fundamentally abandoning such essential backward-looking practices, then this would provide strong grounds to reconsider or reject this approach.

Reis-Dennis attributes a "forward-looking accountability" strategy within the just-culture approach to Virginia Sharpe and Sidney Dekker (Sharpe 2003, 2004; Dekker 2016). On this view, accountability is rendered in the form of *future responsibilities* for action, specifically "preventative steps to design for safety, to improve on poor system design, to provide information about potential problems, to investigate causes, and to create an environment where it is safe to discuss and analyze error" (Sharpe 2004 13). Agents and agencies are held accountable, then, not by looking back to past choices and actions that deserve blame or punishment, but instead by looking ahead to who bears responsibilities for making systems and processes safer and more effective for patients. Importantly, wrongful actions and unfortunate accidents are neither disregarded nor unaddressed by "forward-looking accountability"; they are acknowledged as undesirable, their causes are actively investigated, and actions are taken in response. However, all of this is done with an eye toward meeting victims' present and future needs (Berlinger 2005, 66) and preventing such actions and accidents in the future, rather than fixing blame and issuing punishments accordingly.

Reis-Dennis argues that the fundamentally "forward-looking" just-culture approach must reject the "backward-looking" accountability that "essentially communicates resentful blame" (Reis-Dennis 2018, 740). Although restorative just culture's commitment to responding to victims' needs could be construed as a backward-looking response to prior actions, he argues that the sense of "backward-looking" that is morally required for just punishment is less concerned with its target than with its aim and function. In other words, for a form of accountability to be "backward-looking," on Reis-Dennis's view, is for present action not simply to respond to past wrongdoing, but to do so in a distinctive way; namely, by communicating resentful blame toward offenders by or on behalf of the victims of wrongdoing.

Reis-Dennis argues that an approach to patient safety that lacks backward-looking accountability—specifically, in the form of practices of blame and punishment for wrongful medical error—fundamentally disrespects patients, providers, and wrongdoers. He appeals to norms of fairness, justice, and respect that pertain to cooperative endeavors for mutual benefit. The cooperative endeavor at play here is "a good healthcare system . . . defined for the mutual benefit of all parties" (Reis-Dennis 2018, 740). Within such a system, "patients receive care," and "practitioners make a livelihood providing it" (Reis-Dennis 2018, 740). However, these benefits do not fall like manna from heaven; they are conditioned on all parties accepting "certain burdens in the form of rules that constrain their conduct" (Reis-Dennis 2018, 740). And a central "rule" constraining the conduct of clinicians is to provide competent professional care that benefits, or at least does not harm or injure, their patients and to not engage in reckless or malicious behavior.

When participants within the system "knowingly violate these rules and principles without a good excuse," they create "a social and moral imbalance" (Reis-Dennis 2018, 740). According to Reis-Dennis, following Herbert Morris (1968), backward-looking practices of blame and punishment are morally required for adequately addressing this imbalance. In a key passage, Reis-Dennis summarizes the connection this way:

> A just system of punishment aims to restore the equilibrium wrongdoing disturbs. It endeavors to fairly redistribute benefits and burdens, assuring that participants feel their investment in the organization is not naïve, and that they are not being taken advantage of. These levelling ambitions are expressions of moralized resentment, a desire to bring offenders down (and/or raise up the diminished) to an even plane. When moralized in this way, these desires are not only morally permissible, but laudable. An unfair distribution of benefits and burdens is fundamentally at odds with a conception of community members as moral equals. In punishing wrongdoers, we insist that everyone deserves the respect of fair treatment.
>
> (Reis-Dennis 2018, 741)

As such, just (i.e., proportionate, backward-looking, equilibrium-restoring) punishment connects in two important ways to norms of fairness, justice, and respect for persons: first, by "[communicating] the message that unfairness is unacceptable," and, second, by "[restoring] equality by (at least symbolically) erasing the unfairness that necessitated it" (Reis-Dennis 2018, 741).

Absent backward-looking practices of blame and punishment for wrongdoing, then, a health-care system fundamentally disrespects all who participate. Most obviously, victims of wrongdoing—that is, the patients harmed by wrongful rule violations—are disrespected; their participation in the system leaves them worse off than before, and the failure to punish the offender communicates that this loss is acceptable, implying the victim's lack of equal moral consideration and status. Similarly, rule-following clinicians are disrespected; they accepted burdens to make possible the system's benefits, and the failure to punish free-riding offenders communicates that they, at best, are naïve and, at worst, that they are not moral equals. Finally, even wrongdoers themselves are disrespected, as the failure to punish becomes a failure to "[treat] them as persons who can, through free expressions of their values, become proper objects of the distinctively human reaction of resentful blame" (Reis-Dennis 2018, 741).

Ultimately, Reis-Dennis concludes that the just-culture approach to patient safety and medical error fundamentally disrespects patients, providers, and wrongdoers, leaving the "moral field tilted towards wrongdoers" (Reis-Dennis 2018, 741). It treats victims and dutiful clinicians in a manner that diminishes their "dignity and self-respect," providing no mechanism even for having resentful feelings acknowledged as reasonable at all, let alone expressed in a manner that restores moral equilibrium among system participants. Similarly, it treats wrongdoers in a manner that diminishes their agency and humanity, providing no mechanism for expressing feelings of guilt, repaying debts to society, apologizing, or being forgiven. In all cases, such mechanisms "belong to a logic of resentment, blame and punishment," which this view's "forward-looking" orientation renders impossible.

A Rejoinder to the Objections

These two strands of objection are closely related in that both endorse practices of assigning blame and punishment to individual clinicians and others when certain deviations from ideal medical practice occur; they simply differ in the particular feature they emphasize in their respective accounts. In this section, we will address both objections in turn, seeking to challenge the underlying accounts on which they rest, as well as to defend restorative just culture against the charges rendered. Given the interrelation between the two objections, much of what we will argue against each particular objection would apply to the other objection as well.

A Rejoinder to the Individual Accountability Objection

Pellegrino's concerns about systemic approaches to patient safety are quite sensible on balance. In their early zeal, proponents of significant reform efforts both within and outside medicine often overestimate the ability of one big idea to solve a diverse set of problems. In particular, there is a danger that systemic efforts will neglect or abandon parallel efforts to develop and support individual professional commitments. Pellegrino makes a convincing argument that systemic efforts are destined to fail if individual health-care providers are not motivated by their own professional commitments to endorse the system and help monitor and improve it. The shift to, and implementation of, a systemic approach to patient safety requires caution and careful planning to avoid undermining the moral motivation of health-care providers.

Moreover, Pellegrino's emphasis on the need to preserve individual discretionary space is particularly compelling. Indeed, this insight aligns Pellegrino firmly with proponents of just-culture approaches to medical error. Robust and nuanced accounts of how restorative just cultures work explicitly establish trust in the provider as the foundational commitment of the system. Effective systems work "because of the capacity of your people to recognize problems, adapt to situations, [and] interpret procedures so that they match the situation" (Dekker 2016, 51). Restorative just culture is built upon a foundation of trust—the organization must trust providers to make good decisions and report errors, providers must trust that they will be treated fairly by the organization, and providers must trust each other to fulfill their roles in the system (Dekker 2016, 23–24).

Nevertheless, in other places, Pellegrino's critique overlooks or fails to engage seriously with the cardinal insights of the systemic approach to patient safety. His emphasis on maintaining individual moral culpability for medical errors fails to adequately account for at least three morally significant factors: (1) the influence of hindsight bias, (2) the difficulty of untangling causal factors and relationships that lead to error within complex systems, and (3) the alternative options for facilitating accountability.

First, many instances of medical error result from a number of "complex coincidences" that no individual provider is positioned to notice, either because she is literally not involved in the decisions being made or they only lead to harm in this particular context (Kohn, Corrigan, and Donaldson 2000, 52–53). Unfortunately, human beings are subject to hindsight bias—if one knows the outcome of a combination of factors and events, then the causal connections seem obvious, even though they may have been impossible to predict at the time the event was occurring (Kohn, Corrigan, and Donaldson 2000, 53; Dekker 2016, 55–57).[3] When this general bias combines with the traditional medical approach to error—find the provider in closest proximity to the error and punish her—it fuels the "natural" and "obvious" conclusion that one person's decision led directly to the error and the harm it caused. This distorted view of error is particularly alarming given Pellegrino's insistence that individual culpability depends on the "expected operation" of all agents in executing their complex roles within often complex circumstances (Pellegrino 2004, 87). Appreciating the significance of hindsight bias makes *post hoc* evaluations of such "expected" *pre hoc* behavior ethically perilous.

Second, even if the humans analyzing errors in complex systems after the fact were not fundamentally limited by hindsight bias, it would still be a Herculean task to, in a precise, thorough, and reliable manner: (1) inventory and untangle all contributing variables, in order to (2) determine degrees and kinds of contribution made by human and non-human factors, in order to (3) assign proportionate blame and punishment to individuals. (All three conditions seem necessary, though perhaps not even jointly sufficient, for ethically responsible practices of blame and punishment.) Pellegrino seems to recognize this at moments. He notes, for example, that there is a certain "inherent" fallibility of medicine such that "adverse outcomes at certain levels of occurrence can be expected even in the 'best hands' following the best procedures" (Pellegrino 2004, 87). The vital matter of how precisely to distinguish this inherent fallibility from (blameworthy) preventable adverse events is not discussed in any detail, let alone resolved convincingly. Pellegrino admits as well that "assigning individual or system responsibility is a difficult task sometimes . . . impossible to accomplish with any degree of certitude" and that "bright-line distinctions are also difficult to make with respect to the moral gravity of an error" (Pellegrino 2004, 89–90). Here again, though, no effort is made to flesh out the matter or grapple with the implications of failing to do so. Finally, Pellegrino emphasizes the fact that modern medical practice is fundamentally team-based and that "we must factor in the intricate interdependence of a group of health professionals who are essential to any complex procedure" (Pellegrino 2004, 91). He even goes on to endorse the validity of some notion of shared group agency that further complicates the moral landscape in which decisions are made and accountability is rendered. And, yet, he does not make any attempt to indicate how a large complex health system might try to practically operationalize this insight.

Third, even if those charged with determining moral culpability for medical error were not prone to hindsight bias and could precisely, thoroughly, and reliably manage a fair system for assigning blame and punishment, an open question remains as to why that, and only that, approach to accountability is morally adequate. We can agree with Pellegrino that "preventable adverse action is a moral failure," however complex and of whatever sort it may be, without accepting a decidedly individualistic model of blame and punishment as the only morally sufficient form of accountability. Traditional medical-ethics principles—such as beneficence and non-maleficence, or the clinician's "act of profession"—do not unequivocally and exclusively point in that direction. Indeed, the model of accountability that best promotes beneficence, arguably, is the model that best identifies and prevents error, which is precisely the claim that restorative just culture makes for itself (though admittedly needs to defend, as we are attempting to do in this chapter).

In all three ways, then, Pellegrino's overemphasis on individual culpability raises serious concerns. Moreover, it also may undermine the very goals of systemic approaches to patient safety that he himself has largely endorsed. An approach that sees the primary post-error task as determining whom to blame and/or punish is ripe for overlooking or misapprehending many important details. Once an individual has been identified as culpable for a medical error by virtue of hindsight bias, the impetus to figure out what other factors contributed to the error greatly diminishes (Kohn, Corrigan, and Donaldson 2000, 53).

Meanwhile, restorative just culture deftly avoids or manages all three sources of weakness in Pellegrino's account. The inescapable influence of hindsight bias in error analysis is less concerning for restorative just culture, since its thrust is forward-looking, focused on repairing trust and preventing future recurrence. The need to have a conceptually rigorous system for parsing proportionate blame and punishment to individuals does not arise since restorative just culture is primarily interested in understanding what happened, rather than who to blame for it. And its alternative model of accountability limits the focus on individual culpability and, therefore, makes room for people to identify and investigate more fully system failure, not just individual failures.

Finally, in addition to these three weaknesses with Pellegrino's account of individual professional accountability, the overall guiding principle of the account fits poorly with what looks to be a genuine effort to take systems-level insight seriously. Pellegrino insists that the principle of beneficence must be maintained at the center of medical morality. He argues that, like individual providers in traditional accounts of medical morality, systemic approaches to patient safety also must be motivated and measured by an unyielding commitment to "the primacy of the good of the patient." However, systems are unlike individual health-care providers, who develop distinct relationships with and, therefore, obligations to each patient (though even this construction of the individual clinician's moral obligations is debatable). *Systems by definition must serve not just many patients every day but numerous and diverse stakeholders.* Conflicts arise among obligations of beneficence to current patients, future patients, family members, providers, regulators, vendors, the community at large, and on and on. Crucially, *appeals to individual beneficence itself cannot resolve these conflicts or determine which system design to choose.* Instead we must choose a system design based on the benefits and burdens it creates and whether these are fairly distributed amongst many different stakeholders. Only an account of justice can resolve these conflicts or recommend a choice among system options, and it is precisely here that a restorative just-culture framework is well-equipped to guide microsystems and macrosystems in their approach to medical error.

A Rejoinder to the Backward-Looking Accountability Objection

Reis-Dennis's critique of forward-looking views of accountability might appear, on its face, to be even more threatening to restorative just culture than Pellegrino's concerns with overemphasizing systems. Indeed, if sound, Reis-Dennis's backward-looking accountability objection entails significant implications for a just-culture approach to patient safety and medical error. At the very least, the objection implies that a radical revision of the approach would be necessary if just culture is to avoid fundamentally disrespecting persons. Interpreted more strongly, the objection calls into question whether even radical revision can save just culture; fitting backward-looking practices into a thoroughgoing forward-looking view may be the conceptual equivalent of squaring a circle.

Fortunately, there is good reason to conclude that Reis-Dennis is talking past just-culture approaches here, and that his just-punishment account, at best, applies to a fundamentally different category of action. To see this in the starkest terms, consider an important qualification in Reis-Dennis's discussion of just punishment—namely, that it is confined to "clear cases of recklessness and malice" (Reis-Dennis 2018, 740, fn. iv). Making a qualification like this to weaken one's argumentative burden is fine in itself, and Reis-Dennis's model of just punishment may well provide sound ethical guidance for a certain (rarely instantiated) category of purposeful patient harm. However, it arguably does not apply at all to *medical error* as such. As anesthesiologist, lawyer, and patient safety expert Brian Liang emphasizes:

Medical error can be defined as a mistake, inadvertent occurrence, or unintended event in a health care delivery which may, or may not, result in patient injury. This definition in no way includes purposeful or reckless actions intended to directly or indirectly harm the patient. The distinction is critical. Purposeful or reckless actions are malicious and volitional—not the result of error; moreover, they are the source of a small minority of patient injuries in the health care systems. Instead of focusing on bad actors, a focus of safety should be directed to the much more frequent problem of error by individuals who are in good faith trying to perform effectively, but are working in systems where mistakes can and do occur.

(Liang 2004, 61)

If Liang's clinically informed framework is conceptually adequate, then two important implications follow. First, Reis-Dennis's model of just punishment simply *does not apply* to the most frequent sort of deviation that causes patient injury within complex health-care systems: *unintentional medical error*. Instead, it applies *only*, by self-imposed limitation, to "clear cases" of a highly infrequent sort of deviation that causes patient injury: intentional—or at least readily foreseeable—harm arising from "recklessness and malice" (Reis-Dennis 2018, 740, fn. iv). Second, since the overall thrust of restorative just culture clearly centers on medical error, Reis-Dennis's critique falls flat. It is no objection to the just-culture approach to say that it fails to give space to practices that, by the critic's own admission, do not apply within the relevant domain of concern.

Moreover, were Reis-Dennis to extend his critique beyond "clear cases of recklessness and malice" to include all or most cases of *genuine* medical error, his backward-looking account of resentful blame and punishment would immediately face all three of the challenges we posed to Pellegrino's individual accountability view: (1) the influence of hindsight bias, (2) the difficulty of untangling causal factors and relationships that lead to error within complex systems, and (3) the alternative options for facilitating accountability.[4] Additionally, it is unclear whether several of Reis-Dennis's central claims can withstand scrutiny.

First, though a forward-looking orientation is *emphasized* by all accounts of just culture as having considerable value for uncovering and responding to the vast majority of medical error, it does not follow that it is the *only* kind of orientation possible within the model. Again, just-culture thinking is not rigidly committed to a single blueprint, but rather a flexible set of tools for transforming distinct and already existing institutional cultures toward greater justice. Reis-Dennis sets up his critique on the assumption that there are *only two possible views* of accountability under just culture. However, this is plainly false, both of existing accounts and conceivable accounts. Dekker, for example, spends an entire book detailing how just culture might look more retributive or more restorative depending on particular design choices. He emphasizes that "the line between retribution and restoration is not entirely clear," that we should not "overstate the contrast" between them, and even that a given culture might "actually do some of both, at the same time" Dekker 2016, 21). For organizational cultures that may feel locked within a more retributive model, just culture has resources to guide these cultures toward better versions of themselves:

> A just culture can only be built from *within* your own organization's practice. The various ideas need to be tried, negotiated, and bargained among the people inside your organization. And you need to test them with the various stakeholders that surround your organization, who want their voices heard when things go wrong.
>
> (Dekker 2016, 21)

In other words, specific attempts to develop just culture around medical error will look different for each system depending on dozens of variables, but should never be rigidly imposed from above on a group of stakeholders.

Second, whatever else is true about just-culture approaches to medical error, there is clearly room (and multiple possible mechanisms) "to restore the equilibrium wrongdoing disturbs" and respect persons as moral agents. Indeed, the very label chosen to describe the view is instructive here: *restorative* just culture. At the heart of this approach is an understanding that error often leads to harm, harm creates needs, and needs create obligations (Dekker 2016, x). Armed with this understanding, restorative just culture seeks systematically to consider those needs (recognizing that they often include needs far beyond those of the "first victims" of error) and work out "collaboratively whose obligation it is to meet them" (Dekker 2016, x). Importantly, "reaching a restorative agreement requires that all affected people are involved and have their voices heard," which results in a very different process: one not merely "limited to a boss and an employee," but also involving first (and "second") victims of the incident, colleagues, and other stakeholders." Ultimately, the end of "restoration" is not meeting "hurt" with "more hurt," but rather meeting "hurt" with (1) "healing" (e.g., exchanging perspectives, expressing remorse, making amends, acting to repair trust, etc.) and (2) "learning" (e.g., exploring "why it made sense for the person to do what they did," investigating "organizational, operational, or design issues that could set up others for failure too," etc.; Dekker 2016, x).

Finally, in addressing Reis-Dennis's concern about addressing an "unfair distribution of benefits and burdens," we cannot help but think this is a point *in favor* of just culture rather than against. As we just noted, restorative just culture is fundamentally concerned with, and shaped by, its commitment to restore communities to their moral equilibrium. Moreover, unlike a model that features resentful blame and punishment as the proverbial carrot and stick for addressing all deviations from ideal medical care, restorative just culture appreciates how unfair it would be to distribute burdens of blame and punishment on the basis of luck. It also takes seriously the complex environment and non-neutral playing field of medical hierarchies, recognizing the power differentials that exist among various clinical and administrative staff and the patterns in which nursing staff, in particular, are victimized and scapegoated by punitive safety cultures and overly demanding workloads. This connects with another important point: even if Reis-Dennis is right about the appropriateness of a *patient* who has been (recklessly or maliciously) harmed blaming a distinct individual believed to be at fault, it is unclear that this point transposes to the appropriateness of a *colleague, supervisor, or institutional committee* blaming that same individual for medical error (which, again, does not include reckless or malicious actions).

All of this is especially salient when appreciating how many errors arise from "workarounds" in the system—that is, organic and widely used, but unsanctioned, pathways that respond to inefficiencies, inconveniences, and overly demanding expectations. Consider an example from Dekker in which nurses adapt to the poor quality of medication scanners by printing out a single high-contrast barcode and using it to get reliable scans quickly, rather than struggling with technology to complete the procedure properly (Dekker 2016, 5). When such "normalization of deviance" takes hold (Kohn, Corrigan, and Donaldson 2000, 55–56), all relevant parties are using these workarounds, and all consider them as necessary for getting their jobs done. Any of those parties could have been the unfortunate person who used the workaround at the time that a unique combination of factors led to harmful error. It would be unjust for others utilizing the same, or a relevantly similar, workaround to individually blame and punish the particular person involved in that isolated incident, rather than address the larger issues that are affecting everyone and leading each of them to choose unauthorized workarounds.

Neither Angels Nor Demons: Designing a Medical Safety Culture With Humans in Mind

Taking systems seriously fundamentally changes how we think about the ethics of preventing and responding to medical error. It forces us to re-evaluate what justice and fairness demand of our policies and procedures, considering the interests of all stakeholders and the ways in which particular system designs distribute the benefits and burdens of patient safety. The vast majority of medical errors involve significant systemic factors. The traditional model for addressing medical error does not acknowledge systemic factors, but rather blames and punishes the provider in closest proximity to the error. This approach both fails to accurately identify the cause of the error—missing any opportunity to correct it—and unfairly punishes the provider for an error she could not have foreseen or prevented on her own. Restorative just culture provides an ethically superior approach to medical error. It emphasizes system failures, rather than individual failures, fosters an environment in which providers can report error without fear of unjust punishment, and responds to the needs of all victims—first and second victims, individuals and communities. Under these conditions, the root causes of error can be identified, and the system can be improved.

In reflecting on the larger issues at stake here, we are reminded of Kant's famous distinction between states designed such that they could work *only if* populated by a "nation of angels" and states designed to function effectively *even if* populated by a "race of devils" (Kant 2017, 16). The former rely on the sufficiency of individual virtue, while the latter presupposes the sufficiency of good system design. Clinicians and administrators are, of course, neither angels nor devils, but mere humans. However, what the IOM concluded two decades ago has not changed in our experience: "People working in health care are among the most educated and dedicated workforce in any industry. The problem is not bad people; the problem is that the system needs to be made safer" (Kohn, Corrigan, and Donaldson 2000, 49). A restorative just culture will give them the best chance to do what the overwhelming majority of them set out to do every day—help people and protect them from harm—and treat them fairly when errors inevitably occur.

Notes

1. Reis-Dennis also discusses a second view of accountability he refers to as the "deterrence" approach, which he attributes to David Marx. We are focusing on his discussion and critique of the "forward-looking accountability"

approach, as it more closely aligns with the view of restorative just culture we seek to defend here.

2. See also Chapter 11, "Rehabilitating Blame" by Reis-Dennis.

3. Of course, human beings are subject to a number of cognitive biases in addition to hindsight bias, including future optimism bias, in which comparison with a false standard or norm leads individuals to underestimate their risk for a non-desired outcome. In the health-care setting, then, future optimism bias might balance out hindsight bias when assigning blame for errors. However, it seems equally likely that hindsight bias and future optimism bias would work together to exacerbate the problem. Future-optimism bias would likely be rampant in a punitive culture in which the source of error is identified with an individual's personal failing rather than systemic features. Colleagues simply must compare themselves favorably with the person who committed the error to fall victim to this bias. Because we are also subject to overestimation bias—which leads us to evaluate ourselves more highly than others—a punitive culture will produce conditions in which health-care professionals overestimate their own abilities compared with others and then have their bias confirmed when errors are attributed to personal failings in others. In contrast, a just-culture approach encourages everyone to recognize that they are at the same risk of making errors as everyone else because systemic forces intervene on individual decision making.

4. For Reis-Dennis's most recent work attempting to reckon with medical error with his account, see Chapter 11.

Works Cited

AAP, Steering Committee on Quality Improvement and Management and Committee on Hospital Care. 2011. "Policy Statement—Principles of Pediatric Safety: Reducing Harm Due to Medical Care." *Pediatrics* 127 (6): 1199–1210.

Bates, David, and Hardeep Singh. 2018. "Two Decades Since *To Err is Human*: An Assessment of Progress and Emerging Priorities in Patient Safety." *Health Affairs* 37 (11): 1736–1743.

Beauchamp, Tom, and James Childress. 2009. *Principles of Biomedical Ethics, Sixth Edition.* New York: Oxford University Press.

Beecher, Henry. 1970. *Research and the Individual.* Boston: Little-Brown.

Berlinger, Nancy. 2005. *After Harm: Medical Error and the Ethics of Forgiveness.* Baltimore, MD: The Johns Hopkins University Press.

Bhimji, Steve, and Yevgeniya Scherbak. 2018. "Medication Errors." In *StatPearls.* Treasure Island (FL): StatPearls Publishing. Retrieved from www.ncbi. nlm.nih.gov/books/NBK519065/.

Dekker, Sidney. 2016. *Just Culture: Restoring Trust and Accountability in Your Organization, Third Edition.* London: CRC Press.

Herranz, Gonzalo. 2002. "Why the Hippocratic Ideals are Dead." *British Medical Journal* 324: 1463. https://doi.org/10.1136/bmj.324.7351.1463

Jonsen, Albert. 1977. "Do No Harm: Axiom of Medical Ethics." In Stuart Spicker and Tristram Engelhardt, Jr. (eds.), *Philosophical Medical Ethics: Its Nature and Significance.* Dordrecht: D. Reidel Publishing Co: 27–41.

Joseph, Anjali, Kerm Henriksen, and Eileen Malone. 2018. "The Architecture of Safety: An Emerging Priority for Improving Patient Safety." *Health Affairs* 37 (11): 1884–1891.

Kant, Immanuel. 2017. *Toward Perpetual Peace: A Philosophical Sketch*, Trans. Jonathan Bennett. *Some Texts from Early Modern Philosophy*. Retrieved from www.earlymoderntexts.com/assets/pdfs/kant1795_2.pdf

Kohn, Linda, Janet Corrigan, and Molla Donaldson (eds.). 2000. *To Err Is Human: Building a Safer Health System*. Washington, DC: National Academy Press. Retrieved from www.ncbi.nlm.nih.gov/books/NBK225182/.

Liang, Bryan. 2004. "Error Disclosure for Quality Improvement: Authenticating a Team of Patients and Providers to Promote Patient Safety." In Virginia Sharpe (ed.), *Accountability: Patient Safety and Policy Reform*. Washington, DC: Georgetown University Press: 59–82.

Marx, David. 2001. *Patient Safety and the Just Culture: A Primer for Health Care Executives*. New York, NY: Trustees of Columbia University. Retrieved from www.chpso.org/sites/main/files/file-attachments/marx_primer.pdf.

Morris, Herbert. 1968. "Persons and Punishment." *The Monist* 52 (4): 475–501.

National Academies of Sciences, Engineering, and Medicine. 2015. *Improving Diagnosis in Health Care*. Washington, DC: The National Academies Press. https://doi.org/10.17226/21794.

Pellegrino, Edmund. 2004. "Prevention of Medical Error: Where Professional and Organizational Ethics Meet." In Virginia Sharpe (ed.), *Accountability: Patient Safety and Policy Reform*. Washington, DC: Georgetown University Press: 83–98.

Ratwani, Raj, Erica Savage, Amy Will, Allan Fong, Dean Karavite, Naveen Muthu, Joy Rivera, Cori Gibson, Don Asmonga, Ben Moscovitch, Robert Grundmeier, and Josh Rising. 2018. "Identifying Electronic Health Record Usability and Safety Challenges in Pediatric Settings." *Health Affairs* 37 (11): 1752–1759.

Rawls, John. 1971. *A Theory of Justice*. Cambridge, MA: Harvard University Press.

Reis-Dennis, Samuel. 2018. "What 'Just Culture' Doesn't Understand about Just Punishment." *Journal of Medical Ethics* 44 (11): 739-742.

Sharpe, Virginia. 2003. "Promoting Patient Safety: An Ethical Basis for Policy Deliberation." *Hastings Center Report Special Supplement* 33 (5): S1-S20.

Sharpe, Virginia, and Alan Faden. 1998. *Medical Harm: Historical, Conceptual, and Ethical Dimensions of Iatrogenic Illness*. Cambridge: Cambridge University Press.

Sharpe, Virginia. 2004. "Accountability and Justice in Patient Safety Reform." In Virginia Sharpe (ed.), *Accountability: Patient Safety and Policy Reform*. Washington, DC: Georgetown University Press: 1–26.

4 Rehabilitating Blame

Samuel Reis-Dennis

Introduction

Much of the work on medical error and adverse events is forward-looking. It focuses on how to reduce the risk of future errors and how to make hospitals safer for future patients. As a moral philosopher interested in the psychology and ethics of what philosophers have called the "reactive attitudes" (blame, pride, hurt feelings, gratitude, etc.), my interest is different. My project is backward-looking. It asks: what kinds of attitudes should doctors, patients, and families take toward errors that have already occurred, and what kinds of interactions should we encourage between these parties in the wake of harmful mistakes?

It is widely agreed that physicians should disclose professional errors to patients.[1] But difficult ethical questions arise once an error has been disclosed or discovered. What happens next? In this chapter, I argue that, to adequately face and respond to certain kinds of medical mistakes, we should cultivate a culture of blame. The suggestion will strike many as surprising, even scandalous. After all, the current consensus is just the opposite: blame is thought to be corrosive, counter-productive, and even unjust.[2] It is understood to be an obstacle on the way to improved patient safety practices and a cause of deep distress among providers and patients.[3] Consider, for example, a passage from Nancy Berlinger's *After Harm: Medical Error and the Ethics of Forgiveness*:

> It is difficult to imagine anyone in contemporary medicine who would argue in favor of the traditional 'blame-and-shame' approach to the aftermath of medical error, which holds that mistakes are made by "bad apples" who can be isolated and punished. Yet rooting out the remnants of blaming and shaming attitudes within professional and institutional cultures continues to be a challenge for physicians and others involved in patient-safety efforts. In this, medicine is no different from society in general. It's easier, and perhaps more satisfying psychologically, to pin blame on an individual rather than to do the hard work of facing and addressing systems problems.
>
> (Berlinger 2009, 97)

In vindicating blame as a response to medical error, I will not advocate a return to such a "bad apple" blame culture. I will, however, defend the targeted feeling and expression of angry, resentful, and even vindictive blaming attitudes toward health-care providers who culpably fall short of the standard of care. Only by validating such attitudes in response to such behavior, I claim, can we create a culture that takes victims' fitting resentment seriously as one part of the process of facilitating respect, accountability, and healing.

In the next two sections, I will sketch and respond to some influential, but misguided, arguments against blame as a response to medical error. In doing so, I hope to give the reader a sense of what I mean by "blame," how it differs from shame, and how we might understand the relationship between personal blameworthiness and one's role in an institutional structure. Later, I make the positive case for blame, emphasizing its ability to help us stand up for ourselves and others, thereby facilitating self-respect. In the final section, I raise and respond to what I take to be the most serious objections to a culture of blame in health care and then offer some brief concluding remarks.

Blame and Shame

Some of the resistance to blame in health care stems from a tendency, both in the bioethics literature and in everyday life, to conflate blame and shame.[4] In vindicating a "blame culture," I mean to defend, as Susan Wolf puts it:

> A range [of attitudes] that includes resentment, indignation, guilt, and righteous anger—they are emotional attitudes that involve negative feelings toward a person, arising from the belief or impression that the person has behaved badly toward oneself or to a member (or members) of a community about which one cares and which tend to give rise to or perhaps even include a desire to scold or punish the person for his bad behavior.
>
> (Wolf 2011, 336)

One source of disagreement in the contemporary philosophical literature on blame is the question of whether blame, at its core, is a judgment, or whether the essence of blame is to be found in the feeling and/or expression of "reactive" attitudes, such as anger and resentment. My own position is that this question is somewhat misguided. We use the word "blame" in various contexts to describe a wide range of reactions. In some cases, blaming may involve only a judgment of culpability with no reactive sentiment ("I blame the Secretary of Treasury for the economic downturn."); other times, it seems to involve resentful or angry feelings

("I can't be around Jones. I still blame him for the way he disrespected my mother.").

Here, I do not wade into the debate over the essence of blame. Instead, I have stipulated that I will be focusing on the ethics of a set of emotional blaming attitudes. These attitudes depend upon, but go beyond, judgments of sub-standard conduct. I have chosen to focus on these emotional blaming attitudes for two reasons: First, because they are more difficult to justify, and in greater need of moral vindication, than mere judgments of impropriety. Second, because they seem to lie at the core of the most ethically interesting controversies surrounding blame. After all, even some strong "anti-blame" advocates will no doubt agree that judgments of culpability are sometimes apt and even necessary (for purposes of training and education, for example). What they will not sanction, however, are the angry, resentful, and punitive impulses associated with the kind of "reactive" blaming I am interested in here. These emotional blaming responses are, I think, at the heart of the dispute about the propriety of blame and "blame culture."[5]

These blaming attitudes are responses to wrongful harm; they are appropriate reactions only to the violation of a good standard of interpersonal conduct, or to a wrongful frustration of a reasonable expectation. Shame, by contrast, is characteristically a response to the perception of one's own character or self as deficient or sub-standard.[6] As such, it focuses on the transgressor rather than the transgression, and inspires hiding, isolation, and inwardness. (Consider some classic shame reactions, such as hiding one's head in one's hands or wanting to disappear.)

Unlike shame, blame inspires guilt, which characteristically prompts confession and apology. Blame is an invitation to a kind of moral dialogue: it aims to draw the offender in.[7] Shaming, on the other hand, pushes the offender away, sending the message that the offender may only be fully welcomed back into the community when he is a better person. This is why the philosopher Herbert Morris wrote that blame calls for restoration but shame calls for creativity (Morris 1976, 62).

I will return to the connections among blame, guilt, apology, and forgiveness later. For now, I only wish to emphasize the simple point that shaming and blame can, and should, come apart. In the medical context, this means that a blame culture need not be a shame culture. The fact that a clinician has committed a blameworthy mistake does *not* necessarily mean that he is a bad person, that he should lose his job, that he should be looked down upon or ostracized by his peers, or even that he is a substandard doctor. It means that he culpably violated a reasonable standard of behavior and has perhaps harmed a patient as a result.

The conclusion, then, that making a place for blame as a response to medical error would amount to endorsing a "bad apple," "blame-and-shame" approach to the aftermath of medical error would too hasty (Berlinger 2009, 97). Blaming attitudes—even in their angry, resentful, and vindictive forms—can single out without isolating, aiming to draw wrongdoers in rather than cast them out. And, because they focus on the transgression rather the transgressor, they are deeply antithetical to the "bad apple" model.[8]

Blame, Control, and Accountability

Even if one accepts that blameworthiness does not imply rottenness, one may still have a lingering sense that blame culture is "bad apple" culture in another sense. The fear is that when we place "the blame" for a mistake on a single individual, we exonerate ourselves. One might suspect that the urge to blame others expresses an objectionable desire to avoid or ignore the reality of our own complicity, or to (mis)understand error and failure as results of human agency, rather than more insidious, systemic factors. One might worry, then, that determinations of blameworthiness would block thorough inquiry, preventing us from addressing root causes.

This objection to blame can seem especially significant when paired with worries about agency (or lack thereof) in institutional contexts. That one cannot be blameworthy for what one cannot control is a widely held moral principle. It would be unjust—even cruel, one might think— to blame someone who had lacked control over her actions.[9] In fact, I think that there are reasons to be suspicious of this principle,[10] but I will suppose in this chapter that it is true that control is a necessary condition of blameworthiness. Do clinicians who make mistakes lack the sort of control that would make them proper targets of blame?

Sidney Dekker has suggested that they may for what appear to be two distinct reasons. The first is supposed to follow from the observation that many medical failures are "systems errors" that resist easy attribution to any single agent. Dekker sees the urge to blame as an expression of a human tendency to exaggerate our own agential powers in an effort to maintain an illusion of control. He writes:

> Features of people's tools, tasks, and organizational context all constrain control and limit freedom of choice over good or bad outcomes. The ideal of rational, regulative human action is circumscribed by design and operational features. Design things in certain ways and some errors become almost inevitable.
>
> (Dekker 2013, 31)

It is true that we often overestimate the extent to which agents control outcomes, but surely there is room to admit this fact while leaving some space in the picture for human agency. In other contexts (sports teams, orchestras, corporations, academic departments), we are able to distinguish between actions and outcomes attributable to rational agents, and ones better thought of as products of non-human causes. A trumpet player who arrives to the concert without having practiced his part, for example, is rightly held accountable when he plays poorly. In this respect, medicine is no different from these other arenas. The fact that the causal history of a medical mistake is complex, involving, perhaps, multiple agents operating under varying degrees of institutional constraint, does not in itself imply that these agents are not morally responsible for their behavior.

Of course, in certain cases, when the constraints are especially severe, responsible agency may fall out of the picture entirely, but not all mistakes and failures occur under such extreme conditions. Indeed, even many actions that express a deeply entrenched institutional culture may be blameworthy. Consider, for example, the thesis, defended by Lucian Leape et al., that disrespectful behavior is common in many health-care institutions and poses a grave threat to patient safety (Leape et al. 2012). Patients who are treated disrespectfully, it seems to me, are right to blame disrespectful practitioners for that mistreatment, especially when the dismissive or degrading behavior results in a harmful error. The fact that such behavior may be normal within a given institutional context is not exculpatory—in fact, blaming, and taking actions that express blame, may be the best way to begin the process of changing such a culture.[11]

Dekker's second reason for pessimism is more general. Medicine and its practitioners are imperfect. Human error, especially under conditions of stress and fatigue, is not something that one could reasonably expect to fully avoid, especially over the course of a long career. Everyone makes mistakes occasionally. This is true, but the fact that failure is part of a normal, even good, medical career does not mean that agents are not blameworthy for some of the mistakes they do make. That one could not reasonably be expected to be perfect over a lifetime does not imply that a patient is not entitled to expect her clinician to operate within the standard of care in each instance. Again, we should resist the urge to hold medicine apart from everyday life. It is not reasonable for two friends to expect to go through life without ever failing to live up to the standards that shape and govern their friendship; nevertheless, when one breaks a promise, forgets an appointment, or otherwise falls short of the reasonable expectations friends have for one another, she is rightly blamed for her failure. The fact that being a perfect friend is nearly impossible does not imply that friends lack the control required for responsibility and blameworthiness when they fall short.

It is significant, I think, that these concerns about control seem most pressing in the context of blame that flows "downhill," from powerful people at the top of social or institutional hierarchies to less powerful blamed agents. The CEO of a large hospital system might, for instance, eagerly pin "the blame" for a botched procedure on a young nurse to convince stakeholders not to worry about more serious underlying problems that put the nurse in a position to fail. If we understand blame culture to always involve a funneling of angry feelings toward individual agents at the expense of a complete understanding of contextual factors, then we should reject it. But blame culture need not involve such narrow-mindedness. The assumption that it does, has, I think, been unfortunately pervasive in medicine. Well-meaning scholars and practitioners, though rightly emphasizing the power of systems and the need for accountability up the "chain of command," have thrown the baby out with the bath water in embracing the "no blame" model.

Blame, Status, and Self-Respect

Thus far, I have mostly been concerned to relieve some common, but misguided, worries about blame. Now I will make a positive case for it. I have already discussed some ways in which blame can go wrong: when it veers into unwarranted shaming that does not draw the offender back into the moral fold, when it allows the powerful to deflect responsibility onto socially weaker agents, and when it distracts from deeper systemic problems. My goal in this section will be to explain why and how blame works when it works *well*, and what we would gain by rehabilitating it. My central claim is that we should make a place for blame in our toolbox of responses to medical error because it is a social-leveling mechanism allowing victims and their families to communicate a laudable fighting spirit. To get a sense of how it does so, we will need to understand the distinct social role that feelings and expressions of blame play in moral life.[12]

Let us consider the feeling first. Various philosophers have convincingly argued that resentment is a defensive passion, one that arises in response both to personal disrespect and to threats to the moral order.[13] As Jeffrie Murphy and others have noted, a resentful person cares deeply about how she, and others, are thought of and treated and, as a result of her feeling resentment, is likely to feel motivated to do something about such mistreatment (2005, 19). Feelings of resentment reflect a belief, not only that one has been wronged, but that the wrong cannot stand, that moral order must be restored.[14]

Feelings of resentment are most clearly fitting when a moral agent communicates a disrespectful, degrading, or otherwise morally unacceptable message through his behavior. When this kind of wrongdoing is allowed to stand, it changes what I'll call the *de facto* social statuses of both the victim and the wrongdoer, especially when the victim is harmed. Victims become, in some sense, people whom wrongdoers can insult, disrespect, or otherwise mistreat, while wrongdoers become people who stand "above the law."[15]

Sometimes, perhaps especially when we read philosophy, it can be tempting to tell ourselves that we all have equal moral worth, that nothing anyone does can change that, and that we ought not to indulge our fragile egos by caring so much about our *de facto* statuses. In fact, I think *de facto* social standing is worth caring about, too. A certain kind of concern about where one stands in a social or moral hierarchy is a sign of genuine investment in the project relating to others in a way that does not compromise the dignity of the parties. It is a product of the desire to enjoy the kinds of good relationships that call for social and moral equality. When one's *de facto* status is threatened by culpable wrongdoing, it can often be permissible, and even good, to defend oneself.

For purposes of illustration, suppose a patient presents in the emergency room with burns, and the attending physician fails to wash his hands before treating them. As a result, the patient is infected with sepsis and endures a terrifying hospital stay before recovering. As she is preparing to finally leave the hospital, a resident informs her that she suspects the infection was a result of the physician's failure to follow protocol. Through his actions, the physician reveals a disregard, or at the very least a lack of concern, for the patient's safety. His actions reflect objectionable priorities. Making matters worse, the patient trusted this doctor and had the right to expect better treatment.

In cases like this one, blame is well-suited to the task of standing up for oneself and righting status imbalances. To see why, it will be helpful to contrast blame with another reaction one might have to being wronged: disappointment. Disappointment, though not exactly out of place as a response to disrespect and/or wrongdoing, reflects a distinctive understanding of the event and the relationships at stake. This is because disappointment characteristically goes beyond resentment by revealing a kind of despair, signaling re-evaluation or withdrawal. Consider the distinctive pain of knowing you have disappointed a close friend or family member: if the disappointment is justified, you have not only failed to live up to the standards that govern the relationship. Rather, you have failed to be or become the kind of person the wronged party thought you were or could be. These kinds of shortcomings inspire shame instead of, or in addition to, guilt. As a result, they are in general harder to undo than transgressions that would prompt anger, which do not necessarily imply re-evaluation of character or a weakening of the relationship. In fact, in many cases an angry reaction implies the opposite; namely, that the offender, through humbling himself and apologizing, can more or less set things right, or at least start on a path toward forgiveness and reconciliation.

Angry, blaming emotions are distinctive because they signal a willingness to act rather than to withdraw. In anger and blame, we *fight back* in an effort to right the status imbalances that gave rise to our angry feelings. Expressed blame, then, communicates both vulnerability and resolve. To fight for a relationship, rather than reconsidering it or withdrawing from it, can be a sign of trust and investment. Expressing blame, as opposed to disappointment or sadness, allows us to communicate our faith, or at least hope, that the episode that gave rise to the blame will not force us to reassess or terminate the relationship.

Equally, signaling one's willingness to fight can be an act of bravery, a way to assert or restore one's status, dignity, and self-respect. And because blaming attitudes are fighting attitudes, there is a boldness to anger that sadness and disappointment lack. Anger often triggers anger in return; in expressing it, victims risk potential backlash. But one's willingness to provoke is itself a sign of strength, and demonstrating such courage can facilitate self-respect and the restoration of status.

This analysis helps to explain the significance patients place on apology in their narratives of medical mistakes.[16] I have claimed that blame is a leveling emotion, one that seeks to right social and moral imbalances that arise as a result of wrongful harm. Apology is a humbling act. In saying "I'm sorry," wrongdoers announce that they do not see themselves as above the law, that they understand their victims as worthy of respect and consideration, and that they wish to repair the relationship that their actions altered or jeopardized. In other words, apology is an apt and productive response to one's own *blameworthiness*. In fact, to fully understand apology, we must seriously face the resentful feelings that help shape its meaning and give it significance.

In good relationships between moral and social equals, all parties are able to safely make justified resentful feelings felt and understood in a way that could lead to apology, forgiveness, and reconciliation. Unfortunately, provider–patient relationships—which are usually characterized by imbalances in status—often fall short of this ideal. The rejection of "blame culture" is both a symptom and a (partial) cause of these power disparities. It is a symptom insofar as people who already feel powerless may reasonably feel afraid to express blame for fear of retribution from their powerful targets. Worse yet, it may not even occur to patients to express such attitudes: absent a context in which being heard and understood appears possible, expressions of blame will seem out of place.

The rejection of blame is a partial cause of these power imbalances as well. Not being held accountable for one's mistakes can entrench feelings of superiority, a sense that one is above the law. In victims, discouraging blame reinforces the impression that there is nothing they can do about being disrespected, that they do not deserve, or at least could never hope to achieve, the sort of status that would make expressions of blame safe and effective. The result is that many patients, especially socially disadvantaged ones, may emerge from their interactions with the health-care system feeling frustrated, alienated, and resigned. Rather than fighting to repair and continue relationships with providers as moral equals, they may withdraw in disappointment and despair.[17]

Avoiding Blame's Pitfalls

Until this point, I have mostly focused on the features of blame that allow victims to protect their dignity by expressing a willingness to stand up for themselves. But what about the effects of blame on practitioners who make mistakes? Many providers who act negligently are racked with guilt and shame over their mistakes, and one might reasonably wonder whether an institutional culture that made space for blame, and, by extension, encouraged feelings of guilt, would be professionally and personally devastating. The first thing to say in response to this worry is that feeling guilty in response to one's culpable mistakes is good. It is a psychologically normal, and morally laudable, reaction for a person invested in a lifelong project of healing. Of course, excessive guilt can be pathological, but a culture that aimed to eliminate guilt, or even tried to minimize it, would be artificial and inhuman.

How, then, can we embrace guilt without allowing it to devolve into pathological self-loathing? The key, I think, is to provide a productive outlet for guilt so that it motivates efforts to seek forgiveness and reconciliation rather than solitude. The process that provides such an outlet, that allows wrongdoers to move from guilt to forgiveness, belongs to the logic of blame. In fact, I suspect that it is in large part the *rejection* of the ethics of blame that leads practitioners to internalize their mistakes and misdeeds as crushing, shameful traumas. The point may strike some as counterintuitive, but the thought is an extension of the earlier observation that guilt and blame (as opposed to shame and shaming) characteristically draw offenders *in*, inviting them to participate in moral dialogue. Blame culture—with its almost ritual procession from anger to confession to apology to forgiveness to reconciliation—can provide both victims and authors of error a process through which to heal and move forward. Consider the following passage from David Hilfiker's classic piece "Facing our Mistakes":

> The drastic consequences of our mistakes, the repeated opportunities to make them, the uncertainly about our own culpability when results are poor, and the medical and societal denial that mistakes must happen all result in an intolerable paradox for the physician. We see the horror of our own mistakes, yet we are given no permission to deal with their enormous emotional impact; instead, we are forced to continue the routine of repeatedly making decisions, any one of which could lead us back into the same pit. . . . The only real answer for guilt is spiritual confession, restitution, and absolution. Yet within the structure of modern medicine, there is simply no place for this spiritual healing. . . . It simply doesn't fit into the physician-patient relationship.
>
> (1984, 21)

My suggestion is that a blame culture is uniquely well-suited to provide the sort of structure that would make such redemptive healing possible. Practitioners need to be able to move on, to be resilient, and to forgive themselves in the wake of costly mistakes. Blame offers us a logic within which this resilience could be tasteful, and self-forgiveness could be earned.

Still, one might wonder whether expressions of blame are truly the best way to register that one has been hurt or disrespected. We all know, after all, that blame can often spiral out of control, turning into bullying and abuse. It can also provoke backlash and retaliation, straining relationships and driving people apart. This is a serious and important objection to making room for blame in health care, but I do not think it is fatal. It is no accident that feeling the force of blame is jarring and unpleasant. In fact, in order to fully understand the power of blame, we must acknowledge (and even endorse) its connection to action. The fact that blame can so often be unsettling, loud, and even threatening, is what allows it to do its characteristic work, both of prompting offenders to rethink their behavior and apologize, and of fostering self-respect in victims. I am not claiming, however, all blaming reactions are, or should be, scary and threatening (though in some cases they may be). And, crucially, I am *not* defending blame that is bullying or abusive. Rather, I have mostly been trying to explain why blame works when it works well, and to give the reader a sense of what we would gain by making some space for it in health care.

Full appreciation of blame's dangers does, however, underscore the need for virtues and rules that would help patients and providers feel, express, and receive blame well. The task of developing the virtues and rules necessary to *prevent* blaming interactions from degenerating into corrosive chaos, is both philosophical and practical: Philosophically, we must explicate the virtuous traits of character and the appropriate normative constraints; practically, we must do the everyday work of cultivation and enforcement.

At this point, some readers may suspect that such institutional overhaul is impossible, or at least highly unlikely. Are not hospital administrators and risk managers likely to reject anything even involving the *word* "blame" out of sheer instinct?[18] Is it not likely that doctors will hide their mistakes for fear of being blamed?[19] Where would we even begin the task of cultivating the necessary virtues and establishing the necessary institutional rules? Perhaps these obstacles will ultimately prove insurmountable, but such pessimism and cynicism is no place to begin. Although I do not wish to gloss over the difficulty of cultivating the virtues of character that will allow us to blame well (at the right times, in the right ways, toward the right people) and be good recipients of blame (willing to acknowledge our blameworthiness and apologize without lapsing into defensiveness or self-hatred), my hope is that these challenges will not be overwhelming. Cultivation of virtue is famously difficult, requiring instruction, perseverance, and luck. But we are not totally in the dark: as we aspire to make sweeping changes, we may draw from a wealth of successful cases of interpersonal blame outside of health care as models for a more general practice.[20] In establishing such a practice, we would acknowledge and accept the role blame can play in constructive responsibility exchanges—prompting and facilitating honest and sensitive interactions that acknowledge the ruptures medical mistakes cause personally and socially and that actively seek to mend them.

Specifying exactly what it would mean to give and receive blame well in concrete cases, and offering a more complete outline of a good blaming practice, are important tasks that lie outside the scope of this chapter. The details of both will vary depending on the cases and institutions in question. In some instances, an ethics committee might have a role to play in determining blameworthiness and in moderating a successful blaming interaction; in others, the ideal response to a culpable error could involve respected colleagues encouraging a physician who had behaved negligently to listen to his patient's justified complaints and apologize.

This sort of practical application, though, is not best left solely in the hands of philosophers. I suspect that the most successful blaming practices would be developed locally through a deliberative process that allowed physicians, nurses, administrators, legal experts, patients, and scholars from a wide range of disciplinary backgrounds to express their needs, reservations, and aspirations. My goal in this chapter has not been to offer a comprehensive blueprint for good blaming practices. While I have tried to explain the need for such practices and lay some conceptual groundwork for them, I do not pretend to know exactly how blame could be most justly and productively integrated into the institutional fabrics of specific health-care institutions. This is work that I envision scholars and stakeholders taking up together.

I do hope to have shown that, though daunting, the task of making space for blame in health care is worthy of our best efforts. Rehabilitating blame would help us to bring provider–patient interactions into line with an ideal of human communication that many of us aspire to in our best and most significant personal relationships, and it would give those who have suffered as a result of culpable medical error the opportunity to fight for respect and affirm their dignity with authenticity and force.

Notes

1. See, for example, Tello (2016), Fryer-Edwards (2016), and Berlinger (2009).
2. For two examples of anti-blame sentiment, see: Khatri, Brown, and Hicks (2009), and Bell et al. (2011).
3. One notable exception is the work of Edmund Pellegrino, who, in persuasively arguing that even actors within large systems can be personally accountable for their failures, writes that a blame-free approach opens the

door for "complacency and dulling of the moral sensibilities" (88) and that a "no-blame system could . . . often be a travesty of social and commutative justice" (89). See: Pellegrino (2004). In this chapter, I extend Pellegrino's arguments by defending a blame culture that would promote and facilitate the kind of accountability he has in mind.

4. Berlinger in *After Harm*, for instance, often deals with blame and shame together. For another example, see Liang (2004).

5. For readers interested in the philosophical debate about blame's nature, the essays collected in Coates and Tognazzini's *Blame* are a good place to start. See: Coates and Tognazzini (2013).

6. My thinking about shame has been shaped by Herbert Morris's "Guilt and Shame." See: Morris (1976).

7. For an influential defense of a "conversational" model of blame, see McKenna (2013).

8. This is not to say that some sorts of errors do not reveal their authors to be "bad apples." Some medical failures express contempt for patient safety, shocking arrogance, or other shameful vices.

9. Moral luck seems to put pressure on such a principle. See Chapter 2: "Medical Error and Moral Luck" by Allhoff.

10. For arguments against a control condition on blameworthy agency, see Adams (1985) and Smith (2008).

11. I explain why this may be the case in the next section.

12. This section, particularly my discussion of the differences between blame and disappointment, draws heavily from Reis-Dennis (2018b). In that paper, which does not focus on health care, I explore the psychology and ethics of angry feelings and the scary outbursts that express them, and I respond to some prominent anti-anger arguments in the contemporary philosophical literature.

13. For more on investment in the moral order, see chapter two of Murphy (2005).

14. Murphy, for example, writes, "I am, in short, suggesting that the primary value defended by the passion of resentment is *self-respect*, that proper self-respect is essentially tied to the passion of resentment, and that a person who does not resent moral injuries done to him . . . is almost necessarily a person lacking in self-respect" Murphy (1988, 16).

15. As Murphy (1988, 28) puts the point: "Wrongdoers attempt (sometimes successfully) to degrade or insult us; to bring us low; to say 'I am on high while you are down there below.' As a result, we in a real sense *lose face* when done a moral injury—one reason why easy forgiveness tends to compromise self-esteem. But our moral relations provide a ritual whereby the wrongdoer can symbolically bring himself low (or raise us up—I am not sure which metaphor best captures the point)—in other words, the humbling ritual of *apology*, the language of which is often that of *begging* for forgiveness. The posture of begging is not very exalted, of course, and thus some symbolic equality—necessary if forgiveness is to proceed consistently with self-respect—is now present."

16. See chapter three of Berlinger's *After Harm* for examples of such narratives.

17. For research on the pervasiveness of lack of trust in health care, as well as its implications for patient health, see: Armstrong et al. (2006).

18. I have not mentioned the legal implications of allowing blame back into medicine, though the ways in which blame, apology, and the law interact will obviously be central to the success of a real-life blaming practice. My concern is this chapter has been to establish a moral basis for the rehabilitation of blame rather than to address these important practical legal questions.

19. This is an empirical question that would be difficult, perhaps impossible, to answer without first successfully establishing the kind of "blame culture" I have suggested here. For more on the tension between backward-looking respect for victims and forward-looking safety considerations, especially as it relates to the ambitions of the "Just Culture" movement, see Reis-Dennis (2018a).
20. I have in mind everyday instances of blame between friends and family members. Imagine, for example, that a roommate repeatedly fails to do his share of communal chores. His roommates' forceful but respectful expressions of blame could both help them stand up for themselves and prompt the offender to think harder about the impact of his actions on others. Blame, from patients, families, and even colleagues, could function similarly in health care, at least in response to certain kinds of transgressions.

Works Cited

Adams, R. 1985. "Involuntary Sins." *The Philosophical Review* 94 (1): 3–31.

Armstrong, Katrina, Abigail Rose, Nikki Peters, Judith Long, Suzanne McMurphy, and Judy Shea. 2006. "Distrust of the Health Care System and Self-Reported Health in the United States." *Journal of General Internal Medicine* 21 (4): 292–297.

Bell, Sigall, Tom Delbanco, Lisa Anderson-Shaw, Timothy McDonald, Thomas Gallagher. 2011. "Accountability for Medical Error: Moving Beyond Blame to Advocacy." *Chest* 140 (2): 519–526.

Berlinger, Nancy. 2008. "Medical Error." In Mary Crowley (ed.), *From Birth to Death and Bench to Clinic: The Hastings Center Bioethics Briefing Book for Journalists, Policymakers, and Campaigns*. Garrison, NY: The Hastings Center: 97–100.

Berlinger, Nancy. 2009. *After Harm: Medical Error and the Ethics of Forgiveness*. Baltimore, MD: Johns Hopkins University Press.

Coates, D. Justin, and Neal A. Tognazzini (eds.). 2013. *Blame*. New York: Oxford University Press.

Dekker, Sidney. 2013. *Second Victim: Error, Guilt, Trauma, and Resilience*. Boca Raton, FL: CRC Press.

Fryer-Edwards, Kelly. 2016. "Tough Talk: Medical Error." In *Tough Talk: A Toolbox for Medical Educators*. Retrieved from https://depts.washington.edu/toolbox/toc.html.

Hilfiker, David. 1984. "Facing Our Mistakes." *New England Journal of Medicine* 310: 118–122.

Khatri, Naresh, Gordon Brown, and Lanis Hicks. 2009. "From a Blame Culture to a Just Culture in Health Care." *Health Care Management Review* 34 (4): 312–322.

Leape, Lucian, Miles Shore, Jules Dienstag, Robert Mayer, Susan Edgman-Levitan, Gregg Meyer, and Gerald Healy. 2012. "Perspective: A Culture of Respect, Part 1: The Nature and Causes of Disrespectful Behavior by Physicians." *Academic Medicine* 87 (7): 845–852.

Liang, Bryan. 2004. "Error Disclosure for Quality Improvement: Authenticating a Team of Patients and Providers to Promote Patient Safety." In Virginia Sharpe (ed.), *Accountability: Patient Safety and Policy Reform*. Washington, DC: Georgetown University Press: 59–82.

McKenna, Michael. 2013. "Directed Blame and Conversation." In D. Justin Coates and Neal Tognazzini (eds.), *Blame*. New York: Oxford University Press: 119–140.

Morris, Herbert. 1976. *On Guilt and Innocence*. Berkeley, CA: University of California Press.

Murphy, Jeffrie. 1998. "Forgiveness and Resentment." In Jean Hampton and Jeffrie Murphy, *Forgiveness and Mercy*. Cambridge: Cambridge University Press: 14–34.

Murphy, Jeffrie. 2005. *Getting Even: Forgiveness and Its Limits*. Oxford: Oxford University Press.

Pellegrino, Edmund. 2004. "Prevention of Medical Error: Where Professional and Organizational Ethics Meet." In Virginia Sharpe (ed.), *Accountability: Patient Safety and Policy Reform*. Washington, DC: Georgetown University Press: 83–98.

Reis-Dennis, Samuel. 2018a. "What 'Just Culture' Doesn't Understand About Just Punishment." *Journal of Medical Ethics* 44: 739–742.

Reis-Dennis, Samuel. 2018b. "Anger: Scary Good." *Australasian Journal of Philosophy*, forthcoming, Available online.

Smith, Angela. 2008. "Control, Responsibility, and Moral Assessment." *Philosophical Studies* 138 (3): 367–392.

Tello, Monique. 2016. "Medical Errors: Honesty is the Best Policy." *Harvard Health Blog*. Retrieved from www.health.harvard.edu/blog/medical-errors-honesty-is-the-best-policy-2016100310405.

Wolf, Susan. 2011. "Blame, Italian Style." In R. Jay Wallace, Rahul Kumar and Samuel Freeman (eds.), *Reasons and Recognition*. New York: Oxford University Press: 332–347.

Part II
Communication and Risk

5 A Communication-Based Approach to Safeguarding Against Medical Errors

The Case of Palliative Care

Leah M. Omilion-Hodges

Setting the Stage: Complexities in the Modern Medical System

Preventable medical errors have become so pervasive that some have suggested that they have reached epidemic proportions (Makary and Daniel 2016, i2139). What is equally problematic is that clinicians and researchers continue to trace preventable errors back to routine practices and organizational structures that serve as the scaffolding of modern medicine. More specifically, complex and fragmented health-care systems, faulty or non-existent communication, power differences, and hierarchies all contribute to lapses and mishaps in patient care (Lingard et al. 2002; Lingard, Whyte, and Regehr 2009; Omilion-Hodges and Swords 2017b; Sutcliffe, Lewton, and Rosenthal 2004).

Part of the challenge stems from the ubiquity of the long-established biomedical approach to medicine. This traditional interpretive model stresses provider expertise, technological innovations, and striving to prolong life at all costs. The more contemporary biosocial model centers on transdisciplinary care teams, integration of patients and their loved ones into the development of care plans, and death as a natural part of life. Though these models should work in concert and borrow standardized processes from one another when helpful, more commonly they spark deep divides between specialties and wedge tension between providers (Omilion-Hodges and Swords 2017b, 2017a). Palliative care, or care for those with serious or chronic illnesses or those near end of life, serves as a useful paragon for how providers can integrate small, but meaningful, communication processes to facilitate coordinated patient care while also embedding safeguards against medical mishaps.

Although still a relatively new specialty, the demand for palliative care has skyrocketed over the last 15 years, leading to a recent shift in health-care centers (Dumanovsky et al. 2016). Palliative care teams operate from the more modern biosocial approach, which has prompted a number of dialectical tensions and stressors for providers, especially concerning peer relationships and collaborations with those in other specialties. Because palliative care teams care for those in critical condition, they are often in a position to communicate about patient needs with cardiologists, oncologists, and neurologists. These long-established specialties have traditionally operated from the biomedical model, in which providers may see death as a failure, sparking tension with palliative care providers and often leading to ill treatment or an absence of communication about patient needs (Omilion-Hodges and Swords 2017b).

Drawing from a collection of research gathered from national award-winning palliative care units, this chapter highlights common organizational obstacles and tensions imbued within the medical system (Omilion-Hodges and Swords 2017b; Omilion-Hodges and Swords 2017a). Palliative care is used as a lens to illustrate provider and team challenges, and communication-rooted solutions implemented by these providers are articulated for use across specialties, teams, and units. Shifting attention to intentional and feasible communication processes naturally integrates several layers of checks or safeguards against otherwise preventable medical errors.

After providing a thorough introduction of palliative care, this chapter reviews commonplace organizational obstacles that contribute to medical errors. Although there are a number of ways in which teams can break down and messages can go awry, there also are numerous empirical communication-rooted solutions that may serve as defensive mechanisms against mishaps. Storytelling, cultivating and respecting individual and specialty identity, and enacting personal leadership are pragmatic suggestions for preventing medical errors. The discussion offers pragmatic advice for engineering effective communication processes and integrating them into extant organizational and team practices.

Palliative Care

In the late 1950s, Dr. Cicely Saunders suggested that "only an interdisciplinary team could relieve the 'total pain' of a dying person in the context of his or her family," which remains a foundational principle of palliative care today (Loscalzo 2008). Practitioners continued to question customary approaches to death and dying. Elisabeth Kubler-Ross suggested that end-of-life patients had a right to expect honest and respectful communication. In the 1970s, the term "palliative care" was suggested as a means to separate care for those with serious illness from hospice care. Since 2008, practitioners can become board-certified in this rapidly growing specialty.

Palliative care delivers holistic care addressing physical, psychological, emotional, practical and spiritual needs for those with serious illnesses or nearing end of life. Unlike hospice, palliative care can be delivered in concert with curative treatment. This progressive medical specialty employs individualized communication to provide relief and help alleviate the stress or confusion that may be associated with chronic or serious illness and medical procedures. Palliative care providers also help to mitigate family dynamics when necessary. Similarly, practitioners embrace patients' families as part of their charge and, therefore, often become integral components of family end-of-life communication. Part of the reason that the demand for palliative care has risen so steeply is because death has largely moved from private residential settings to health-care facilities. For illustration, roughly 63 percent of Americans die while in hospitals, while an additional 17 percent die in other institutional settings, such as hospice or palliative care (Foley 1995; Isaacs and Knickman 1997). Relatedly, in the Western context, especially in the United States, conversations about death and dying often do not occur until circumstances force loved ones to discuss needs and wishes. Moreover, palliative care providers often become leaders and/or active participants in facilitating conversations with those with serious illnesses and their loved ones because these discussions often do not commence before a health scare pushes the point. Yet when a serious illness has set in, there are often a number of associated challenges that arise simultaneously, such as the strain between addressing curing and caring for a patient. Ideally, patients feel cared for and have their wishes honored during curative treatment, yet in the midst of a serious illness, patients, their families, and providers may find themselves at odds in attempting to navigate the progression of a disease.

In research with award-winning palliative care units and in more recent work considering the intersection of family communication and palliative care (Omilion-Hodges and Swords 2017b, 2017a), the cure–care tension has emerged. As noted, the tension coiled between care and cure can spark a division between providers, patients, and family members, particularly if individuals do not agree on a course of action. This stress is also imbued within the biomedical and biosocial models, in which the former emphasizes cure, and the latter stresses care. The distinctions between the models and continued confusion regarding the purpose and scope of palliative care can be traced back to the fact that one of the primary charges of the specialty was to predict the progression of an illness or disease (Rokach 2005). This early charge has resulted in palliative-care practitioners being called to question for their utility in medicine and being referred to as enforcers of the death schedule, Dr. Death, and the grim reaper (Omilion-Hodges and Swords 2017a). The roots of this often-misunderstood specialty may stem in large part due to the distinctions between the biomedical and biosocial models (Omilion-Hodges and Swords 2017a). Moreover, the divergences between these interpretive models also have placed palliative care providers in trying organizational situations in which they attempt to navigate opposing tensions.

Palliative care is a departure from the traditional, biomedical model in which the physician is often not only the guiding, but also often the sole voice in creating a plan to eradicate a disease. Palliative care does not typically rely on innovative technology to offer care. Instead, providers may use pain inventories and are more likely to offer a homemade quilt, calming music, and (in place of or) listen to patients' wishes in an effort to deliver supportive care (Pres 2012). This is in stark contrast to other specialties in which advances in technology are crucial catalysts for attracting patients and contributing to the overall revenue of health-care centers. The stress coiled between cure and care continues to complicate family end-of-life conversations much in the same way it can hinder the interprofessional relationships between medical providers.

The guiding focus on care has resulted in palliative care clinicians navigating unique opposing tensions: the living–dying dialectic and the practicing–advocating dialectic (Omilion-Hodges and Swords 2017a). The first dialectic reiterates much of the above discussion in the sense that palliative care providers embrace death as a necessary aspect of life and, therefore, providers do not necessarily subscribe to or suggest curative treatment in all scenarios—especially if the patient indicates otherwise. Communication scholars uncovered that part of the challenge is the lack of clarity in terms of the foci of palliative care (Omilion-Hodges and Swords 2017a). As one participant put it, "It's impossible to communicate comprehensively about end of life care or options if you don't know what to do in the absence of a treatment plan" (Omilion-Hodges and Swords 2017b). Moreover, this particular dialectic is associated with others assigning value (or lack thereof) to palliative care in the sense that the nuances of palliative care are confusing, and the specialty does not generate as much revenue as others.

The second dialectic tension is an extension of the first. Considering the confusion surrounding the purpose or scope of palliative care, practitioners report feeling as though they must be practitioners of, but also advocates for, the specialty. In this sense, palliative care practitioners have indicated feeling like specialty cheerleaders or educators because they so frequently have to articulate their role within medicine. That is, the relevant newness of palliative care still requires some context. Madeline, a palliative care physician exemplified this point in acknowledging that

> When you have a heart attack you see a cardiologist, when you're pregnant you see an obstetrician. There is a constant stream of patients and reimbursements. But in PC, I am constantly explaining to my colleagues, administrators, consults and really anyone I interact with what it is, what I do and why it's important.
> (Omilion-Hodges and Swords 2017a, 1279)

Although providers report navigating and assuaging this tension with intentional and instructive communication, these dialectic tensions and those that arise between the biomedical and biosocial models can prompt otherwise preventable accidents.

Researchers have routinely traced medical errors back to miscommunication among members or lapses in communication about patient care (Lingard et al. 2002; Lingard, Whyte, and Regehr 2009; Sutcliffe, Lewton, and Rosenthal 2004). Nestled within the dialectic challenges introduced earlier, when care providers feel they are not valued or have routinely been chastised for offering divergent opinions, they tend to withdraw from teams and withhold their expertise. This stems from the fact that offering opinions, especially those that may be different from higher-status members, requires a level of confidence and vulnerability. It means that a provider has to feel comfortable being able to question the decisions of other providers, regardless of status similarities or distinctions. In fact, communication researchers have found that peers are more pivotal than leaders in creating an environment in which innovation and opinion sharing are encouraged (Omilion-Hodges and Ackerman 2018). When providers stop speaking up and sharing suggestions, communication channels are severed or at the very least strained or ignored. Although these concerns have been couched within the practice of palliative care, they are nestled with the larger practice of medicine. This chapter now looks at challenges embedded within modern medicine that may lead to, or at the very least not prevent against, medical mishaps. Palliative care providers' experiences and solutions for navigating these obstacles are then articulated to illustrate feasible and zero-financial-cost means of safeguarding against errors.

Organizational Obstacles

The delivery of medical care through hospitals and health-care institutes is a societal staple. Yet coordinating and delivering care is a complex and concerted effort that requires multiple departmental and organizational units to function in unity to be successful. Hierarchies often are employed to structure and facilitate the delivery of care. Although hierarchies can be successfully implemented to help to organize complex processes and large organizations, they also can lead to obstructive status and power distinctions that can interfere with the ability to form constructive interpersonal relationships. In turn, large power differences can lead to apprehension with upward communication. When organizational members, such as nurses or techs, feel unable to question a physician's decision, for example, these structural elements coalesce to contribute to faulty communication. Without mindful communication processes embedded throughout the delivery of patient care, the chances for medical errors increase.

Structural Flaws in the Medical System

Similar to the hierarchical and status challenges imbued within medicine, faulty communication has long plagued the delivery of care. Interprofessional communication can be especially challenging because specialties tend to hold divergent ideologies and employ different rhetoric, and these assumptions present when designing care or treatment plans and in the continued delivery of patient care. This can lead to breakdowns in transdisciplinary teams in which siloing and lack of understanding of various specialties can spur negative practices to become part of an organization's culture.

Medicine has long been built, sustained, and practiced as a hierarchy. From the deference afforded physicians to the need for multiple levels of management to maintain the intricacies of organizing and delivering care, hospitals and health-care centers are complex entities. From an organizational perspective, they are among the most sophisticated structures, considering the variance in employee educational levels and wages among those required to meet patient and organizational needs, including janitors, food workers, billing coordinators, social workers, and surgeons. Although the various departments and hierarchies may be necessary, they propagate a status system classified by power distinctions. By their very nature, hierarchies classify individuals in explicit rank roles, which can then lead to implicit expectations for how individuals of various ranks are expected to interact. Naturally, when some organizational members are in formal leadership positions or possess more expertise, individuals in lower-status positions may feel apprehensive speaking up or questioning the decisions of higher-ranking peers. Some have referred to hierarchical differences, concerns with upward influence, and interpersonal power and conflict as "latent flaws throughout the [medical] system" (Sutcliffe, Lewton, and Rosenthal 2004, 186).

Through a series of in-depth interviews with 26 medical residents, researchers uncovered approximately 70 medical incidents (Sutcliffe, Lewton, and Rosenthal 2004, 186). Even more concerning than the number of errors unearthed is the fact that, without the latent flaws imbued within the medical system, the majority of these mishaps could have easily been prevented. Often these oversights began with the ubiquitous hierarchical system in terms of the resident–attending physician relationship. Although attending physicians serve as teachers and sounding boards, the resident physician often provides the hands-on patient care and designs patient treatment plans. This system is intended to empower new physicians, but the fear of being judged or being perceived as incompetent can prompt residents to withhold information or refrain from asking questions. Sutcliffe et al. found that residents were especially hesitant to call attendings in the middle of the night in order to avoid conflict or perceived retribution, even if protocol deemed the call necessary. Dyadic hierarchical challenges do not stop at the resident–attending relationship, but also occur between residents–community physicians, residents–specialists, and residents–nurses. Additional research also indicates status challenges between physicians and nurses (Apker, Propp, and Ford 2005).

Unfortunately, hierarchical concerns do not remain confined to the parties in the dyadic relationship. Rather, the social structure in place leads to lower-status actors fearing judgment and, therefore, refraining from asking necessary questions, withholding or massaging information that they feel may reflect poorly on them, or communicating in ways that make a provider—virtually always the lower-status actor—feel intimidated or incompetent. A palliative care nurse with over 30 years of experience disclosed that she "still has physicians that come up to me and ask 'who have you killed lately?'" Relatedly, other palliative care providers indicated enduring frequent name calling by being referred to as "the death squad," "angels of death," "grim reaper," or "the hounds of hell" (Omilion-Hodges and Swords 2017b, 1276). Such treatment hardly encourages interprofessional collaboration and can leave necessary patient information in limbo.

Misinterpreting information or not providing enough information are more than just suboptimal practices. Returning to the Sutcliffe et al. study, the researchers found that a lack of continuity in care—such as shorter hospital stays, shift changes, or moving patients between units—often came with a lack of information, missing medical reports, and a dearth of instruction in terms of next steps (Sutcliffe, Lewton, and Rosenthal 2004). Moreover, because of the complexity and scope of hospitals, medical professionals may receive information from other units, such as the emergency department, that is upwards of 12 hours old because of the variety of tests and procedures that a patient may have undergone in the meantime.

Taken together, foundational aspects of the medical system may in fact be the impetus for approximately 10 percent of deaths in the United States (Makary and Daniel 2016). Medical professionals Makary and Daniel see preventable patient deaths due to medical errors as an under-recognized epidemic (2016). Martin Makary, a professor of surgery and health policy at Johns Hopkins University of School of Medicine, indicated that "People don't just die from heart attacks and bacteria, they die from system-wide failings and poorly coordinated care" (Sternberg 2016). Lapses in coordination of care, provider judgement, and system failures are contributors of otherwise avoidable deaths. These latent flaws are rooted in miscommunication or absences in communication, leading researchers to label communication failures as insidious contributors to medical mishaps (Sutcliffe, Lewton, and Rosenthal 2004). Effective communication among medical professionals may be the most efficient route to changing the fact that medical errors are the third leading cause of death in the U.S. (Makary and Daniel 2016).

An experienced palliative care provider exemplified the pivotal role communication plays in the delivery of patient-centered care: "It was then that I realized that as much as I am a physician, I am also a communicator. I couldn't, we [the unit] couldn't, provide care like this without being mindful and intentional with our communication" (Omilion-Hodges and Swords 2017a, 331).

Faulty Communication

Although there are system-wide flaws and shortcomings that make the delivery of holistic care challenging, especially across units and providers, it is the inability to communicate effectively that contributes most readily to preventable surgical and medical errors (Mackles 2014). This realization has led to the Triple Aim initiative, which includes better health, improved care, and reduced costs. These foci rest on the ability of individuals, teams, and health-care systems to practice adept communication and integrate safeguards at each level to ensure that providers have accurate and timely information and that proper handoffs occur between providers. Before turning to empirical solutions for helping to guard against medical oversights, this section explores additional common communication mistakes.

One such issue is the lack of experience many clinicians have working in interdisciplinary and transdisciplinary care teams. Multifaceted care teams are better equipped to provide holistic patient care and naturally infuse a system of checks and balances, as providers have to dialogue to plan complementary courses of care. Such conversations help to guard against duplicative tests, but can also raise red flags before potential adverse medical interactions or conflicting advice occur. Yet, the exchange of ideas from experts in different specialties and positions requires collaboration and interdependency, which can be challenging in light of power, status, and hierarchical differences (Rose 2011). Moreover, each discipline comes with its own "conceptual framework, what it believes, assumes, and takes for granted, its specific ways of thinking, observing, measuring, judging and evaluating" (Frank 1961). Thus, approaches among the specialists can lead to breakdowns in transdisciplinary teams, even though multifaceted medical teams are best positioned to provide a comprehensive care plan and the coordinated care required by those with serious illnesses.[1] Again, part of the challenge with transdisciplinary teams is that fact that each specialty has been trained in a specific area and tends to focus on areas "which the profession has selected for observation and concern," often overlooking points that are contrary to its own training (Frank 1961, 1799).

Transdisciplinary teams are positioned to provide the most comprehensive patient care because of the scope and strength of the care teams. However, if teams are thrown together haphazardly, members often do not know their specific role in the team or how they are expected to work collaboratively with other members. Moreover, without clear team guidelines and shared expectations in place, these multifaceted teams can lead to individuals treating patients as they would individually, abandoning the basic principles of transdisciplinary care by retreating to their individual silos and operating unilaterally outside of the boundaries of a multifaceted team. Researchers have found that members of interprofessional medical teams tend to refer to the "other" in the operating room where clinicians' constructions of other professions' roles, values, and motives were often dissonant with those professions' constructions of themselves (Lingard et al. 2002). Novices, in particular, tend to simplify and distort others' roles and motives.

Part of this issue may stem from the fact that medical education does not provide adequate training on the complexities of teamwork. Without discussion of the fluidity of team roles, rotation, and adept use of communication, new medical providers are ill-equipped to work well collaboratively. Scholars have suggested Activity Theory and its extension, Knotworking, as helpful ways to conceptualize transdisciplinary communication (Varpio, Schryer, and Lingard 2009; Engestrom 2000). The researchers use the theories as a way to illustrate that each medical professional should see him/herself as a defense against errors and can use multiple forms of communication (e.g., electronic medical records, text messages, routine team meetings, hallways conversations) as means to ensure that every provider has access to all relevant information.

Organizational Culture

In addition to receiving limited training on communication or complex team processes, medical professionals are often at the mercy of the culture of the organization they enter. This can be particularly challenging, as traditional approaches to medicine have long favored the biomedical model that has emphasized a more individual approach to treatment. Traditional approaches also have privileged certain revenue-generating specialties, such as cardiology and neurology, in terms of access to resources (e.g., space, new hires, marketing materials; Omilion-Hodges and Swords 2017b). Recent research has demonstrated the community desire for comprehensive care, especially in terms of palliative care, and rules and resource allocations are changing. However, there still are some organizational challenges that may block or hinder effective communication.

Apker and Eggly found that physician identity is developed through ideological discourse that produces and reproduces dominant approaches, while marginalizing more humanistic approaches (2004). Put simply, medical cultures have inadvertently helped to propagate a system that emphasizes more individual approaches to expertise, emphasizing that life should always be prolonged; these elements, in turn, can set physicians up to view death as failure. However, providers working within the biosocial approach to medicine may experience knowledge, communication, and value gaps from providers in other models.

A knowledge gap implies a surface-level challenge, such as the idea that palliative care physicians let patients die while other specialists save patients. A fissure in understanding can be alleviated through education, whether in terms of CME courses or dialogue amongst peers. A communication gap burrows slightly deeper, assuming that individuals have been exposed to accurate information, but remain unaware of idiosyncrasies of the topic. In a 2017 study, Ahmed, a palliative care nurse, described a communication gap as "an outsider's stereotypes of the profession" (Omilion-Hodges and Swords 2017b, 1227). That is, someone may possess a rudimentary understanding of palliative care, but remain unaware of the benefits of the specialty, how it differs from hospice care, or the day-to-day duties of a palliative care clinician. A value gap, in contrast, implies that, regardless of the knowledge one possesses regarding a topic, the area is still viewed as insignificant or trivial. Unfortunately, this coincides with numerous palliative care providers' experiences with medical peers who pose questions such as, "Everyone dies. So what do you do?" "Why do I need a doctor to help me die?" and "Why are there death doctors?" These questions reiterate the tension coiled within the living–dying dichotomy (Omilion-Hodges and Swords 2017b, 1227).

Knowledge, communication, and value gaps serve as useful illustrations of Apker and Eggly's finding that medical discourse tends to benefit the dominant majority whose specialties focus on innovative technology, treatment plans, and medical interventions (2004); these are prized as the gold standard (Sutcliffe, Lewton, and Rosenthal 2004). However, reaffirming certain discourses and privileging certain specialties over others create an environment in which transdisciplinary conversations are far and few between because of the associated knowledge, communication, and value gaps. Returning to the Sutcliffe and colleagues article, communication lapses are major contributors to otherwise avoidable medical errors (2004). Yet, communication-rooted research offers empirical solutions that may help to provide scaffolding for safeguarding against medical errors.

Communication-Rooted Solutions to Guard Against Medical Errors

Considering that communication errors are a major contributor to medical errors, adept and mindful communication becomes part of the solution. Storytelling, intentional transdisciplinary teams, and a focus on individual leadership are discussed as empirical interventions that may help to reorient health-care providers to more deliberate discussions about patient safety and the delivery of holistic care.

Storytelling has emerged as an empowering practice and an effective means for palliative care providers to articulate and contextualize their specialty (Omilion-Hodges and Swords 2017b). Stories are important sense-making devices, and the narrative structure of stories can appeal to others' emotions. Palliative care clinicians reported using vibrant imagery to create narratives to preserve a patient's medical story, which should start at the initial consult. A registered nurse in a palliative care unit suggested that the specialty of palliative care provides "a new twist to an old story," in terms of allowing patients to largely guide the end of their stories via choice and entitlement (Omilion-Hodges and Swords 2017b, 1279). A leader in a palliative care facility, Derrick, suggested that, in terms of the standardized patient consult:

> We don't go into these consults with a script. My rule is no script, new people, new story. Every person demands a fresh take and our time in asking questions, getting to know them, and helping to continue and finalize their story as they intend.
> (Omilion-Hodges and Swords 2017b, 1279)

Part and parcel with storytelling is the foundational role of communication. As a means to provide comprehensive care across a large medical system, one palliative care unit adhered to guidelines that emphasized the pivotal role of communication. Providers were asked to do "everything we can to promote continuity of care and information in our very fragmented health care system including: calls and notes to PCPs [primary care physicians] and the appropriate specialists (when in doubt: Communicate!) and handoffs to colleagues" (Omilion-Hodges and Swords 2017b, 1279). This commitment to communication among health-care providers not only saves patients from having to recount their own medical histories, but also embeds several levels of informal safety checks so providers are able to collectively care for patients asynchronously and across a dispersed medical system.

In addition to applying the idea of storytelling to delivering concerted care across providers, storytelling can also empower practitioners. In this sense, palliative care providers were able to craft a narrative that illustrated how they care for patients and families in a way that honors end of life while articulating the nuances of their profession. Palliative care leaders also have reported using storytelling as a means to earn a spot on the agenda at a senior leadership or board of directors meeting. Jeanine, a California-based palliative physician, exemplified this point through the following quote:

> I learned early on that if I don't clearly articulate what I do and why it's important, that I'm treated like a leper. I've learned to tell a really

good story. People don't like to talk about dying, but they do like stories.

(Omilion-Hodges and Swords 2017b, 1279)

Similarly, Steven, a geriatric palliative care clinician, found that telling stories of patients who have passed (with their consent or that of their families) has also been an effective means of empowering providers and securing organizational resources:

> I used to think of myself as a cheerleader, but now I just think of myself as the storyteller—the intermediary. I get to know my patients and their families, and many times they are so appreciative of our services that they ask how to help. I ask for their permission to tell their story and oftentimes they will ask, "What else?" But once you have a face, a name, a life to tell, it becomes a lot easier to get approval for the brochures or the physical space or people you need.
>
> (Omilion-Hodges and Swords 2017b, 1279)

In this way, taking the time to consider how to thoughtfully and strategically respond to the ubiquitous "What do you do?" question allows providers to leave others with a realistic idea of their role in the medical world. Although the research discussed has been done with palliative-care providers, the idea can easily be adopted by any medical provider—and is especially recommended for those who are new to medicine or find themselves in positions in which they feel they are treated as lower status than others. In this sense, residents and nurses, for example, could craft a strategic narrative about their specific role in patient care. This could be especially helpful for surgical nurses so that they can illustrate their agency in a way that shows other team members, including physicians, what they do, what they are responsible for, and why they need to be in the room. Demonstrating agency through mindful and clear communication can help to minimize power differences and clarify any confusion about any one member's role or contribution. Feeling empowered to perform their roles to their fullest can allow medical personnel to voice concerns or make suggestions for patient care.

Another means of assuaging status differences and minimizing concern with upward communication is to create intentional transdisciplinary teams. This means that, instead of haphazardly throwing a group of specialists together and calling them a team, that members are given time to consider the role of the team, the culture of the team, and guiding principles for the team. Having the space to consider these key elements, and doing so before patient care begins, allows teams to work out any differences and begin on common ground. Moreover, recognition of the unique expertise and contribution of each member can help lessen perceived status distinctions and allow the team to engineer an effective process for the delivery of patient care. To this end, members are not duplicating each other's efforts, nor are essential aspects of patient care overlooked because members are making assumptions about others' roles.

One way to establish effective guiding principles is through structured routine team meetings. Although often considered a time drain, when designed with clear expectations, meetings can be instrumental to the delivery of exemplary patient care. Successfully orchestrated meetings can also serve as a means for a team to develop a shared sense of purpose and identity. Part and parcel with effective meetings are guidelines for length, for rotating through roles of timekeeper and devil's advocate, and procedures for addressing conflict when it arises. Adhering to these guidelines provides members the architecture necessary to tactfully navigate potentially challenging communicative encounters, such as when two or more team members disagree on a course of treatment. Yet, continually cycling through the team roles and working within the parameters established by the group allows members to demonstrate self-leadership.

In addition to storytelling and intentional transdisciplinary teams, committing to a culture of self-leadership and accountability also helps to guard against medical errors. Influence is the heart of leadership. Therefore, engaging in conversations and behaviors that encourage others to act in a certain way suggests one is leading. The challenge then becomes helping organizational members to be reflective about their actions and communication to demonstrate prosocial and inclusive behaviors. Thus, if an attending physician is short with residents or shows new physicians that they can disrespect nurses and techs, then this attending is propagating behavior that emphasizes the dominant majority and is overlooking the strengths and contributions of other personnel. One way for all medical employees to demonstrate positive self-leadership and to serve as exemplars for others is through their use of powerful communication. This means speaking in assertive, declarative sentences (e.g., the dose prescribed is incorrect given the patient's weight) rather than hedging or using justifications (e.g., I am new at this and could be wrong, but are you sure that dose is right?). Powerful language is an immediate way to illustrate one's expertise. Although fear of speaking up has continually been flagged as a source of medical errors, teaching and exemplifying powerful language and personal accountability allow providers to assert themselves and safeguard against preventable mishaps. The following section focuses on how transdisciplinary teams and medical institutes may implement small changes to work processes to prevent medical errors.

Implementing Meaningful Changes to Simplify the Modern Medical System

Today's medical systems are complex and often fragmented, and it may be impossible to prevent all medical errors. As Sutcliffe and colleagues noted, in some ways medical errors are woven into the fabric of modern medicine (2004). However, as medicine continues to shift from the biomedical to the biosocial, the focus on communication may help to prevent unnecessary oversights.

Empowering providers to purposefully craft narratives of their expertise and their unique contributions to patient care allows them to articulate an identity and exemplify leadership. Storytelling has emerged as a means to address negative peer treatment in palliative care and has helped providers in this rising specialty to articulate the nuances of their profession (Omilion-Hodges and Swords 2017b). Other medical providers may take a cue from palliative care practitioners to consider how they can use storytelling to position their role while also applying the idea of storytelling to preserve patients' medical histories. Though this may seem like a minor overture, focused narratives—especially in terms of how providers deliver exemplary patient care or how they see their role in a care team—establish confidence and reiterate providers' expertise. Because this is a communication skill, the more it is practiced, the easier it becomes for individuals to use powerful language as they navigate encounters with patients, families, and other medical providers.

Interprofessional communication has been a challenge for as long as providers have been attempting to connect across specialties (Frank 1961). Yet one way to minimize or eradicate these challenges is by focusing on peer relationships and group cohesion. When individuals feel valued for their contributions to the group, they begin to develop trust and a sense of community. By implementing and following team guidelines and meeting rules, especially how to address conflict within the team, cohesion and sense of community remain even in trying moments. These small steps help to prevent individuals from retreating to silos during times of stress and instead encourage members to turn inward to the team to address the concerns at hand.

Communication is a powerful defense against medical errors. An initial means to activate communication as a preventative measure is to reflect on individual, group, and organizational practices. This includes reflecting on what is done well, and perhaps more important, intentionally looking for gaps in patient handoffs, shift changes, between units, within teams, and in the organization as a whole. To be taken most seriously, this charge should be written into an organization's strategic plan and unit and individual charges. Moreover, personnel should be given time and a deadline to complete these assessments. Without a focused task, it can be easy to shirk the responsibility and evaluate one's own communication or one's group communication as satisfactory or better. However, awarding units for finding flaws in processes or for suggesting alternatives can increase participation and member buy in. Additionally, this brainstorming and problem-finding process requires individuals of all ranks to be a part of engineering more effective solutions. For example, employees working in patient transport may realize that information communicated between providers on one unit is not being received by medical professionals on the next unit. This is extremely problematic and, unfortunately, all too common. However, charging all associates with the task to fill communication gaps and suggest alternative and safer ways of providing care stresses provider agency and expertise. When providers embody their role expertise, speaking up against possible errors or concerns would not be looked down upon, but rather, rewarded.

Note

1. This is emphasized as a possible solution in Chapter 3: "Toward a Restorative Just Culture Approach to Medical Error" by Garrett and McNolty.

Works Cited

Apker, Julie, and Susan Eggly. 2004. "Communicating Professional Identity in Medical Socialization: Considering the Ideological Discourse of Morning Report." *Qualitative Health Research* 14 (3): 411–429.

Apker, Julie, Kathleen Propp, and Wendy Ford. 2005. "Negotiating Status and Identity Tensions in Healthcare Team Interactions: An Exploration of Nurse Role Dialectics." *Journal of Applied Communication Research* 33 (2): 93–115.

Dumanovsky, Tamara, Rachel Augustin, Maggie Rogers, Katrina Lettang, Diane Meier, and Sean Morrison. 2016. "The Growth of Palliative Care in US Hospitals: A Status Report." *Journal of Palliative Medicine* 19 (1): 8–15.

Engestrom, Yrjo. 2000. "Activity Theory as a Framework for Analyzing and Redesigning Work." *Ergonomics* 43 (7): 960–974.

Foley, Kathleen M. 1995. "Pain, Physician Assisted Dying and Euthanasia." *Pain* 4: 163–178.

Frank, Lawrence. 1961. "Interprofessional Communication." *American Journal of Public Health and the Nations Health* 51 (12): 1798–1804.

Isaacs, Stephen L., and James R. Knickman. 1997. *To Improve Health and Health Care.* San Francisco, CA: Jossey Bass.

Lingard, Lorelei, Richard Reznick, Sherry Espin, Glenn Regehr, and Isabella DeVito. 2002. "Team Communications in the Operating Room: Talk Patterns, Sites of Tension, and Implications for Novices." *Academic Medicine* 77 (3): 232–237.

Lingard, L., S. Whyte, and G. Regehr. 2009. *Safer Surgery: Analysing Behaviour in the Operating Theatre.* Surrey, UK: Ashgate Publishing: 283–300.

Loscalzo, Matthew. 2008. "Palliative Care: An Historical Perspective." *ASH Education Program Book* 1: 465–465.

Mackles, Arnold. 2014. "The Pivotal Role of Communication in Healthcare Reform and Risk Reduction." *Risk Rx*, October—December, Accessed March 29, 2019. Retrieved from http://flbog.sip.ufl.edu/risk-rx-article/the-pivotal-role-of-communication-in-healthcare-reform-and-risk-reduction/.

Makary, Martin, and Michael Daniel. 2016. "Medical Error—The Third Leading Cause of Death in the US." *BMJ* 353: i2139.

Omilion-Hodges, Leah, and Crystal Ackerman. 2018. "From the Technical Know-How to the Free Flow of Ideas: Exploring the Effects of Leader, Peer, and Team Communication on Employee Creativity." *Communication Quarterly* 66 (1): 38–57.

Omilion-Hodges, Leah, and Nathan Swords. 2017a. "Communication Matters: Exploring the Intersection of Family and Practitioner End of Life Communication." *Behavioral Sciences* 7 (1): 15.

Omilion-Hodges, Leah, and Nathan Swords. 2017b. "The Grim Reaper, Hounds of Hell, and Dr. Death: The Role of Storytelling for Palliative Care in Competing Medical Meaning Systems." *Health Communication* 32 (10): 1272–1283.

Pres, Heidi. "Pain and Palliative Care Program Awarded Accreditation." *St. Joseph Mercy Oakland Press Release*, January 25, 2012, Accessed March 29, 2019. Retrieved from www.stjoesoakland.org/body_pontiac.cfm?id=2898&action=detail&ref=5348.

Rokach, Ami. 2005. "Caring for Those Who Care for the Dying: Coping with the Demands on Palliative Care Workers." *Palliative & Supportive Care* 3 (4): 325–332.

Rose, Louise. 2011. "Interprofessional Collaboration in the ICU: How to Define?" *Nursing in Critical Care* 16 (1): 5–10.

Sternberg, Steve. 2016, May 3. "Medical Errors Are Third Leading Cause of Death in the U.S." *U.S. News and World Reports*, Accessed March 29, 2019. Retrieved from www.usnews.com/news/articles/2016-05-03/medical-errors-are-third-leading-cause-of-death-in-the-us.

Sutcliffe, Kathleen, Elizabeth Lewton, and Marilynn Rosenthal. 2004. "Communication Failures: An Insidious Contributor to Medical Mishaps." *Academic Medicine* 79 (2): 186–194.

Varpio, Lara, Catherine Schryer, and Lorelei Lingard. 2009. "Routine and Adaptive Expert Strategies for Resolving ICT Mediated Communication Problems in the Team Setting." *Medical Education* 43 (7): 680–687.

6 Communicating About Technical Failures in Assisted Reproductive Technology

Rashmi Kudesia and Robert W. Rebar

Technical Failures in Reproductive Medicine

The practice of clinical medicine requires detailed communication between members of the health-care team as well as between medical providers and patients. Though this dogma applies to all fields of medicine, different specialties and settings present unique medical, scientific, and ethical challenges. Recently, two highly publicized laboratory failures occurred within the field of reproductive medicine, resulting in the loss of thousands of cryopreserved eggs and embryos. Analysis of these events offers a window into the ethical sticking points of technological failures in the world of reproductive medicine. To fully understand and query these events, we begin by reviewing the science of assisted reproductive technologies (ARTs) and unique aspects to the clinical practice of reproductive medicine. We then consider the ethical issues posed by ARTs, the details of these two specific cases, and how they were handled. We summarize with a guide to planning and executing conversations around errors in reproductive medicine.

Understanding ARTs

In the United States, 10–15 percent of heterosexual couples face infertility (Martinez, Daniels, Febo-Vazquez 2018). Those that fail less aggressive therapy make up the bulk of those utilizing ARTs. However, an increasing number of women are pursuing fertility preservation via oocyte cryopreservation (Petropanagos, Cattapan, Baylis, and Leader 2015), either because of anticipated delayed childbearing or growing utilization of oncofertility treatment, namely the option for fertility preservation before or during radiation or chemotherapy for the treatment of cancer (Barlevy, Wangmo, Elger, and Ravitsky 2016). LGBT individuals may also electively utilize ARTs to allow for oocyte preservation prior to oophorectomy in transmen or to allow for reciprocal IVF in lesbian couples, in which both women can participate biologically by one donating eggs to the other, who then carries the pregnancy. In 2016, 263,577 ART cycles were started in the United States, with 25 percent (65,840) being egg or embryo banking cycles (CDC 2018). With 76,930 infants born in that same year conceived via ART, out of 3.9 million liveborn deliveries, ART cycles accounted for 1.9 percent of births in that same year, continuing a general upward trajectory of ART births as a percentage of all U.S. births (Martin et al. 2018).

Undergoing ARTs requires numerous steps, with multiple interventions that may be part of the treatment plan. At the minimum, ARTs are defined as requiring extracorporeal manipulation of eggs and sperm, which is done via in vitro fertilization (IVF). In an IVF cycle, injectable medication taken by a female partner stimulates the ovaries to produce multiple eggs at once. During this process, which takes at least seven to ten days, the patient is monitored via transvaginal ultrasound and bloodwork for the measurement of circulating estrogen levels at one- to three-day intervals. After this stimulation phase, the eggs are retrieved, usually under sedation, via ultrasound-guided transvaginal aspiration. At this point, the eggs can be frozen for later use or fertilized by conventional insemination (each egg placed in a pool of sperm) or by intracytoplasmic sperm injection (ICSI, where a single sperm is injected directly into each egg). If necessary, a variety of patient circumstances may call for the utilization of donor eggs or sperm, which can come anonymously from a bank, or via directed donation from a friend or family member.

The resulting embryos are cultured in the laboratory and can be transferred back into the uterus two to six days after the egg retrieval, termed a "fresh embryo transfer." Alternately, the embryo can be biopsied for preimplantation genetic testing (PGT). PGT can screen the embryos for chromosomal aneuploidy (having the incorrect number of chromosomes, therefore, being at risk for failed implantation, miscarriage or birth defects) or single-gene mutations (in the case of parents who carry an inheritable genetic mutation that would impact resulting afflicted children). The embryo is cryopreserved after biopsy, and so "frozen embryo transfer" refers to an embryo that is subsequently thawed and transferred. Frozen embryo transfers can also occur for untested embryos that were preserved after a prior ART cycle. On occasion, either for women with history of uterine disease, recurrent miscarriage, congenital anomalies or serious health co-morbidities, or for gay or single fathers, a gestational carrier is contracted to carry the pregnancy for the intended parent(s).

Thus, the process of ARTs can require months of testing and preparation, months to years of treatment, repeated injections and blood draws, invasive procedures, emotional anxiety and stress, and disruption to one's daily routine. In addition, the average cost of an IVF cycle in the United States is $12,000, with state-to-state variation of any insurance coverage (Henne and Bundorf 2008). In short, undergoing ARTs is a time-consuming, expensive, and stressful endeavor.

In addition to these burdens on patients, the staff also have many responsibilities. Providing high-quality reproductive care requires extensive detailed communication between many individuals. In addition to the intended parent(s), the list of individuals participating in the treatment might include the primary physician, covering physician partners, nurses, medical assistants, front desk and billing staff, embryologists, phlebotomists, other laboratory staff, lawyers, mental-health consultants, and gamete donors or a gestational carrier. Given the high complexity of these technologies, it is unsurprising that mistakes occur; some errors are minimal with no permanent fallout, but others can prove absolutely devastating. We will briefly review the most common categories of error in the management of ARTs.

Sources of Error in ARTs

Many errors relate to the communication of certain requirements, processes or results between different participants in an ART cycle. For example, certain tests should be done prior to treatment, whether bloodwork to ensure one's health is optimized prior to treatment or procedures to confirm a normal uterine cavity or sperm parameters. Health-care teams can miss an indicated test, overlook a patient who has not yet completed an ordered test, or fail to communicate important results back to the patient. Once treatment begins, ART cycles require many medications, many of which are injectable, requiring subcutaneous or intramuscular administration, and some of which arrive in powdered form and require reconstitution by the patient prior to injection. Reconstituting and injecting can easily be performed incorrectly by a nervous or poorly counseled patient. Medication dosing might be handled incorrectly in terms of the dose selected, instructions given, or patient administration.

Communication Errors

On a larger level, communication can break down among a variety of involved parties. The stress of the fertility treatment process is on occasion enough to cause severe marital discord or even divorce (Kjaer et al. 2014). On a more mundane level, however, clinics often rely on one partner to communicate responsibilities or decisions to the other, and incomplete communication—or changes of heart—can lead to substantial grief. The highly publicized case of actress Sofia Vergara, whose ex-fiancé attempted to claim custody of embryos they had created while romantically involved, serves as a reminder of how custodial and "right to life" arguments come into play in ARTs (Holpuch 2015). In such cases in which one partner wants to utilize embryos in joint custody for the purpose of having a child, but the other partner does not, the dilemma has been whose claim is greater—the right for one partner to become a parent, particularly if those embryos represent the only option for genetic parenthood; the right of the other partner to not be forced into parenthood; or the right to life of the embryo. Thus far, legal precedent has upheld that the embryo does not have rights, and that, out of the two partners, the superior claim is that of the partner not wishing to be forced into parenthood (Smajdor 2007).

On another front, "wrongful birth" or "wrongful life" lawsuits have originated in the context of children born with genetic diseases that couples allege should have been detected prior to conception (Caulfield 2001). The concept here is that, with available testing, the specific child with a severe (often fatal) illness "should not" have been born. The corollary of this argument is typically that, if appropriate testing had been applied, the parent(s) would have been able to choose a different, unafflicted embryo, and had a healthy child. Couples and individuals undergoing ARTs expect a "perfect" child, which is, unfortunately, not commensurate with the scientific reality (Damiano 2011).

Communication between intended parent(s) and directed gamete (egg or sperm) donors or gestational carriers can also become contentious, with contracts in this setting having limited legal enforceability. Indeed, after a spate of lawsuits including the infamous Baby M case, the industry moved sharply away from the practice of traditional gestational surrogacy, in which a woman contributed her oocytes and carried the pregnancy for an infertile couple (Krim 1996).

Communication within the embryology laboratory is also critical. Using or discarding the wrong gamete or embryo or thawing or transferring an incorrect number of embryos can lead to devastating outcomes. Other procedural complications can occur as well, at the time of surgery prior to ART or during an egg retrieval or embryo transfer. One of the most undesirable outcomes is ectopic pregnancy, where the embryo implants outside of the uterus, a complication with a prevalence known to be slightly elevated in ART cycles (Chang and Suh 2010). Ectopic pregnancies, uncontrolled hemorrhage after a procedure or surgery, and severe ovarian hyperstimulation during the ovarian stimulation phase of an ART cycle are the highest-risk complications that have the potential to end in fatality. Fortunately, severe morbidity and mortality are rare in this specialty (Venn et al. 2001).

Technological Errors

These types of errors typically affect one patient or couple, or potentially a few, if embryos or gametes were switched. Without proper systems and checklists in place, these mistakes can be repeated, affecting more patients. However, the class of error that has the potential to quickly impact a high volume of patients is general technological failures affecting the IVF laboratory. The environment within the lab is sensitive to fluctuations in temperature, air quality, fumes, and other environmental exposures, including severe weather events, such as flooding or fire. Individual storage tanks are additionally subject to electrical outages, mechanical failures and human error due to incorrect maintenance. Thus, there are multiple events that can impact all gametes or embryos in storage; in a large clinic, the number of affected gametes or embryos can number into the thousands and tens of thousands.

Recent Laboratory Failures

Thus, we can see that an error, or series of errors, that lead to outcomes, such as those experienced in Ohio and California, are among the gravest that can occur in reproductive medicine. However, these two situations do not seem to have unfolded in identical fashion. Both clinics had up-to-date inspections by the College of American Pathologists (CAP), a commonly used accreditation body. However, in Ohio, the University Hospitals (UH) Cleveland Medical Center acknowledged an element of human error (Buduson 2018). In that incident, the clinic reported a loss of 4,000 eggs and embryos, likely impacting at least 700 individuals or couples. (Buduson 2018). The tank in question had had prior malfunctions and was undergoing a maintenance process under the direction of the manufacturer. However, its alarm had been manually turned off, and it remains unknown why this happened, or for how long the alarm had been deactivated. As such, UH has taken responsibility for the failure, acting to rectify the situation, offering packages of free cycles, refunding and waiving storage fees, etc.

In contrast, the Pacific Fertility Center in San Francisco—where affected eggs and embryos are estimated at 2,000, impacting 400–500 individuals or couples—has not offered public details about any explanations behind the tank failure and what remuneration they are offering, if any (Nestel and Reshef 2018). Indeed, multiple lawyers working on lawsuits related to the two clinics have noted that the clinics have responded in very different fashions, with more transparency attributed to UH's response (Scutti 2018). Regardless, multiple individual and class-action lawsuits have been filed against each clinic (Scutti 2018). Indeed, in subsequent court proceedings, even UH has denied negligence, so the legal defenses between the two clinics may end up unfolding similarly (Serino 2018).

Embryos: Property or Life?

In considering these cases, one of the central questions is whether to treat affected embryos as property loss or as loss of life. A number of the lawsuits allege "wrongful death," thereby assigning the embryo personhood. To answer this question, we must examine the ethical and legal statuses of gametes and embryos and assess whether their loss is equivalent to human morbidity or mortality. From the scientific perspective, the traditional biological criteria for being considered "alive" includes qualities such as the independent ability to react and adapt to environmental stimuli, reproduce, maintain independent metabolism, etc. (McKay 2004). Biologically, though the loss of preserved sperm or eggs might be equally devastating in terms of eliminating the possibility of future genetic parenthood for patients affected by these cases, in applying this definition, there is no case to be made for personhood of single sex cells. As for embryos, though all living people were once embryos, the vast majority of embryos do not become living individuals. In this regard, it is more appropriate to regard embryos only as "potential lives." Many eggs fertilized *in vivo* fail to implant, and one in every four pregnancies that implants ends in miscarriage, ectopic pregnancy or something other than a live birth (American College of Obstetricians and Gynecologists 2018). Legal pregnancy terminations are similarly not generally viewed as interrupting life. Thus, society does not typically treat embryos as living persons.

Further, there are serious consequences to designating embryos as alive. Namely, it allows for the criminalization of miscarriage, certain forms of birth control, and pregnancy termination (American Society of Reproductive Medicine 2018). Such designation would also complicate the ability to manage ectopic pregnancies, as treatment to save the woman's life necessitates preventing the pregnancy from developing further. Additionally, this stance would severely limit options for managing ARTs in a number of ways. First, if discarding these embryos were illegal, the alternate approaches would have lower success rates, and likely take longer and cost more, as fewer eggs could be fertilized at any given time. Second, the typical IVF cycle results in extra embryos that may ultimately be discarded due to abnormalities or completed family-building. These options would be prohibited if embryos were treated as living individuals. Even more extreme, as the PGT process involves embryo biopsy, a personhood designation implies the need to obtain embryonic consent for this invasive procedure, which could jeopardize the ability to continue using this technology.

The basis for a claim of embryonic personhood appears to be emotional or religious, as has been the case in many recent legislative bills introduced by ostensibly "pro-life" organizations, such as Personhood USA (Legislative Tracker 2018). This organization remains active in all 50 states, and legislation attempting to codify embryonic or fetal personhood has been put to the ballot in multiple states, including Colorado, Mississippi, and Alabama. The Alabama bill passed, but has relatively weaker language that does not criminalize any treatments, medications or behaviors. Many more states have rejected ballot initiatives or proposed amendments to their state constitutions. Thus, even in conservative states, the legislative precedent and ongoing sentiment of the general public has been to treat embryos as property. The American Society for Reproductive Medicine Ethics Committee regards embryos as "deserving of special respect, but they are not afforded the same status as persons" (Ethics Committee of the American Society for Reproductive Medicine 2016a).

Safeguarding Reproductive Property

If we accept the premise of embryos as property, then we can move forward to considering what each clinic's responsibility must be for safekeeping these incredibly valuable assets. To a certain extent, there is no limit to how many backup systems one could put in place, and so ideally, an objective consensus of what expectations are appropriate might assist clinics in making these determinations. Fortunately, the American Society for Reproductive Medicine (ASRM) does provide such guidelines (The Practice Committee of the American Society for Reproductive Medicine and the Practice Committee of the Society for Assisted Reproductive Technology 2008).

Currently, ASRM guidelines list certain agencies that can provide certification and accreditation. However, these bodies vary substantially from one to another in their stringency, with the ASRM/College of American Pathologists (CAP) inspection being considered "the gold standard" (Dubey 2012, 478). However, labs can also apply for accreditation to the Joint Commission or New York State, and each of these has its own checklists and protocols. From the clinic's side, the individual tasked with overseeing the inspection process is the laboratory director, a position mandated by the ASRM guidelines. The qualifications for a laboratory director stipulate at least six months of training with 60 ART cycles, which can overlap with two years of clinical experience. Furthermore, a laboratory director can serve as an off-site director to up to four additional laboratories, each of which he or she must visit at least once monthly. Thus, one can easily imagine that infrequent contact with a director, or a director early in her career or who has managed fewer cases, could lead to substantial variation between laboratories.

The remainder of the guidelines provide details about the management and conduct of laboratories. They cover additional staff, the ratio of staff to clinical volume, elements of laboratory space and design, equipment and procedure manuals, laboratory safety and infection control, quality control and assurance, and satellite facilities. However, typical guidance includes the types of protocols and manuals that should be in place while allowing for individual differences among clinics. In many cases, the specific proprietary products, techniques, and protocols to be utilized are left to the staff to determine. Certainly, the various topic areas that a laboratory director should consider are all listed in the document, but there is room by design for substantial variation in interpretation and implementation.

As such, given these two cases, there are some specific questions we may wish to reconsider. First, what kind of oversight is appropriate, and by whom? Currently, the main governing body is the Society for Assisted Reproductive Technologies (SART), which collaborates with the Centers for Disease Control and Prevention (CDC) to track and report ART outcomes (CDC 2018). However, it is not mandated that a clinic report to SART, and 5 percent of clinics choose not to do so (Adamson 2002). Additionally, there are many ways of presenting the data, and clinics can be selective about which patients they care for, making it difficult to compare one clinic to another (CDC 2018). Of course, it will never be possible to prevent individual clinics with bad actors from choosing to disregard appropriate safeguards. Despite numerous ASRM guidelines on clinical practice, there are no legal consequences to flouting accepted standards of care or recommendations (Dubey 2012). The main recourse one has against flagrant violations of ethics or standards of care would be to report a physician to the medical board or perhaps to alert one of the accrediting bodies. Given these limitations, some commentators have questioned whether these regulations are inadequate (Adamson 2002). However, the U.S. government has been reluctant to assume this role in the practice of medicine and limit the autonomy of patients and providers in making health-care decisions.

Even if no changes are made to the current requirements, and despite best attempts to safeguard against recurrence of such events, another laboratory failure may occur again in the future. Given this possibility, what is the responsibility of the field of reproductive medicine to disclose this risk to patients? In thinking about how and when to deliver this message, we can apply the four ethical principles—beneficence, non-maleficence, autonomy, and justice—to weigh the arguments for and against pre-emptively raising the specter of future technological failures.

Pre-Emptive Disclosure of Risk

From a beneficence perspective, the presumption of ART cycles is that they are undertaken in order to help the patient. In the case of infertility patients who have failed other treatment, this presumption seems appropriate. In these circumstances, it appears likely that, even if clinics were proactively forthcoming about the potential for a technological failure, infertile patients would still opt to move forward with treatment because of the lack of alternative family-building options. However, we can more concretely consider whether it would benefit the patient to be explicitly informed of rare catastrophic outcomes, such as a tank failure. In analyzing this question, we turn to an example with an analogous catastrophic outcome. If we consider the similarly rare outcome of intraoperative mortality in a healthy patient, we can ask a parallel question: should preoperative counseling of a patient for low-risk surgery always mention the risk of dying during the procedure? In this situation, the ethical literature provides conflicting opinions. Some argue that the surgeon should verbally explain risks that are common, but not necessarily serious, and those that are uncommon, but serious. However, others have argued that, in cases in which risk seems nearly negligible, mentioning it actually distorts its probability to the patient and is misleading (Van Norman 2019; Rialon et al. 2012). Thus, it seems one could make an ethics-based argument for or against preemptive discussion of rare catastrophic risks.

Prior to these two 2018 events, one would have thought that a large-scale laboratory failure was essentially impossible, and one could ethically take either of the analogous stances on preemptively discussing lab failure. Though there could be an ethics-based argument either way, it is likely that most ART consent forms included verbiage about rare laboratory failures. In light of these recent events, should common practice shift toward pre-emptive verbal disclosure of risk? Certainly, some patients may ask questions about these cases to confirm they are not also at risk, and these inquiries should be thoroughly answered. However, if each clinic critically assesses its equipment, alarm systems, staff training, etc., and concludes that the chance of a catastrophic technological failure remains low, the underlying reasoning defending either approach would remain identical, and a change in policy may not be warranted.

Next, we consider the principle of non-maleficence, colloquially rephrased as "do no harm." In this context, this concept may apply in two different ways. First, labs must truly ensure they have taken reasonable steps to prevent such outcomes. Unfortunately, this paradigm is vague—different laboratory directors may have varying degrees of risk tolerance, and substantial variation in clinic procedures and protocols can persist even when following guidelines and accreditation standards. Stricter, more detailed guidelines would increase uniformity of practice, but at the risk of reducing each clinic's autonomy. Complicating this discussion is the observation that available storage tanks for frozen embryos clearly have definitive lifespans. Tanks utilized for this purpose were originally developed for the livestock industry, with little change over the last 20–30 years to match the pace of growth in ART utilization (Pomeroy 2018). Technologically, there are many possible ways a tank failure can occur, and the likelihood of such events may increase as many tanks in current use age. As they age, failures may become more frequent, even if clinics implement planned replacement of storage tanks prior to their achieving obsolescence. The purchase of new tanks is an expensive undertaking, and without clear standards in place both from the ASRM and the manufacturers, it remains a clinic's independent choice as to when to replace an aging tank. Moreover, from a practical standpoint, the manufacturers may not have sufficient new tanks available to replace all of those nearing the end of their functional lifespan.

An additional layer to the non-maleficence principle is as follows: many patients seek ART cycles for fertility preservation. The explosion in the number of patients seeking to cryopreserve gametes and embryos is beginning to outstrip the capacity of existing tanks and the capability of manufacturers to provide new tanks. Will some system of rationing be required in the future? No matter the circumstances, individuals choosing to undergo fertility preservation do so with a belief in the integrity of the clinic's technology and protocols to safeguard their valuable reproductive property. When physicians or embryologists are aware of, or suspect, deficiencies in their storage system, they are doing a disservice by encouraging any patient to pursue cryopreservation.

However, even if there is no such known concern, there has already been a great deal of societal consternation over the idea of fertility preservation, and whether, in particular, women freezing eggs are being sold a product that has greater social ramifications than they may realize since the procedure is not quite an "insurance policy" to rely upon (Petropanagos et al. 2015). The distribution of fertility practices in the United States has shifted sharply toward for-profit clinics over the past decade or more, with an influx of venture capital, and many companies are trying to push egg freezing as an option to preserve future fertility (Research and Markets 2018). These tank failures throw into question the paradigm of fertility preservation—namely, that if a woman knows she would like to become a mother, and is aware that her biological ability to do so is waning, egg freezing offers the freedom from the primary alternative of simply getting pregnant at that time. If she does freeze eggs, she forfeits her ability to try for pregnancy at that time. If those eggs are all rendered non-viable due to a technological failure before she returns to use them, she would be right to claim that she may have made a completely different decision had she understood this risk. Such a patient may have been robbed of her ability to have genetic offspring. Thus, it appears that the chance of tank failure should be a critical consideration for those interested in fertility preservation, and in understanding whether it is an investment worth making.

This hypothetical, but highly plausible, situation links directly to the third ethical principle of autonomy. Depending on one's view, it seems defensible to argue that failure to inform patients of these possibilities robs them of their autonomy to make an informed decision on how to best preserve their ability to have a child in the future—indeed, autonomous decision making on the part of an individual or couple undertaking any medical treatment, including ARTs. How can patients make appropriate decisions autonomously if we haven't alerted them to the possibility of these catastrophic possibilities? Thus, the autonomy principle seems to fall more favorably on the side of pre-emptive disclosure of risks, no matter how rare they may be. There is no consensus, however, on whether such disclosure must be—as discussed earlier—in writing or with verbal explanation.

Finally, we step back to look at the fourth principle of justice. On a societal level, the impact of ART failures circles back to the controversial question of a right to reproduction. Many have claimed that all individuals should have the right to reproduce in the fashion that befits them (Silvers and Francis 2017). This claim, if accepted, puts a responsibility on society to support individuals who require reproductive technology to build their family, and indeed, many European countries and Israel do have such policies. As would be expected, with financial support, utilization of ARTs increases with government subsidization of the expense (Ethics Committee of the American Society for Reproductive Medicine 2015). However, in the case of catastrophic technological failures, it is unclear what a nation or society's responsibility should then be. More specifically, as society increasingly relies on technology to assist in reproductive endeavors, if the technology fails, especially in a manner that may completely preclude genetic parenthood, what is owed to the affected individuals? Currently, these two cases do not demonstrate a pattern that puts any particular group at elevated risk, but if such circumstances manifested in the future—in which, perhaps, individuals seeking low-cost treatment more often chose clinics with higher risk for technological failures—they could change our current understanding of a just approach to counseling and managing oversight of ARTs.

As we consider what society's investment in reproduction is or should be, we also indirectly query how society gains or suffers from the birth, or lack thereof, of certain individuals? With 10–15 percent or more of couples being infertile, and increasing numbers using ARTs to achieve pregnancy, it seems clear that, if such failures occurred on a recurring basis, the numbers might quickly become substantial enough to result in societal outrage and demand for some intervention. However, if years pass again without further incidents, we might calculate that the effect is very small indeed: approximately 1,000 couples or individuals were impacted, with some already having children or being able to undergo new cycles to regain what was lost. Thus, the number of people that might have been barred from genetic parenthood purely because of these incidents is likely in the mid-hundreds. In other words, approximately 0.0001 percent of the current U.S. population of 325.7 million was impacted (United States Census Bureau 2019). Though the loss to individuals involved was devastating, the likely impact to society was quantitatively negligible.

Making Reparations

It is, however, entirely appropriate to ask what is owed to those impacted individuals. The staff at University Hospitals in Cleveland initially admitted to human error, while the Pacific case was attributed purely to technological failure. Are the responsibilities different in these two circumstances? Indeed, it appears that UH may be doing more to offer compensatory cycles for affected patients. For Pacific, if its consent process had not included the possibility of tank failure, a patient's claim to compensatory treatment may have been stronger. However, in any circumstance in which it seems some reparations are indicated, the next question is how extensive should the reparations be? Would it be one treatment cycle, a set number of cycles, the number previously required to obtain the eggs or embryos, or something else? If, due to the passage of time, genetic motherhood is no longer possible for women affected by these tank failures, is the clinic further obligated to cover ovum donation cycles to allow these women to achieve pregnancy?

Another component of making reparations and caring for the patient would be resources geared toward their mental suffering in the wake of this loss. Some patients have held memorial services for their lost embryos, and in doing so, also faced criticism of their grief over "just" embryos (Cha 2018). Thus, perhaps arranging support groups and therapy sessions may help affected patients cope with these events.

From an ethical standpoint, answering these questions is no easy feat. Given the unique nature of reproductive medicine, there are no clear analogous situations or legal precedents from which to draw parallels and conclusions. It seems defensible to fall back upon one's consent forms, if they included the possibility of storage tank failure, and offer the patient nothing. Yet this course of action may permanently harm the clinic's reputation. If one concludes that the patients are owed, how does that conflict with the clinic's need for financial solvency? Depending on how extensive the treatment offered is, the total cost of treatment could easily exceed millions of dollars. In the case of UH, it appears the finances of the practice may be linked to those of the hospital system, which allows deeper financial pockets, but a smaller private clinic could easily go bankrupt by having to offer uncompensated treatment on this scale. As with medical errors in general, it may be that the manner of the physicians, embryologists, and leadership in handling the situation may ultimately determine patient response (Petronio et al. 2013). The pending lawsuits, however, will be a separate matter, and it remains unclear what the disposition of the legal proceedings will be.

Thus, there is no one clear ethically superior manner of handling these situations. Nonetheless, as the ASRM Ethics Committee Opinion on "Disclosure of medical errors involving gametes and embryos" describes, clinics should "promote a culture of truth telling and should establish written policies and procedures" regarding disclosure (Ethics Committee of the American Society for Reproductive Medicine 2016b). As do the technical guidelines, this document emphasizes the need for rigorous procedures meant to eliminate such errors. However, this document expounds upon the next steps, which should include a root-cause analysis to uncover systemic failures and an ethical obligation to report errors based on "respect for patient autonomy and in fairness to the patients."[1]

The document reiterates the view that the method of disclosure, including its timeliness and sincerity, can have an important salutatory impact upon the patient's perception and recovery from the error. The topic of whether the burden of compensatory treatment should be borne by the patient or clinic remains unmentioned.

Avoiding Future Tragedies

In summary, the two ART tank failures from 2018 served as a wake-up call for the field about a class of catastrophic outcome that most considered essentially impossible. The shocking nature of these unexpected cases occurring independently on the same weekend and the societal fascination with embryos and reproduction contributed to the wealth of media coverage. Though the legal outcomes remain unknown, these events provide the context for a stimulus for all practices to consider their own room for improvement in equipment, training, and communication policies. It also may be time for the industry and society to perhaps reconsider what legislative safeguards are appropriate. From an ethical standpoint, the only dictum that seems unassailable is the need for transparency and integrity in the face of a medical error, whether human or technological.

However, the situation offers the opportunity for the community to explore anew challenges within reproductive medicine: the legal standing of embryos, the appropriate rigor for storing reproductive tissues, and the fairest methods of handling catastrophic errors. Further, we must forge a responsible path forward for the field, an effort that will require grappling with a few key dilemmas: the impending need to innovate and replace technology that individuals and couples increasingly rely upon, the high cost of doing so, and the divided sentiment in the United States regarding who should bear the cost for such investments. Continuing onwards with mere oversight of basic regulatory principles, and leaving such decisions in the hands of individual physicians and practices—who are currently disincentivized to take on the high cost of updating technology or routinely address technological failures with patients—opens the door for tragic repetition of these catastrophic outcomes.

Though venture capital and private investors have flooded the fertility market, they have primarily focused on targeting new potential patients with expendable income, not on expanding access among those of lower socioeconomic means or on improving the fundamental technology upon which we rely. Leaders in the field of reproductive medicine may consider a call to action, with dedicated task forces to study these questions and develop proactive and comprehensive strategies to mitigate future risk and improve the protection of patients' invaluable cryopreserved gametes and embryos.

Note

1. Communication issues might be one such root cause that is eminently preventable. See Chapter 5: "Communication as a Safeguard against Medical Errors" by Omilion-Hodges.

Works Cited

Adamson, David. 2002. "Regulation of Assisted Reproductive Technologies in the United States." *Fertility and Sterility* 78 (5): 932–942.

Alison, Venn, Elina Hemminki, Lyndsey Watson, Fiona Bruinsma, and David Healy. 2001. "Mortality in a Cohort of IVF Patients." *Human Reproduction* 16 (12): 2691–2696.

American College of Obstetricians and Gynecologists. 2018. "Early Pregnancy Loss." ACOG Practice Bulletin No. 200. *Obstetric Gynecology* 132: e197–207.

American Society of Reproductive Medicine. 2018. "ASRM Position Statement on Personhood Measures." Retrieved from www.asrm.org/ASRM_Position_Statement_on_Personhood_Measures/.

Barlevy, Dorit, Tenzin Wangmo, Bernice Elger, and Vardit Ravitsky. 2016. "Attitudes, Beliefs, and Trends Regarding Adolescent Oncofertility Discussions: A Systematic Literature Review." *Journal of Adolescent and Young Adult Oncology* 5 (2): 119–134.

Buduson, Sarah. 2018. "Human Error Blamed for Ohio Fertility Center Malfunction, Says 4,000 Eggs and Embryos Lost." *WXYZ Detroit*. Retrieved from www.wxyz.com/news/national/human-error-blamed-for-ohio-fertility-center-malfunction-says-4000-eggs-and-embryos-lost.

Caulfield, Timothy. 2001. "Liability in the Genetic Era: Wrongful Birth and Wrongful Life Lawsuits." *Journal SOGC* 23 (2): 143–147.

Centers for Disease Control and Prevention, American Society for Reproductive Medicine, Society for Assisted Reproductive Technology. 2018. "2016 Assisted Reproductive Technology National Summary Report." Atlanta, GA: US Department of Health and Human Services.

Cha, Ariana. 2018. "These Would-Be Parents' Embryos Were Lost. Now They're Grieving—and Suing." *The Washington Post*. Retrieved from https://wapo.st/2NeMTIB?tid=ss_mail&utm_term=.082974b13f2b

Chang, H., and C. Suh. 2010. "Ectopic Pregnancy After Assisted Reproductive Technology: What Are the Risk Factors?" *Current Opinion in Obstetric Gynecology* 22 (3): 202–207.

Damiano, Laura. 2011. "When Parents Can Choose to Have the 'Perfect' Child: Why Fertility Clinics Should be Required to Report Preimplantation Genetic Diagnosis Data." *Family Court Review* 49 (4): 846–859.

Dubey, Anil. 2012. *Infertility: Diagnosis, Management and IVF*. New Delhi, India: Jaypee Brothers Medical Publishers.

Ethics Committee of the American Society for Reproductive Medicine. 2015. "Disparities in Access to Effective Treatment for Infertility in the United States: An Ethics Committee Opinion." *Fertility and Sterility* 104 (5) 1104–1110.

Ethics Committee of the American Society for Reproductive Medicine. 2016a. "Defining Embryo Donation." *Fertility and Sterility* 92 (6): 1818–1819.

Ethics Committee of the American Society for Reproductive Medicine. 2016b. "Disclosure of Medical Errors Involving Gametes and Embryos: An Ethics Committee Opinion." *Fertility and Sterility* 106 (1): 59–63.

Henne, Melinda, and Kate Bundorf. 2008. "Insurance Mandates and Trends in Infertility Treatments." *Fertility and Sterility* 89: 66–73.

Holpuch, Amanda. 2015. "The Fight over Sofia Vergara's Embryos: Ex-Fiance Makes Right-to-Life Argument." *The Guardian.* Retrieved from www.the-guardian.com/us-news/2015/apr/30/sofia-vergara-embryos-nick-loeb-editorial.

Kjaer, Trille, Vanna Albieri, Allan Jensen, Susanne Kjaer, Christoffer Johansen, and Susanne Dalton. 2014. "Divorce or End of Cohabitation Among Danish Women Evaluated for Fertility Problems." *Acta Obstetricia et Gynecologica Scandinavica* 93 (3): 269–276.

Krim, Todd. 1996. "Beyond Baby M: International Perspectives on Gestational Surrogacy and the Demise of the Unitary Biological Mother." *Annals of Health Law* 5 (1): 193–226.

Legislative Tracker. 2018. "Personhood." *Rewire News.* Retrieved from https://rewire.news/legislative-tracker/law-topic/personhood/.

Martin, Joyce, Brady Hamilton, Michelle Osterman, Anne Driscoll, and Patrick Drake. 2018. "Births: Final data for 2016." *National Vital Statistics Reports* 67 (1). Hyattsville, MD: National Center for Health Statistics.

Martinez, Gladys, Kimberly Daniels, and Isaedmarie Febo-Vazquez. 2018. "Fertility of Men and Women Aged 15–44 in the United States: National Survey of Family Growth, 2011–2015." *National Health Statistics Reports.* Hyattsville, MD: National Center for Health Statistics: 113.

McKay, Chris. 2004. "What Is Life—And How Do We Search for It in Other Worlds?" *PLoS Biology* 2 (9): e302. https://doi.org/10.1371/journal.pbio.0020302.

Nestel, M., and Erielle Reshef. 2018. "San Francisco Fertility Clinic Experiences Cryostorage Malfunction on the Same Day as Cleveland Hospital." *ABC News.* Retrieved from https://abcnews.go.com/US/san-francisco-fertility-clinic-experiences-cryostorage-malfunction-day/story?id=53669584.

Petronio, Sandra, Alexia Torke, Gabriel Bosslet, Stephen Isenberg, Lucia Wocial, and Paul Helft. 2013. "Disclosing Medical Mistakes: A Communication Management Plan for Physicians." *Permanente Journal* 17 (2): 73–79.

Petropanagos, Angel, Alana Cattapan, Francoise Baylis, and Arthur Leader. 2015. "Social Egg Freezing: Risk, Benefits and Other Considerations." *CMAJ* 187 (9): 666–669.

Pomeroy, Kimball. 2018. "Liquid Nitrogen Storage Tank Failure: Can We Improve the Current System?" *Fertility & Sterility.* Retrieved from www.fertstertdialog.com/users/16110-fertility-and-sterility/posts/33372-pomeroy-consider-this.

The Practice Committee of the American Society for Reproductive Medicine and the Practice Committee of the Society for Assisted Reproductive Technology. 2008. "Revised Guidelines for Human Embryology and Andrology Laboratories." *Fertility and Sterility* 90 (5S): 45–59.

Research and Markets. 2018. "U.S. Fertility Clinics & Infertility Services: An Industry Analysis." Retrieved from www.researchandmarkets.com/research/5sk7kf/u_s_fertility?w=5.

Rialon, Kristy, Dan Blazer, Amy Abernethy, and Paul Mosca. 2012. "Surgery and the D-Word: Approaching the Topic of Death and Dying with Surgical Patients." *Journal of Palliative Care & Medicine* 2: 108. https://doi:10.4172/2165-7386.1000108.

Scutti, Susan. 2018. "Fertility Clinic Embryo Failures Are a 'Tale of Two Cities' Lawyer Says." *CNN*. Retrieved from www.cnn.com/2018/04/04/health/fertility-center-lawsuits/index.html.

Serino, Danielle. 2018. "UH Denies Wrongdoing in Fertility Failure Case in Latest Court Filing." *WKYC News*. Retrieved from www.wkyc.com/article/news/health/uh-failure/uh-denies-wrongdoing-in-fertility-failure-case-in-latest-court-filing/95–570437613.

Silvers, Anita, and Leslie Francis. 2017. "Reproduction as a Civil Right." *The Oxford Handbook of Reproductive Ethics*. https://doi.org/10.1093/oxfordhb/9780199981878.013.9.

Smajdor, Anna. 2007. "Deciding the Fate of Disputed Embryos: Ethical Issues in the Case of Natallie Evans." *Journal of Experimental & Clinical Assisted Reproduction* 4 (2). doi:10.1186/1743-1050-4-2.

United States Census Bureau. 2019. Retrieved from www.census.gov/popclock/.

Van Norman, Gail. 2019. "Informed Consent in the Operating Room." Retrieved from https://depts.washington.edu/bioethx/topics/infc.html.

7 Respecting Patient Autonomy in Radiation Oncology and Beyond

Megan Hyun and Alexander Hyun

The Problem of Limited Autonomy in Radiation Oncology

In contemporary biomedical ethics, it is widely accepted that health-care providers have a strong *prima facie* moral duty to respect the autonomy of patients. We will argue that this *prima facie* duty to respect autonomy generates a strong moral case for increasing patient education through direct consultations with a medical physicist throughout treatment. This chapter is structured as follows. First, we offer an argument for the conclusion that the way in which cancer patients are currently informed about the nature of their radiation treatment is morally problematic in virtue of some considerations about patient autonomy. Second, we present our proposal for the use of consultations with medical physicists and argue that it is a particularly attractive solution to this problem of autonomy, particularly in view of the potential for error in this medical field. Finally, we conclude by explaining why the argument of this chapter has important implications for many medical fields beyond Radiation Oncology.

Radiation Oncology is the field of medicine that encompasses the treatment of cancer (as well as a few non-cancerous conditions) with radiation. Radiation therapy is an extremely complex process and, as such, can be prone to error without proper safety measures. Currently, most cancer patients[1] are not educated about these safety measures and potential errors prior to deciding whether, where, and how to receive radiation therapy.

Once a patient is referred to a Radiation Oncology department, he/she will have a consultation with the radiation oncologist (see **Figure 7.1**). At this consultation, the physician will typically discuss treatment options as well as indications for, potential benefits of, and potential risks of radiation. The potential benefits may include pain management, local or regional control, progression-free survival, or overall survival.[2] Risks will include potential side effects (both acute and chronic),[3] but current standard of care does *not* include a discussion of possible medical errors or the associated risk of these errors occurring.

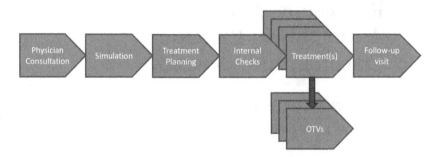

Figure 7.1 Radiation Oncology workflow diagram, not including events occurring outside the department, such as diagnosis, referral, and previous or concomitant treatments (e.g., chemotherapy).

Consultation often will include a description of the process of radiation therapy. This would cover anything related to the patient experience, such as: how the body will be positioned and immobilized, why contrast agents will be injected during imaging, where the radiation is going and what parts of the body will be avoided, the importance of making each treatment reproducible, etc. At some institutions, this description may be tailored to the patient based on what he/she wants to know. For example, a patient who is a nuclear engineer might ask more technical questions than one who is a philosophy professor, so the engineer will enter treatment with more detailed knowledge. The patient's decision regarding whether to receive radiation therapy will typically (but not always) occur at consultation. The physician will then obtain the patient's written consent prior to simulation (see **Figure 7.1**). The consent form will contain written acknowledgment of the benefits and risks that have been discussed, and much of the information given at consultation will be repeated to ensure the patient is informed.

To summarize the above current practices regarding patient education prior to radiation therapy: physicians give patients an explanation of the benefits and risks of radiation, as well as some information about what patients will experience. They typically do not discuss possible treatment errors, associated risks, or the safety measures in place to prevent such errors. Additionally, they provide few technical details regarding the nature of the treatment unless patients explicitly request them.

Our view is that the current practices of patient education prior to radiation therapy are morally problematic for reasons that have to do with patient autonomy. For our discussion, we will adopt the dominant account of the nature of autonomy in medical ethics, namely the one developed by Tom Beauchamp and James Childress in *Principles of*

Biomedical Ethics. According to this account, an action is autonomous only if it meets three conditions. First, the action must be done intentionally. Second, it must be sufficiently free from "controlling influences," such as coercive pressure exerted by family members and doctors (Beauchamp and Childress 2009, 101). And third, the act must be done with "a substantial degree of understanding" (Beauchamp and Childress 2009, 101). This last condition will be particularly important in what follows, so it is worth explicating in more detail. Persons act with understanding if "they have acquired pertinent information and have relevant beliefs about the nature and consequences of their actions" (Beauchamp and Childress 2009, 127). When the action in question is consent to a kind of medical treatment, pertinent information will include information about the nature and purposes of the treatment, alternatives to the treatment, and the treatment's risks and benefits.

Consider an example. Some cancer patients must decide not only whether to pursue radiation therapy, but also how aggressive their treatment will be. Aggressive radiation treatment may involve receiving a higher dose of radiation in a shorter period of time. A patient's decision to undergo aggressive radiation treatment is autonomous only if that patient makes her decision with an adequate understanding of the relevant facts about the treatment and its alternatives. For instance, the patient must understand (a) the major benefit of aggressive treatment (e.g., higher chance of survival), (b) the added risks (e.g., more dose delivered in a short period of time means that, if something goes wrong during one of the treatments, more damage can be done), (c) any difference in expected side effects, and (d) any differences in the patient experience of the treatment (e.g., how many treatments and how long the patient will need to lie still for each treatment). Note that the autonomy of an action comes in degrees, and this is because understanding comes in degrees. Suppose that one patient understands only (a) and (b), whereas a second patient understands (a), (b), and (c). Both patients have some level of understanding of the nature and consequences of the decision to undergo aggressive radiation treatment, but the latter patient's understanding is greater. As a result, the second patient's decision to undergo aggressive radiation treatment would be more autonomous than the first patient's decision to undergo this treatment, all else being equal.

In contemporary biomedical ethics, it is widely accepted that healthcare providers have a strong *prima facie* moral duty to respect the autonomy of patients. A *prima facie* moral duty to perform an action is a moral consideration in favor of doing that action that has some weight, but that may be outweighed by competing moral considerations. To illustrate, suppose that I promise to meet you at the library, but on the way there, I come across someone who urgently needs to be taken to the hospital. If I take her to the hospital, I cannot make our meeting at the library. There is a *prima facie* moral duty to go the library, since there is something to be said in favor of keeping one's promises, from the moral point of view. But this *prima facie* moral duty is outweighed by a stronger *prima facie* moral duty to forego the trip to the library in order to take the person to the hospital. The standard view in biomedical ethics is that there is always a *prima facie* moral duty, or some moral consideration, that favors respecting patient autonomy.

What does it mean to respect a patient's autonomy? As Beauchamp and Childress observe in their influential statement of the principle, it requires "actions that foster autonomous decision making"—actions such as disclosing relevant information to the patient and ensuring that patients understand the relevant medical facts (Beauchamp and Childress 2009, 104). As we understand it, this principle implies that there is a *prima facie* moral duty for a health-care provider to perform those actions that would increase the level of autonomy of a patient's medical decisions. To illustrate, consider informed consent requirements, which are by far the most prominent application of the principle of respect for autonomy within medicine. Below is a statement from the American Medical Association's Principles of Medical Ethics:

> In seeking a patient's informed consent (or the consent of the patient's surrogate if the patient lacks decision-making capacity or declines to participate in making decisions), physicians should:
>
> (1) Assess the patient's ability to understand relevant medical information and the implications of treatment alternatives and to make an independent, voluntary decision.
> (2) Present relevant information accurately and sensitively, in keeping with the patient's preferences for receiving medical information. The physician should include information about:
>
> The diagnosis (when known)
> The nature and purpose of recommended interventions
> The burdens, risks, and expected benefits of all options, including forgoing treatment
>
> (3) Document the informed consent conversation and the patient's (or surrogate's) decision in the medical record in some manner. When the patient/surrogate has provided specific written consent, the consent form should be included in the record.
>
> (American Medical Association 2019)

The principle of respect for autonomy provides the standard moral justification for these informed consent requirements. When a physician fulfills requirements (1) and (2), for example, this can be expected to deepen the patient's understanding of the nature and consequences of the prospective treatment. Consequently, the level of autonomy of a patient's decision to undergo this treatment will be greater as a result of the physician's fulfilling these requirements. The principle of respect for autonomy, therefore, implies that it is good, from the moral point of view, for physicians to satisfy requirements (1) and (2).

We have now presented all of the concepts needed to explain why we think the status quo in Radiation Oncology is morally problematic on the grounds of autonomy. As noted above, cancer patients often receive little or no information about possible treatment errors, associated risks of such errors, and the safety measures in place to prevent these errors.[4] It is, therefore, safe to assume that many patients have a poor understanding of these matters.[5] And it is surely the case that such matters are directly relevant to some medical decisions that cancer patients must make. These include the decision to undergo the doctor's recommended treatment, rather than to undergo no treatment or an alternative treatment, as well as the decision to undergo the recommended treatment at one hospital rather than another. Because the facts about possible treatment errors, their associated risks, and the relevant safety measures are relevant to these medical decisions, and because cancer patients typically lack understanding of these facts, we should conclude that important medical decisions regularly made by cancer patients are significantly less autonomous than they could be. Because the principle of respect for autonomy implies that there is a *prima facie* moral duty to perform those actions that would increase the autonomy of patients' medical decisions, this principle implies that there is a *prima facie* moral duty to favor modifying those practices and policies that do not optimize patient autonomy. Because the current practices of patient education prior to radiation therapy result in medical decisions being made that have an unnecessarily low level of autonomy, the principle of respect for autonomy implies that there is a moral duty for health-care providers to favor altering current practices in such a way as to increase the autonomy of cancer patients' medical decisions. We conclude that the status quo is morally sub-optimal.

There may be multiple solutions to the problem of autonomy in Radiation Oncology. However, we propose what we believe is the optimal solution: patient consultations with medical physicists. To understand why this proposal is ideal, it will be useful to first explain the role of medical physicists in Radiation Oncology.

Consultations With Medical Physicists as a Solution to the Problem

Medical physicists' primary duties are clinical service, research and development, and teaching (American Association of Physicists in Medicine 2019a). In Radiation Oncology, clinical service typically includes creating and checking treatment plans, performing quality assurance (QA) tests for imaging and treatment equipment, designing and testing radiation shielding installation, and otherwise collaborating with physicians and other colleagues to ensure the safe and effective delivery of radiation therapy. Research and development covers a wide array of activities that vary depending on the environment (e.g., university or community hospital), as well as the specialization of the department and its physicists. However, all medical physicists will lead or participate in numerous projects, whether basic science, translational research, clinical improvement, product design, and/or procedure implementation. Teaching duties also will vary depending on the environment. For example, a faculty physicist in a department with physics residents may have more formal teaching responsibilities than a solo physicist at a small community hospital. However, all physicists must communicate with service engineers, nurses, managers, technologists, physicians, and other groups, often educating them on matters of radiation safety and technical details of quality management and machine operation.

Figure 7.1 shows that, according to the current status quo, patients do not typically interact directly with medical physicists. Exceptions include any treatments involving radioactive material or special cases in which patients' questions about the treatment machines may be referred to the physicist. Physicist-patient consultations could easily be added into the workflow shown in **Figure 7.1**. We propose these consultations take place prior to simulation, as well as immediately after the treatment plan is approved, with additional consultations as needed per patient request.

The purpose of the first consultation (prior to CT simulation) would be to provide general, layperson-appropriate education regarding the radiation therapy equipment and process, as well as to explain possible treatment errors, associated risks, and the safety initiatives in place to keep patients safe during their treatments. This consultation would increase understanding relevant to decisions regarding where and whether to undergo radiation therapy. For example, if a physicist at Hospital 1 explains several initiatives in place to keep patients safe, and Hospital 2 does not (or the Hospital 2 procedures seem less thorough), a patient may choose Hospital 1 for treatment, much like choosing an airline based on its safety record. The second consultation would focus on the patient's individual treatment plan, ideally including images and other graphics, to increase patient understanding prior to beginning treatment. Although the patient will have already signed a consent form at this point, this consultation may help patients make the decision whether to continue treatment.

We have several reasons to think that medical physicists are particularly well-suited to increase the level of patient understanding in Radiation Oncology. Because we have already drawn the connection between patient understanding and patient autonomy, the following also serve as evidence that our proposal would significantly increase the autonomy of relevant medical decisions:

- **Medical physicists have the technical expertise.** Physicists have cultivated a deep understanding of the interactions of radiation in matter, treatment planning complexities, radiation safety, risk, quality assurance, etc. Physicists are not only trained in didactics related to radiation therapy physics, health physics, radiobiology, etc.; they are also required to do residency training and are certified by a physician board (the American Board of Radiology).
- **Medical physicists have the communication skills.** Part of a physicist's job description is communicating with physicians, technologists, nurses, residents and students about medical physics on various levels. The way they talk about technical details with a student might differ widely from how they discuss the same topic with a physician. They have experience reducing complex topics to their simplest form and are ideally suited to give technical explanations to patients.[6]
- **Increasingly, medical physicists have the time.** Medical physicists' time in the clinic is as precious as the radiation oncologists'; however, current advances in health-care automation are reducing the burden of many routine clinical tasks, which can free up physicists' schedules for other activities, such as research or direct patient care (Laberta 2017; Yaddanapudi et al. 2017; Zwan et al. 2017). The same cannot be said for radiation oncologists. Although automation of chart checks, QA and plan optimization are a current reality, automation of target delineation and clinical decision making (both a large part of physician workload) are much further away.
- **Medical physicists have the movement.** This proposal is offered just as a new movement is taking shape within the medical physics community. Called Medical Physics 3.0, this movement aims to "re-define and re-invigorate the role of physics in modern medicine" (American Association of Physicists in Medicine 2019b). According to Ehsan Samei, one of the chairs of the initiative within the American Association of Physicists in Medicine, "Medical physicists have the skills, background and desire to improve the practice of evidence-based medicine while keeping patients safe. They just need the chance to step out from behind the scanners and introduce themselves" (Samei 2017b). The movement is about more than just physicist-patient consultations, but these are clearly a part of this initiative (Samei 2017a).

In light of these four facts, it is clear that our principle of respect for autonomy implies that we have moral reason to implement our proposal.

Objections and Replies

In this section, we respond to five objections against our position. The first objection targets the version of the principle of respect for autonomy that we have espoused. Recall that this version implies that there is a *prima facie* moral duty for health-care providers to perform any action that would increase the level of autonomy of a patient's medical decisions. Because the autonomy of a medical decision increases with the degree to which the patient has understanding of the facts relevant to the medical decision, and because there are millions of facts that are relevant to every medical decision, it follows that our favored version of the principle implies that health-care providers have a *prima facie* moral duty to explain to each patient millions of facts. Many of these facts will be only barely relevant to the medical decisions. For example, consider a patient with severe back pain who needs to decide whether or not to pursue radiation therapy for her breast cancer. Relevant facts she would need to consider include: radiation has been shown to improve overall survival rates for breast cancer patients, treatments will require the patient to lie still on her back or stomach for 15–20 minutes at a time, and a common side effect is reddening of the skin over the treated area. Barely relevant facts that would be a waste of time to explain include: this radiation procedure resulted in a medical error 20 years ago due to a mistake made by a physician who no longer works at the hospital, a clinic 30 minutes away has a negligibly higher safety record (e.g., 1 fewer incident for every 100,000 procedures) when performing this treatment, and this radiation oncologist has performed 200 of these procedures, whereas a colleague at another hospital has performed 205. There is a sense in which it would be understandable to consider these facts during decision making. However, it would be silly for a physician to take the time to share such facts with her patients. Our principle of respect for autonomy implies that there is a *prima facie* moral duty for health-care providers to share these and countless other facts with every patient. Critics may insist that it is intuitively implausible that health-care providers have a *prima facie* moral duty to explain millions of barely relevant facts to every patient.[7]

We concede that our argument does commit us to thinking that there is a large number of facts that are such that health-care providers have a *prima facie* moral duty to explain them to every patient. But this is not an implausible commitment. First of all, the number of facts that are such that our principle implies that there's a *prima facie* moral duty to explain them to patients will not be in the millions, for patients are more likely to be confused than to be enlightened if medical practitioners overwhelm them with a huge number of facts. As Beauchamp and Childress observe, "information overload may prevent adequate understanding" (Beauchamp and Childress 2009, 130). Health-care providers need to be selective when choosing which information to share with patients because patients can handle only a limited amount of information. Second, those who are inclined to think that it is implausible that there is a *prima facie* moral duty to explain a large number of barely relevant facts to patients may be confusing the claim *that there is a* prima facie *moral duty to explain these facts* with the logically stronger claim *that there is a significantly strong* prima facie *moral duty to explain these facts*. This latter claim is indeed implausible, but we are not committed to it. For on our view, the weight of a *prima facie* moral duty to perform an action that is generated by the principle of respect for autonomy varies with the degree to which performing the action increases the autonomy of patients' medical decisions. If a fact is barely relevant to a medical decision, then a patient coming to understand that fact would increase the autonomy of her medical decision only by a tiny amount, and so we are committed only to the existence of a very weak *prima facie* moral duty to explain that fact to patients. Such a weak *prima facie* moral duty can normally be ignored for all practical purposes. To return to our example, our principle of respect for autonomy does imply that if a clinic 30 minutes away has a negligibly higher safety record when performing a type of treatment that a patient needs to undergo, then there's a *prima facie* moral duty for health-care providers to inform the patient of this fact. But intuitively, this fact is only barely relevant to the decision of whether to undergo the treatment at the patient's current hospital. So, helping her to understand this fact would increase the autonomy of her decision to undergo this treatment only by a tiny amount, and the *prima facie* moral duty to inform the patient of this fact is correspondingly weak. A *prima facie* moral duty that is this weak normally should not factor seriously into our deliberations.

A second objection is suggested by our response to the first. Since *prima facie* moral duties that are generated by the principle of autonomy can be weak to the point of practical insignificance on our view, it may be objected that our conclusions lack practical import. Above, we argued that there is a *prima facie* moral duty of respect for autonomy to change the status quo with respect to the way that patients are informed about facts pertaining to their treatment. We then argued for the further conclusion that there is a *prima facie* moral duty of respect for autonomy to favor the implementation of consultations with medical physicists. But if the reasoning we have offered in response to the first objection is correct, then the *prima facie* moral duties to change the status quo and to implement these consultations could be extremely weak, for all we have shown. If they are extremely weak, then for all practical purposes they should not factor seriously into our deliberations.

In response, we argue that the strength of the *prima facie* moral duty to implement our proposed policy is quite strong. Recall that the issues that we envision being explained by medical physicists include (a) possible treatment errors, (b) associated risks of such errors, and (c) the safety measures in place to prevent these errors. Facts about these issues intuitively bear directly on the sorts of medical decisions that cancer patients will typically need to make, such as decisions about whether to accept treatment for their illness, about which available treatment to favor, and about which hospital and physician to go to for the favored treatment. Because these facts are quite relevant for the medical decisions that cancer patients must make, it is reasonable to think that patients' acquisition of a decent understanding of these facts would increase the autonomy of some of their medical decisions significantly. So, the *prima facie* moral duty to implement our proposed policy is significantly strong.

A third objection relates to the monetary cost of physicist consultations: is the potential increase in patient understanding worth the cost to the patient (which may not be covered by insurance companies)?[8] This question is one that may not be answered for some time because the process of billing for this type of consultation is still under discussion in the field of Radiation Oncology. Currently, there are no billing codes associated with physicist–patient consultations. Our argument that there is a strong *prima facie* moral duty for hospitals to offer these consultations is unaffected by the cost to the patient. However, the hospital's decision on whether to include physicist consultations in the typical treatment workflow for all patients should take into account the added cost. We envision these consultations eventually becoming standard-of-care in Radiation Oncology, in which case it is our hope that they will be bundled into the treatment charges in a way that will be covered by insurance and not substantially increase the patients' financial burden.

The final two objections are more practical in nature and have both been pressed by Dr. Kristi Hendrickson (Schuller, Hendrickson, and Rong 2018). She first argues that physicists lack the communication skills to conduct these sorts of consultations effectively:

> Medical physicists are not trained to interact with patients in the setting of an initial patient consult. Anecdotally, I recall attending an initial patient consult with a member of my family who was considering radiotherapy. I did ask to meet the physicist and asked several questions about their QA processes as it related to the proposed treatment. What I experienced was a "deer in the headlights" reaction and a fumbling response that did not instill in me a confidence in that clinic's radiation safety processes.
>
> (Schuller, Hendrickson, and Rong 2018, 7–8)

Hendrickson then suggests that medical physicists would require more training in "the soft skills of patient interactions" before medical physics consultations of the sort we have proposed would be advisable. We think this is an important concern, and we have three thoughts in response to it.

First, we readily acknowledge that more training in effective interaction with patients should be given to medical physicists. Ideally, this training should be incorporated into accredited medical physics residency programs, but the medical physics community should also make options available for practicing physicists to improve their skills. At a minimum, physicists should receive training to improve general and specific communication skills, as well as simulation-based training with realistic patient interactions. It is also important that these residency or community-offered programs have a standardized method for assessing competency in patient interaction. Such a training program has already been developed at UC San Diego (Brown et al. 2018).

Second, as we mentioned in the previous section, the standard responsibilities of medical physicists provide them with a wealth of experience communicating about medical physics to a wide array of audiences, including students, technologists, nurses, and physicians. We, therefore, have excellent reason to expect that many medical physicists will be particularly skilled at communication with patients once they have received the sort of training in soft skills that we envision.

Finally, the successful implementation of our proposal in a given hospital requires only that there be at least one physicist working at that hospital who has the requisite social and communication skills. This one physicist can be the one who takes on the primary responsibility for these consultations. Because it is typical for there to be multiple medical physicists working at large hospitals, it is likely that large hospitals employ at least one medical physicist with the needed social and communication skills. For this reason, our proposal may be ideal for larger hospital environments.

Hendrickson's second objection to physics consultations is that physicists lack the time required by them. She writes:

> The time commitment required for a medical physicist to routinely be present at every initial patient consult would be substantial. In my clinic, there are 1200–1500 initial patient consults on average per year or 24–30 per week. The meetings are typically 20–60 or more minutes long. Expecting a physicist to be present at each of these patient meetings would be an inappropriate utilization of a limited and expensive resource—physicist time—and would therefore add an inappropriate cost to the present medical care system.
>
> (Schuller, Hendrickson, and Rong 2018, 7)

We are inclined to disagree with Hendrickson on this point. In light of our observation that physics consultations would increase the autonomy of patients' medical decisions, we think that these consultations would be an appropriate use of physicists' limited and valuable time. But, even if Hendrickson is correct that considerations of time show that it does not make sense to begin physics consultations immediately, it will make sense to begin these consultations in the near future. Recall our observation from the previous section that current advances in health-care automation are reducing the burden of routine clinical tasks. As automation continues to improve, we can expect that physicists will have more time to devote to direct patient care, and physics consultations would be a worthwhile way to use this time.

Implications for Other Medical Fields

We will conclude by directing attention to two worthwhile avenues of investigation that are suggested by our discussion. First, we think that it would be fruitful to consider what implications the other widely accepted moral principles of biomedical ethics have for our proposed physics consultations. In particular, we suspect that these consultations receive additional support from the principle of beneficence, according to which health-care providers have a strong *prima facie* moral duty to act for the benefit of their patients (Beauchamp and Childress 2009, 197–239). One reason to think this has to do with these consultations' potential to decrease patient anxiety. Early results from a recent clinical trial at UC San Diego suggest that providing cancer patients with these sorts of consultations may make them less anxious throughout their treatment (Atwood et al. 2018). If confirmed by further investigation, this would suffice to show that the principle of beneficence entails a *prima facie* moral duty to favor the use of these consultations, for anxiety makes one worse off. Further, there is evidence that lower patient-reported distress is associated with higher survival rates in radiation therapy (Habboush et al. 2017). Because one is less distressed when one is less anxious, this bolsters the case for thinking that there is a strong argument from beneficence for physics consultations if these consultations decrease patient anxiety. A second reason to think that the principle of beneficence may support the use of physics consultations is that these consultations may help to decrease the rate of medical errors within Radiation Oncology. Because these consultations could include discussion of possible treatment errors and their frequency, these consultations could make medical errors more transparent to patients than they currently are. This would provide hospitals with even more incentive to minimize the rate of treatment errors, for patients will naturally prefer to receive treatment at hospitals with lower rates of such errors. We intend to develop these lines of reasoning in greater depth in future work.

Second, our argument from autonomy for physics consultations likely has important implications for medical fields beyond just Radiation Oncology. If our argument is sound, then there is a significantly strong *prima facie* moral duty to favor policies that significantly increase patients' understanding of facts relevant to their medical decisions, such as facts about possible treatment errors, associated risks of such errors, and the safety measures in place to prevent these errors. This moral insight implies that there is moral reason to make some changes in any medical field in which patients tend to have a low level of understanding of these sorts of facts. Both general literacy and health literacy have been shown to be low in the United States, which implies that many patients across many fields of medicine may have a low level of understanding regarding facts relevant to their care (Graham and Brookey 2008; Kutner, Greenberg, Jin, and Paulsen 2006). The problem of limited autonomy is far more widespread than the field of Radiation Oncology, so the argument of this chapter has quite broad implications.

Unlike the specific lack of understanding we have laid out for patients in Radiation Oncology, patient health literacy has been an important topic of discussion for many years (Graham and Brookey 2008; Ishikawa and Yano 2008; Baker 2006; Safeer and Keenan 2005; Williams et al. 2002; Berkman et al. 2011; Nutbeam 2008). However, much of this literature focuses on the physician–patient relationship and how physicians can increase patient understanding. We have shown that, in Radiation Oncology, a group of non-physician specialists (i.e., Medical Physicists) is well-positioned to participate in this process through consultations with patients. We suspect that other fields of medicine may have analogous non-physician specialists who are not currently meeting with patients, but who could be similarly well-positioned to improve patient autonomy by increasing patient understanding of relevant facts, such as facts pertaining to medical errors. It would be worthwhile for those with the relevant medical expertise in these fields to explore this possibility further.

Notes

1. In this chapter, when we discuss what information is provided to the patient, it is implied that the patient's family and/or caregivers will be involved. "Patient" may be taken as "patient and his/her caregiver(s)."
2. "Local control" is the halting of growth at the origin of disease, whereas "regional control" is halting growth at the first site where the disease has spread. Patients may be given survival estimates at consultation, such as "progression-free survival," meaning how long they are expected to survive with extant but not worsening disease, or "overall survival," which is how long they are expected to live after finishing treatment.
3. "Acute" side effects are those that occur during treatment, for example, skin reddening ("erythema"), fatigue, etc., and will typically go away within weeks of finishing treatment. "Chronic" side effects are longer-lasting and may develop during treatment or months to years after treatment ends. Examples include fibrosis, infertility, and secondary cancers.
4. Physicist–patient consultations should not focus only on medical error and safety. Rather, they are an opportunity for the physicist to educate patients on a number of facts related to their care, including how the radiation is delivered, how the treatment plan is created, and other technical details. However,

because medical error is the focus of this text, we will primarily discuss the physicist–patient consultations in this context.

5. In treatment and in testing, the concern of whether the criteria of informed consent are met looms large. This chapter will focus primarily on autonomy, however. For more on informed consent in relation to medical over-testing and, to a lesser extent, treatment, see Chapter 8: "Medical Over-testing and Racial Distrust" by Luke Golemon.

6. Preventing errors via communication is a very promising strategy; see Chapter 5: "Communication as a Safeguard against Medical Errors" by Omilion-Hodges.

7. Thanks to Dr. Nathan Bennion for raising this objection.

8. Thanks to one of our anonymous reviewers for raising this objection.

Works Cited

American Association of Physicists in Medicine. 2019a. "Medical Physicist." Accessed January 6, 2019. Retrieved from https://aapm.org/medical_physicist/default.asp.

American Association of Physicists in Medicine. 2019b. "MedPhys 3.0." Accessed January 6, 2019. Retrieved from www.aapm.org/MedPhys30/default.asp.

American Medical Association. 2019. "Informed Consent." Accessed January 6, 2019. Retrieved from www.ama-assn.org/delivering-care/ethics/informed-consent.

Atwood, Todd, Derek Brown, James Murphy, Kevin Moore, Arno Mundt, and Todd Pawlicki. 2018. "Establishing a New Clinical Role for Medical Physicists: A Prospective Phase II Trial." *International Journal of Radiation Oncology*Biology*Physics* 102 (3): 635–641.

Baker, David. 2006. "The Meaning and Measure of Health Literacy." *Journal of General Internal Medicine* 21 (8): 878–883.

Beauchamp, Tom, and James Childress. 2009. *Principles of Biomedical Ethics, Sixth Edition*. New York: Oxford University Press.

Berkman, Nancy, Stacey Sheridan, Katrina Donahue, David Halpern, and Karen Crotty. 2011. "Low Health Literacy and Health Outcomes: An Updated Systematic Review." *Annals of Internal Medicine* 155 (2): 97–107.

Brown, Derek, Todd Atwood, Kevin Moore, Robert MacAulay, James Murphy, Arno Mundt, and Todd Pawlicki. 2018. "A Program to Train Medical Physicists for Direct Patient Care Responsibilities." *Journal of Applied Clinical Medical Physics* 19 (6): 332–335.

Graham, Suzanne, and John Brookey. 2008. "Do Patients Understand?" *The Permanente Journal* 12 (3): 67–69.

Habboush, Yacob, Robert Shannon, Shehzad Niazi, Laeticia Hollant, Megan Single, Katherine Gaines, Bridget Smart, Nicolette Chimato, Michael Heckman, Steven Buskirk Laura Vallow, Katherine Tzou, Stephen Ko, Jennifer Peterson, Heather Biers, Atiya Day, Kimberly Nelson, Jeff Sloan, Michele Halyard, Robert Miller. 2017. "Patient-Reported Distress and Survival Among Patients Receiving Definitive Radiation Therapy." *Advances in Radiation Oncology* 2 (2): 211–219.

Ishikawa, Hirono, and Eiji Yano. 2008. "Patient Health Literacy and Participation in the Health-Care Process." *Health Expectations* 11 (2): 113–122.

Kutner, Mark, Elizabeth Greenberg, Ying Jin, and Christine Paulsen. 2006. *The Health Literacy of America's Adults: Results from the 2003 National Assessment of Adult Literacy (NCES 2006–483)*. Washington, DC: National Center for Education Statistics.

Laberta, Valerie. 2017. "Benefits of Automation in Radiation Oncology." *Oncology Times* 39 (1): 1, 9–10.

Nutbeam, Don. 2008. "The Evolving Concept of Health Literacy." *Social Science & Medicine* 67 (12): 2072–2078.

Safeer, Richard, and Jann Keenan. 2005. "Health Literacy: The Gap between Physicians and Patients." *American Family Physician* 72 (3): 463–468.

Samei, Ehsan. 2017a, September 29. "Stepping Out from Behind the Machines." *Becker's Hospital Review*. Retrieved from www.beckershospitalreview.com/patient-engagement/stepping-out-from-behind-the-machines.html.

Samei, Ehsan. 2017b, October 16. "Medical Physicists Bring New Value to Patient-Centered Care." *Patient Safety & Quality Healthcare*. Retrieved from www.psqh.com/analysis/medical-physicists-bring-new-value-patient-centered-care/.

Schuller, Bradley, Kristi Hendrickson, and Yi Rong. 2018. "Medical Physicists Should Meet with Patients as Part of the Initial Consult." *Journal of Applied Clinical Medical Physics* 19 (2): 6–9.

Williams, Mark, Terry Davis, Ruth Parker, and Barry Weiss. 2002. "The Role of Health Literacy in Patient-Physician Communication." *Family Medicine* 34 (5): 383–389.

Yaddanapudi, Sridhar, Bin Cai, Taylor Harry, Steven Dolly, Baozhou Sun, Hua Li, Keith Stinson, Camille Noel, Lakshmi Santanam, Todd Pawlicki, Sasa Mutic, and Murty Goddu. 2017. "Rapid Acceptance Testing of Modern Linac Using On-Board MV and kV Imaging Systems." *Medical Physics* 44 (7): 3393–3406.

Zwan, Benjamin, Michael Barnes, Jonathan Hindmarsh, Seng Lim, Dale Lovelock, Todsaporn Fuangrod, Daryl O'Connor, Paul Keall, and Peter Greer. 2017. "Commissioning and Quality Assurance for VMAT Delivery Systems: An Efficient Time-Resolved System Using Real-Time EPID Imaging." *Medical Physics* 44 (8): 3909–3922.

Part III
Vulnerable Populations

8 Medical Overtesting and Racial Distrust[1]

Luke Golemon

Medical Overtesting

The phenomenon of medical overuse in general and specifically medical overtesting is well-known and harmful to both the patient and the health-care system (Boland, Wollan, and Silverstein 1996; Shapiro and Greenfield 1987; Bishop, Federman, and Keyhani 2010; Greenberg and Green 2014; Morgan et al. 2015). It is estimated that between 10 and 30 percent of all care is overuse, depending on the definition and method (Berwick and Hackbarth 2012; Morgan et al. 2015; Smith 1991). Overtesting is just one kind of overuse, but a kind I argue is different from its siblings. Unlike other forms of overuse, it is not obvious we should focus significant effort into reducing it. Because minority groups (specifically black Americans) are liable to be victims of medical underuse and physicians' perceptions of underuse and overuse in individual cases can be affected by unconscious bias, these groups do not suffer the harms of overtesting in the same way as others. Furthermore, race-neutral policies aimed at reducing undertesting might further lower treatment they already receive, increasing already-existent health inequities. Finally, if we are to reduce it via some policy, we should strongly consider race-conscious policies. Before I can argue either point, more must be said about overuse and overtesting.

The Nature of Overuse and Overtesting

The reasons overuse occurs are hard to parse. According to some studies, defensive medicine plays some role in this—doctors feel pressure to do more than necessary to avoid liability, including testing (Greenberg and Green 2014; Mello, Chandra, Gawande, and Studdert 2010; Bishop, Federman, and Keyhani 2010). Other and more recent studies indicate that low-value care (some of which includes preventative care, such as medical tests) is driven primarily by local practices, patient expectations, or is idiosyncratic to certain diagnoses (Reid, Rabideau, and Sood 2016; Morgan et al. 2018). Medical overuse increases the cost of healthcare, puts the patients' health at risk, and reduces the amount of time available with medical professionals for everyone (Greenberg and Green 2014; Mello, Chandra, Gawande, and Studdert 2010; Thomasian 2014). This gives us strong reasons to try to reduce medical overuse, of which overtesting is a part (Morgan et al. 2018; Mello, Chandra, Gawande, and Studdert 2010). Although awareness of medical overuse has greatly increased, practice remains largely unaffected (Morgan et al. 2015; Morgan et al. 2018).

Part of the issue is located in the definitions and concepts used to try and probe the problem. Overuse and underuse in a medical setting are typically thought of as paradigm cases of medical error. Medical error is conceptually broad. The Institute of Medicine report on medical error defines it as "Failure of a planned action to be completed as intended or use of a wrong plan to achieve an aim" (Kohn, Corrigan, and Donaldson 2000, 210). It can be usefully thought of as the result of a knowledge-based or practice-based mistake in a medical setting.[2] As Morgan et al. point out, there are multiple overlapping concepts used to describe medical overuse: overutilization, overmedicalization, low value care, and so on (2015).[3] Additionally, there are related concepts like overdiagnosis, overtreatment, and overtesting that are commonly used (Morgan et al. 2015). Many have adopted the Institute of Medicine's definition of medical overuse as "care in the absence of a clear medical basis for use or when the benefit of therapy does not outweigh the risk" (Institute of Medicine 2001). While I intend to focus on overtesting shortly, we should first critically examine this definition.

The primary issue with the definition is that it does not distinguish between two different readings: one is read as subjective while the other reading is objective. Suppose a physician examines a patient and their perception of the patient identifies symptoms that point toward a heart attack. The physician now has a medical basis for care. Suppose also that one of the symptoms that the medical field identifies as a symptom for heart attacks does not actually correlate with heart attack rates, although the medical community is unaware of this. Finally, suppose that the care involves managing this same problematic symptom. Now we have a case in which the physician believes they have a medical basis for care, but, objectively speaking, the benefit of therapy does not outweigh the risk. Under the definition cited earlier, this seems as if it is both a case of overuse and not a case of overuse.

To understand how to resolve this issue, we can draw an analogy to justified beliefs and true beliefs. It is commonly accepted among epistemologists that someone may be justified in holding a false belief. For example, someone might be justified in believing that they saw a zebra when they in fact only saw a cleverly disguised donkey (Alspector-Kelly 2019), or believing "laudable pus" to be healing (Nuland 2011). If "medical basis" is anything like justified belief, then it is possible to have a medical basis despite the therapy's actual costs and benefits being net negative.

It is likely that the definition of medical overuse is consistent, treating both concepts as subjective,[4] but it is important to show that we rely on this subjective reading whether or not the Institute of Medicine conflated the issues. When determining how to reduce overuse, vacillating between readings may seriously hamper efforts. A brief foreshadowing is illustrative: bias can cause one person to perceive a situation in a different way than another; if there is no medical basis for care given a racially biased evaluation, then the physician could believe they are entirely justified in withholding care when they in fact should provide it. While an objective reading of "medical basis" might help us find low-value care elsewhere, it seems to systematically overlook catching instances of subjective bias when evaluating whether something is low-value care by the physician.

This discussion generalizes to overuse's drivers. Overtesting specifically seems to have similar conceptual joints: physicians may overtest despite their perception that it is not necessary, or the community may learn that the benefits of a test do not outweigh the cost and fail to keep its members testing with best practices. The upshot is that we now can identify roughly two ways overtesting might be identified: one in which a physician accurately identifies a case in which "[testing] in the absence of a clear medical basis for use or when the benefit of therapy does not outweigh the risk," and one in which a physician *believes* they have identified such a case, but are incorrect for reasons including unconscious bias. Both of these are likely phenomenologically indistinguishable to the physician at the time.[5]

As with overuse, medical overtesting is regarded as harmful to the patient and the health-care system. On this basis, there has been a push to rather bluntly reduce medical overtesting (Hendee 2010; Morgan et al. 2015; Morgan, Dhruva, Wright, and Korenstein 2016). Once we learn that we use imaging tests much more often than necessary, physicians are encouraged to cut back on the use of such tests (such as the MRI or the CT scan) in addition to major systemic changes to liability and non-legal financial incentives (Hendee 2010). Moreover, the community-wide push to reduce medical overuse and waste likely seeps into individual practice.[6] Notably, many of the anti-overtesting policies argued against here are race-neutral, which often contributes to their blunt nature with regard to problems of racial disparities. I argue that we have assumed too quickly; the basis on which we have made the leap from overtesting to its reduction does not have a strong foundation. Characterizing harm in such a broad way neglects an important factor: racial minorities[7] are not harmed by overtesting in the same way as other groups. To see this more clearly, we should review some major points about medical racism.

Black Experience and Medical Racism

It is beneficial to begin with the facts of racial disparities and center the discussion at the margins before considering policies (Airhihubuwa and Liburd 2006). The history of the United States is plagued with racism. Not only has intentional, interpersonal racism led to horrific acts, racial animus has created structures of power and attitudes that affect its victims in ways that may no longer involve interpersonal racists at all (Bonilla-Silva 2017). Hardly any aspect of society has been left untouched.[8] Medicine has fared no better. For more than a thousand years, black biology and black intellectual ability have been denigrated or assumed to be inferior.[9] From Galen to Avicenna to Carl Linnaeus, the luminaries and founders of medicine have diagnosed darker-skinned peoples with primitivity, savagery, stupidity, or categorized them as wholly subhuman (McBride 2018; Byrd and Clayton 2001). As each new scientific theory was developed, racism was either already present or quickly twisted the theory to support itself. For example, it was not long before Darwinian physicians and natural scientists proclaimed that they had found the missing link between apes and humans: black people (Drake 1987; Byrd 2000).

This inevitably led to healthcare that was entirely inadequate and often pernicious. A lexicon of "Negro diseases" was developed (Byrd and Clayton 2001). Almshouses, medical centers for the "undeserving poor" were built to house black patients (Rosenberg 1987). Hospitals denied service to any but whites or would abuse black patients (Rosenberg 1987). It goes without saying that medical training was an exclusively white privilege.

The Tuskegee experiment is illustrative of these attitudes within the medical field. In the government-approved and government-funded study, 622 poor black men were monitored to study the progression of syphilis. Despite developing an effective cure during the study, the men did not receive any such treatment. Furthermore, none of the men were informed of their illness or of the true timeline of the study. None of them were ever given penicillin, an effective cure for the disease, during the experiment. This study was not halted until 1972, only after its horrors were leaked to the press.

This racist history has not merely influenced the present day—it is continuous with it. As Vanessa Gamble put it, "the problem we must face is not just the shadow of Tuskegee but the shadow of racism that so profoundly affects the lives and beliefs of all people in this country" (Gamble 1997). Many accept that there was racism, even medical racism, up to the 1920s (Hoberman 2012; Byrd and Clayton 2001; Smedley, Nelson, and Stith 2003). The Tuskegee experiment is emblematic of the continuing racism up till its halt in 1972. But this was not the end:

> More than 600 studies have documented racial and ethnic differences in health care dating back at least to the 1980s. These studies

suggested that racial and ethnic differences reflect, in part, underuse by black patients who fail to receive these procedures when their use is clinically appropriate.

(Jha et al. 2005, 690; Hoberman 2012, 235)

In 1999, Schulman et al. found that black patients were less likely to be referred for cardiac catheterization than white patients, and black women less than white men, white women, or black men (Schulman et al. 1999). This revelation sent shockwaves through the medical community, but anyone familiar with the data or the history of medical racism was not surprised (Byrd 2001). It is not that we are shaking off the remnants of racism from the Civil War, or the Civil Rights movement, or anything of the sort (McBride 2018). We are actively—although perhaps unconsciously—engaged in the same, continuous, pejorative, and centuries-long history that has so badly wronged black people in America.

Modern medical racism may be less intentional, but it still exists in both interpersonal and structural forms (Hoberman 2012; Gee and Ford 2011; Massey and Sampson 2009). While intentional interpersonal racism is evil, structural racism and unconscious biases lead to true medical error, which perhaps entails less blame. I will quickly survey some ways these racial divides occur and why doctors propagate them, even if unintentionally, through two fruitful examples. First, physicians refer black patients for cardiac catheterizations less often than their white counterparts (CDC 2017). Second, black women have incredibly high maternal mortality rates in comparison to white women (CDC 2017). These examples are not just paradigm instances of medical racism, but illuminative examples, as we will see.

In a well-publicized study, Schulman et al. showed unequivocally that clinical outcomes are affected by race (Schulman et al. 1999).[10] Physicians are significantly less likely to refer a patient for cardiac catheterizations if the patient is black, and even less likely to do so if the patient is a black woman. Although the study leaves open why the physicians did so, John Hoberman details how this sort of medical malpractice can come about. Medical "gossip," still thrives in the medical field simply by filtering patients and experiences with them through the doctor's personal beliefs (Hoberman 2012, 12–13).[11] Unfortunately, doctors' personal beliefs do not vary much from the public when it comes to racial attitudes. Just like the public, "whites have largely abandoned principled racism.[12] . . .[but] they have not necessarily given up negative racial stereotypes" or other negative attitudes about people of color (Hoberman 2012, 12–13; Massey and Sampson 2009).

This has been further corroborated by studies about pain treatment. It has been well-documented that black patients' pain is both underestimated and undertreated by the medical community, even in cases involving children (Smedley, Nelson, and Stith 2013; Anderson, Green, and

Payne 2009; Cintron and Morrison 2006; Freeman and Payne 2000). The causes of this might be a number of factors, but one of the best explanations is the actual content of medical professionals' beliefs about different races. Many of the researchers studying the phenomenon argue that doctors simply assume that black patients experience less pain than white patients. Consider a study by Staton et al.: patients were asked to report how much pain they were currently experiencing, and doctors were to report how much pain they thought the patients were experiencing. The mismatch was quite large: black patients' pain was significantly underestimated compared to non-black patients (47 percent to 33.5 percent; Staton et al. 2007).

This fits in with other findings adjacent to this point. Many people simply believe biological falsities about black bodies, and medical professionals are no exception. Many believe black people are biologically more athletic as a result of natural selection or even from breeding during slavery (Hoberman 1997; Morning 2011). In a study in 2016, white medical students and residents were found to hold biologically false beliefs about the black body. In this case, their beliefs centered on pain tolerance (Hoffman, Trawalter, Axt, and Oliver 2016).[13] The focus was not just to see if there were widespread false beliefs, but if they led to different treatment recommendations in which the symptoms of black patients were downplayed—which they did. Although these beliefs do not necessarily constitute racism, they can and do have impacts on how black people are treated and also correlate with acceptance of racial disparities and outcomes as unproblematic (Williams and Eberhardt 2008).[14]

Given the data cited here, it seems that we have a fairly straightforward explanation for why treatment and recommendations might differ between white and black patients: physicians falsely believe that black patients simply aren't experiencing what they profess to be experiencing.[15] If patients are experiencing severe chest pain, this is a reason to refer them for heart treatment. If the physician believes patients are only experiencing mild pain, then there is much less reason for the referral. Physicians systematically underestimate the pain of black patients; therefore, it should be no surprise that black patients often receive less treatment when pain is a significant symptom. Of course, there are other explanations along this line. Consider that, for a long time, doctors did not think that African-Americans could develop myocardial infarction (a certain kind of heart disease; Hoberman 2012, 12), or that they believed black people have fewer nerve endings (Hoffman, Trawalter, Axt, and Oliver 2016), or any number of other false biological beliefs that many medical professionals hold (Hoffman, Trawalter, Axt, and Oliver 2016; Hoberman 2012).[16] What is important is that a significant amount of undertreatment is almost certainly due to *biological* beliefs that, unbeknownst to the physicians and other medical personnel who hold them, are false.

W. E. B. DuBois was one of the first to study the white/black disparity in infant mortality rates sociologically, and from which racial injustice is easily inferred (DuBois 1899). At the time, the black infant mortality rate was 340/1000 babies whereas the white infant mortality rate was 217/1000 babies. Although both have decreased significantly, the disparity between black and white infant mortality rates has remained steadfast. Today, a black baby is more than twice as likely to die than a white baby—11.3/1000 compared to 4.9/1000, a statistic that has recently received media attention (Villarosa 2018; Roeder 2019). Intimately related is the maternal mortality rate, which has its own, even more staggering disparity. The white maternal mortality rate is currently 12.4 deaths per 100,000 white pregnant women compared to 40.0 deaths per 100,000 black pregnant women (CDC 2017). Easy alternative explanations such as class or education do not explain the data: black women still die at higher rates than white women even when they have similar educational backgrounds (Schoendorf, Hogue, Kleinman, and Rowley 1992).[17]

A controversial explanation that has garnered considerable interest has been "weathering," a term that describes the effects of toxic stress caused by structural and institutional racism on a black woman's body, which increases the likelihood of high blood pressure, pre-eclampsia, and so on (Geronimus 1987, 1992; Geronimus, Hicken, Keene, and Bound 2006; Kramer and Hogue 2009). Of course, any regular symptom increase is further complicated and exacerbated by pregnancy, which only worsens the consequences of weathering. There are at least two good reasons to think the weathering hypothesis is true. Consider privileged or normally stressed women (e.g., white women in America) who have maternal mortality risks that resemble inverse bell curves—higher risk during teen years, then lower risk during years of prime health before rising again with age. Because there is more time for toxic stress to affect her body, the weathering hypothesis predicts that women who have weathered stress from racism will have a steadily increasing maternal mortality risk (Geronimus 1987). This turns out to be true: it is actually *less risky*—with regard to the mother's life—to have a child as a teenager if one is a black woman than to have a child in one's 20s (Geronimus 1987). Second, allostatic load score analyses measure the amount of the toxic chemicals stress can leave behind in one's body (Geronimus, Hicken, Keene, and Bound 2006). As weathering predicts, we find much higher levels of these chemicals in older black bodies (Geronimus, Hicken, Keene, and Bound 2006).

Weathering links the disparate numbers to black experience—specifically, the medical community's continuing ignorance of it. Not only do medical personnel hold false biological beliefs about black people, they also ignore the reports of black people's symptoms and experiences, consequently poisoning the chances of equitable and fair treatment.

Black women are emblematic of this, as the evidence cited earlier shows (Geronimus 1987, 1992; Geronimus, Hicken, Keene, and Bound 2006; Kramer and Hogue 2009).[18]

Not only are black women more likely to experience the complications associated with weathering, but their experiences are discredited and their symptoms downplayed or ignored. Serena Williams's almost lethal experience after childbirth catalyzed some popular press of the well-documented disparities in the maternal mortality rate. After delivering her baby Olympia, Williams experienced several serious symptoms and told a nurse outside her room that she thought she was experiencing a blood clot, asking for blood thinner and tests. Her experience was at first dismissed—she must be confused from the pain killers. Williams continued to insist on testing, and they relented, allowing an ultrasound which showed nothing. Williams persisted and eventually secured a CT scan, which showed several blood clots (Roeder 2019; Villarosa 2018).

Medical education is no immunization to this dismissal. Shalon Irving was an epidemiologist at the CDC and worked specifically on racial and other health inequities. Despite her concern about her alarming postpartum symptoms, she was reassured that her symptoms were normal. Hours after her latest appointment, she collapsed and died (Roeder 2019; Villarosa 2018).

On top of the black maternal mortality rate, a tragedy all on its own, there are obvious downstream effects. The children must be raised without their mother, which means their family is missing additional income, community involvement, or the loving care of a mother (McLanahan and Sandefur 1994). These and other results might explain why being raised by a single parent is often correlated with worse health outcomes (Jennings and Sheldon 1985).

This is by no means all of the evidence for the medical community's ignorance of black women's lived experience. Take the fact that 26 percent of black women meet their birth attendants for the first time during childbirth compared to about 18 percent of white women. Black women are also less likely to have obstetrician-gynecologists as their birth attendants than white women (Declercq et al. 2013).[19] All of this is just a tiny snapshot of what could be said about the lived experience of being black in America, but these two examples center the discussion around concerns of undertreatment, dismissal, and distrust that motivate the argument to abandon certain policies opposed to overtesting.

Medical Overtesting and Racial Distrust

Black people in America have had little reason to trust white people in positions of power over them. They have been captured, held, and forced to work against their will by and for white people. Later, almost any person of authority would abuse it in one way or another or else totally misunderstand the condition and needs of black people. This has been no different in the medical field. With such a large disconnect in understanding between black patients and white doctors further complicated by historical and present medical abuse, it is easy to see why distrust between black patients and white doctors would grow. We have evidence of this distrust between "free" black patients and white doctors from as far back as the early 1900s, when white doctors' complaints about treating black patients center on, among other things, black patients not coming to the doctor until their illness had already progressed significantly or not following the doctors' orders (Douglas 1926, 736–737; Hoberman 2012, 23; Airhihenbuwa, Ford, and Iwelunmor 2013).

Today, medical professionals often feel that this distrust is unwarranted. "*I* nor anyone I know has done anything to earn your distrust," or "*I* didn't participate in the Tuskegee study," can often be sentiments expressed by doctors who are subjects of distrust to their patients.[20] Nevertheless, individuals usually inherit their values from their community. A history of medical abuse and neglect has shaped the community of black Americans to be wary of the medical profession (Gamble 1993). Although it is partially explainable this way, it is also misleading. Racism has become less conscious and more structural, but it is still ongoing (Gamble 1993, 1997; Hoberman 2012; Massey and Sampson 2009). So, for both historical considerations of abuse and present considerations of medical racism, it seems racial distrust has been well-earned by the medical community.[21]

I have no new policies that I will advocate here, but we can retain an existing practice that might prevent further medical neglect: overtesting. With this in mind, we can turn to principles of justice to see how these goods should be distributed.

A common proposal to combat overtesting is to discourage doctors from testing in cases in which the physician judges the test to be low in value or high in risk (for an example in medical imaging, see Hendee et al. 2010). The measures for this are not merely individual. The medical community must push to educate physicians on the tests that are the most wasteful, that are the lowest in value, and so on (Morgan et al. 2015; Morgan, Dhruva, Wright, and Korenstein 2016; Morgan et al. 2017; Morgan et al. 2018). Furthermore, there should be structural change. One path suggested is eliminating measures that enforce overtesting, such as reducing the need for defensive medicine or eliminating financial kickbacks from ordering tests (Berwick and Hackbarth 2012; Mello, Chandra, Gawande, and Studdert 2010). This solution would only decrease the already-reduced care given to black Americans given the racial biases of physicians in the United States. Even if overtesting is harmful for non-black Americans (or even for all patients), the reduction in appropriate testing that would result from implementing this policy is unacceptable. So, we should not bluntly discourage most overtesting of patients by physicians and therefore avoid increasing the high incidence of harmful medical error inflicted on certain racial minorities.[22]

There are myriad ways for overtesting to occur. Overtesting can be administering the same test more times than necessary, administering different tests but that have little or no reason to suspect will discover anything of importance, and so on. In the discussion that follows, I want to focus on two particular kinds of overtesting. The first is not a case of *actual* overtesting, but instead a case of *perceived* overtesting in which a doctor has formed a belief that further tests are not necessary or help-ful (perhaps because of harmful stereotypes) when they in fact would be helpful or are necessary. In this case, perhaps a physician has some mis-taken perception (due to bias or bad training) that causes them to evalu-ate the situation in such a way that they decrease the odds of a certain cause, taking it out of the range of needing to be tested for.[23] Because of this mistaken evaluation, the physician then decides to withhold the test in order to reduce overtesting.[24, 25] The second is *actual* overtesting, in which the helpfulness and necessity of the tests coincide with the doctor's belief that they would not be helpful or are not necessary. In this case, the physician evaluates the situation as not providing a medical basis for overtesting *and is correct*. If both cases turn out to be beneficial for oppressed minority groups, then we have reason to apply principles of distributive and restorative justice. Consider the following case:

> **Actual Overtesting:** A black male is anxious about a few of his symp-toms. The physician informs the patient that there is no reason to test the patient for any further underlying causes, but the physician administers the tests anyway after the patient persists. The patient is relieved at the test results and returns home. The doctor has shown a willingness to listen to the patient even when there is no reason to think the tests will be helpful or necessary.[26]

There are two benefits of actual overtesting: (1) the patient's personal medical anxieties are relieved; and (2) there is some restoration of trust between the patient and the doctor. (1) is not usually considered to be sufficiently weighty to favor overtesting, since similar anxieties are pre-sent in white patients to the same or nearly the same degree, but few feel this justifies the practice of overtesting. Additionally, some test results will not return to the patient for significant periods of time, during which heightened medical anxiety or other negative mental states can be pre-sent. Thus, (1) is not sufficient for justifying overtesting on an individual basis.

Restoration of trust has not been seriously considered by the medical community, perhaps because most do not believe it is in need of restora-tion or have dismissed it prematurely. There are a few reasons to think it would restore trust. One important reason is that it relieves anxiety not present or not present to the same degree for other patients: fear of with-held care. Because of the long history of withholding care to black Ameri-cans, the appearance of doing so is particularly harmful (Jones 1993; Gamble 1993, 1997; Krakauer and Truog 1997). A second reason is the trust shown by the physician first by listening and believing the patient. An additional consideration is that the transparency of the interaction helps in more than one way, both from a trust-building perspective and to better acquire informed-consent when the test is administered. Trust restoration is not present in the "usual" consideration of this problem because it is *not* present in cases involving overtesting and white patients. Despite this being a case of actual overtesting, it seems *prima facie* good for black communities. Perhaps this can be outweighed by other consid-erations (such as driving up costs), but this and other objections will be addressed later. Consider a different case:

> **Perceived Overtesting:** A black female is anxious about a few of her symptoms. The physician has formed the belief that her symptoms are not the result of anything serious but, aware that she might be misperceiving the situation due to bias, agrees to extra tests regard-less. The tests reveal that the patient has an underlying condition causing the symptoms. The doctor orders the proper treatment, and the condition is resolved without complication.

Like the previous case, the doctor has shown humility and awareness of racial bias in medical practice through her willingness to be open to something she missed regardless of the outcome of the tests. Further-more, if something is found on the tests, the patient is greatly helped by the medical community rather than greatly harmed (as would happen if no test had been run).[27] Therefore, cases of perceived overtesting that nevertheless get "over-tested" can be extremely beneficial to people and communities of color. Furthermore, we have good reason to think there are a great number of perceived overtesting events given the arc of medi-cal history in the United States. Consider again the cases of Serena Wil-liams and Shalon Irving. In perceived overtesting, the result is a welcome one, but consider the resistance Williams and Irving received in response to their concerns, and the lethal result if they are ultimately denied fur-ther testing and care. There is also harder evidence, such as how black women were less likely than white women to receive testing for high blood sugar in a postpartum visit among women with chronic or gesta-tional diabetes (Declercq et al. 2013).[28]

Perhaps more importantly is the harm prevented, however. Physi-cians who are encouraged to cut back on medical overtesting will be looking for occasions to cut back on what they perceive as unnecessary testing. Because both actual and perceived overtesting are phenomeno-logically indistinguishable to the physician at the time of deliberation, the physician will view both as candidate situations for withholding testing. Withholding testing in a case of perceived overtesting can be a great harm, medically and within the context of racial distrust regarding withholding care. Thus, the worry here is not merely losing the extra good that may come from overtesting, but also causing great harm by encouraging physicians to cut back on tests they perceive to be unnecessary or unlikely to help despite their necessity. In fact, Williams's experience is paradigmatic of the harm described in this chapter. There is a push to reduce the use of the CT scan due to its financial cost and its high radiation level (Hendee et al. 2010). Medical personnel thereby become more reluctant to use the test.[29] Couple this with unconscious racial biases such as over-reporting pain and dismissal of black experience and one can easily see how black women can end up untested and untreated in life-threatening circumstances.

There are also cases of testing that do not appear harmful if overlooked. Does this change the calculus of harm? Yes. But in every case, some harm occurs—if a test is justified based on the presentation of the symptoms, then it is overall *better* for the test to be performed than not. Even in cases of the least amount of *physical* harm, there appears to be a certain amount of dignitary harm that comes from not respecting the patient by under-testing them. But many tests *are* intended to help diagnose serious health problems, and so the risk of great harm is present in many cases. If the characterization or policy discouraging overtesting is not sufficiently nuanced, then cases of perceived overtesting will go without the necessary testing, causing serious harm.[30] In fact, cases of actual overtesting can be unequivocally bad, and yet pursuing policies that seek to reduce overtesting can still be outweighed by the risks of cutting back on necessary tests in cases of perceived overtesting.

We have just analyzed the two possibilities in a case of overtesting: actual overtesting and perceived overtesting. In one case, merely the act of testing to alleviate race-based anxiety helps to alleviate the overall phenomenon of racial distrust of the medical community, even if it is at some cost to the doctor or the health-care system at large. In the other case, overtesting actually prevents harm from occurring to the patient, benefitting everyone involved *and* restoring trust between medical and black communities.[31] Notably, it does not matter whether the overtesting is actual or perceived; racial trust is restored. Also noteworthy is the possibility of serious harm if racist medical mythology leads to higher incidence of perceived overtesting and the requisite tests are not administered. There are goods at stake in both cases, then, for people and communities of color. Overtesting that discovers disease, as well as restores trust, is a very great good and plausibly quite commonplace.[32, 33] As mentioned before, however, even if actual overtesting is certainly bad, the harms of perceived overtesting can still be great enough to outweigh the benefits of policies aimed at reducing overtesting.

Cost-Benefit Analysis of Overtesting

Having argued that there are benefits to overtesting, I turn now to whether these benefits outweigh the costs of permitting medical overtesting to continue. First, consider the beneficial effects. We have seen that a confluence of factors including dismissal of black experience, false biological beliefs, and the push to reduce overtesting can result in what I have called perceived overtesting, in which a physician, due to evaluative mistakes or unconscious biases, believes testing would not be of sufficient help when in fact it would be medically appropriate to test. Failing to utilize tests in cases of perceived overtesting can result in great harm to the patient, and this harm becomes racialized if the patients are disproportionately black. Racialized harm is an especially bad kind of harm, one that should be avoided even at the cost of some net gains.[34] Furthermore, current policies advocating for the reduction of overtesting will only discourage administration of tests in cases of perceived overtesting. Knowing this, utilizing tests in cases of perceived overtesting is a great good. We have also seen that, even in cases of actual-overtesting, there is good to be gained. Not only does the patient herself feel relieved, but this contributes to the much greater good of building trust between the medical community and communities of color.

Next, let's consider the costs. The first two are individual costs to overtesting. Considering people of color are often less well-off or impoverished (mostly due to previous racist treatment both interpersonally and structurally), it seems that medical bills could be far too expensive for most poor people of color. This would be a strong reason to *not* order tests that would appear to be unnecessary, since the bill could ruin their life just as well as the disease. Second, it is well-known that radiation has several negative effects: it is a carcinogen, can cause tissue hardening, scarring, discoloration, and so on. Receiving too many radiation-based tests could harm a patient (FDA 2017; Thomasian 2014). The computed tomography (CT) scan is a flagrant offender on this front. Because CT scans are quick and data-rich, they have become commonplace in emergency rooms, but its radiation dosage is the equivalent of 200 chest x-rays (FDA 2017; Thomasian 2014). There is also an increase in costs of healthcare overall when there is a climate of overtesting. Because insurance companies foot most of the bills, they will pass that bill onto their clients, increasing premiums (or taxes, if healthcare is socialized). Finally, we must consider the cost to those who would *not* suffer race-specific harms if overtesting were bluntly discouraged but *would* still bear the burdens of overtesting. In order to weigh these considerations properly, let's consider each in turn.

When patients enter the emergency room, they can refuse almost any test or care. Patients are informed of the risks and costs of each test; otherwise, the physician would not have obtained informed consent.

Therefore, we can hold the variable of the patient understanding the *cost* of overtesting constant.[35] Hence, there are two possibilities that describe patients in cases of individual harm caused by overtesting. The first is a misestimate of the benefits of the test. In these cases, the patient just does not understand the chances of a successful test.[36] Alternatively, the patient may accurately estimate the chances of a successful test and nevertheless thinks it is worth it, despite differing medical opinion (e.g., from opponents of unnecessary testing). The second case is easy to deal with: patients are not impermissibly harmed by overtesting because they would, given their values, prefer the test. In other words, there is not any harm present we would not countenance in any other medical situation, especially given the commitment to the value of autonomy in medical environments. Pursuing aggressive, almost-certainly-futile life-saving therapy is a harm to the patient, but it is a harm we allow the patient to pursue. Overtesting is almost certainly less of a harm than aggressive-yet-futile therapy or dying after months unconscious on a ventilator at an advanced age.

The first case might seem harder to parse at first, but notice that, while overtesting might harm them in some way, the true solution is better communication about the benefits of the test. If they are misestimating just how unlikely it is, then the onus is on the physician (or medical personnel explaining the test's benefits) to communicate more clearly, lest we receive mere uninformed consent.[37] This sort of analysis resolves concerns about both the cost of testing on one's health (radiation risks to one's health versus health benefits of the test results) and one's financial health (monetary cost versus health benefits of the test results).[38] Still, there is a concern about how this communication should be fixed. If the physician has unconscious biases, how does the explanation of their mental state help the patient? Will it not have the same bias and therefore fail to communicate the risks and benefits?

While this is a serious concern, it is not unique to overtesting. Once again, this threatens informed consent in our medical systems in totality. Still, there is hope that simple measures aimed at improving informed consent might help—the physician might have to rethink their assessment of the patient's pain, or confront the fact that their evaluation of the patient is at odds with the patients' testimony, or the odd explanation may indicate to the patient that there is something fishy going on.[39, 40]

Beyond the interpersonal case, there are issues that do not concern the individual patient weighing the costs and benefits. The third part of the concern about overtesting involved the financial situation broadly construed. Although the earlier analysis should deal with both issues, it is worth pointing out that there are alternatives to depriving patients of medical care when they cannot afford it. Programs such as Public Aid, Medicare, Medicaid, and so on help the poor afford medical costs. Should these prove insufficient, it does not seem as if the climate of overtesting is the obvious change to make. One alternative is to make the case for different health-care systems. Drawing on this analysis, one can argue that the poor should not suffer consequences of perceived overtesting simply because they are poor, especially when their poverty might be due to racist institutions or history.[41] The analysis provided here strongly supports crucial premises in traditional arguments for universal access to healthcare.[42, 43]

The final two considerations run parallel. There are those—such as wealthy, white men—who would *not* be harmed by a blunt solution to overtesting but *would* be harmed by the continuance of overtesting. These burdens might include personal financial problems, personal health risks, and overall cost to the system. There are two ways to frame and answer the objection. The first way the objection might be presented would be an individual sense. The answer to this form resides in the arguments provided here involving informed consent.

The second has to do with the balance of harms and benefits as spread across all affected, making it essentially a problem of distributive justice. White, wealthy men are currently harmed by medical overtesting, but black women would be harmed if certain solutions to overtesting are implemented. In order to avoid rehashing debates over the nature of distributive justice, consider how one influential conception balances the harms. Following Rawls, "Social and economic inequalities are to be arranged so that they are both: (a) to the greatest benefit of the least advantaged, consistent with the just savings principle, and (b) attached to offices and positions open to all under conditions of fair equality of opportunity" (1988, 266). Notice that the overall benefits here do not favor the least advantaged. The least advantaged here (racial minorities) would instead be *harmed* by blunt solutions to overtesting. Thus, it would be impermissible under Rawlsian distributive justice principles to implement solutions to overtesting that have this deleterious effect.[44, 45]

Another popular conception of distributive justice is utilitarian. Here, the question faced is just the cost to the system at large if overtesting is maintained. Although the current health-care system is extremely expensive, it is not clear that overtesting is even close to being one of the most significant factors. In a commissioned report, the University of Virginia Miller Center found nine of the most significant drivers of health-care costs in the United States. Although overuse of CT scans was mentioned (about double the average of other developed countries), it is only mentioned briefly as part of a much larger phenomenon of Americans assuming expensive treatments are the same as higher-quality treatments (Thomasian 2014). Berwick and Hackbarth identify six ways to reduce the huge financial cost of medical overuse. Medical testing is mentioned just once: as an example of pricing failures (2012).[46] But, even if overtesting turned out to be a significant driver of health-care costs, there are many other costs that could be reformed before overtesting that would not correspondingly cause further harm to communities of color.[47]

There might be a final concern of achievability. Perhaps the other drivers of health-care costs are simply unachievable relative to lesser costs like overtesting.[48] But this does not bear out in the reports of the authors writing about the drivers of health-care costs. First, the primary drivers of health-care costs are *so* expensive that "achieving even a fraction of that amount in the short run" could result in serious savings, stability, and prevent harm to patients (Berwick and Hackbarth 2012, 1515). There are also state-based alternatives laid out in other reports of a similar kind, with specific steps and recommendations for cutting these drivers of costs (Thomasian 2014). As noted before, these need only be mildly successful to compare very favorably with reform efforts in overtesting. If we are going to focus our solutions due to limited resources, it makes sense to cut out issues that are uncontroversially bad before turning to other, more controversial issues.

Some Helpful Advances

The case against unnecessarily testing patients for conditions is intuitive and widely accepted. It is also wrong. Once we keep the history of medical racism in mind, we see that our climate of overtesting is surprisingly beneficial to communities of color in two ways: (1) it prevents commonplace cases of perceived overtesting from greatly harming the patient, and (2) even in cases where testing is actually unwarranted, it restores trust between the medical community and black people in America as well as avoiding harm caused by perceptions of withholding treatment. Objections to overtesting usually overlook important explanatory features of the medical industry. The nature of overtesting harms and benefits are misconstrued or undertheorized. Similarly, the compromised epistemic position of physicians when determining whether a certain test is necessary is often missed, both in a contemporary and historical context. Finally, there are several other uncontroversially bad problems that could be solved before addressing problems such as overtesting, which has noteworthy benefits for communities of color. Therefore, the distributions of benefits and harms give us a powerful reason to retain our current climate of overtesting.

My argument does not preclude solutions to overtesting; it merely demands that they be nuanced such that the race-specific harms associated with blunt discouragement are not present. There is extensive literature on the risks and benefits of tailoring policies with race as a variable (King 1992; Osborne and Feit 1992; Comstock, Castillo, and Lindsay 2004; Kaplan and Bennett 2003; King 2007; Bonilla-Silva 2017). It distinguishes between "race-neutral" or "colorblind" policies that do not use race as a variable and "race-conscious" policies, which do. Patricia King argues that race-conscious policies risk reifying racial stereotypes but are often the only policies that can properly address racial inequalities

(King 1992, 2007). She proposes some criteria for acceptable race-conscious policies: they should be short-term in nature and no broader in scope than their use demands (King 2007). Moving forward, likely some mix of race-conscious and race-neutral solutions should be carefully considered. Some piecemeal race-neutral solutions that appear to sufficiently address my concerns are already popping up, such as specialty-specific waste analyses documenting the most-used and least-useful tests.[49]

More race-conscious reforms might look like feedback-focused attempts to close racial gaps in testing and diagnosis. Solutions as simple as recording the race, ethnicity, and gender of each patient of a provider, running analyses to see if there are gaps along those lines, and then providing the medical professional with their results appear to work well in the studies led by Hannan (Hannan et al. 2010, 2014, 2018). This sort of feedback could be mandated, and even financial penalties assessed if disparities continue. This would parallel the significant success of a similar policy of mandated measurement of hospital and physician quality of care by the Centers for Medicare and Medicaid Services (U.S. Department of Health and Human Services 2018).[50] Another promising alternative are the community-based participatory research models that have shown some success at reducing racial and ethnic health disparities (Stone, Wallerstein, Garcia, and Winkler 2014). These and other nuanced solutions would work toward ending overtesting without the race-specific harms other common solutions to overtesting threaten.

Overtesting has been thought of as uncontroversially bad, but I have argued that the downsides of the current sentiment to reduce overtesting have unacceptable consequences due to the phenomenon of perceived overtesting. Furthermore, it may have significant and surprising benefits, such as restoring trust between the medical community and racial minorities. Therefore, even assuming overtesting is a significant driver of health-care costs, we should focus our attention elsewhere before advocating for the elimination of overtesting from the health-care system. This is especially true if we have no sufficiently nuanced alternative proposal to restore trust between communities of color and communities of medicine and prevent the medical error that regularly occurs due to racial biases in the medical field. Still, there are solutions that avoid the worries presented here, usually by adapting race-neutral proposals into race-conscious proposals, or by building policies by beginning with the fact of racial disparities. Regardless, the discussion around overtesting must change.

Notes

1. Golemon, Luke. "Medical Over-testing and Racial Distrust." *Kennedy Institute of Ethics Journal* 29: 3 (2019), 273–303. © 2019 Johns Hopkins University Press. Adapted and reprinted with permission of Johns Hopkins University Press.

2. For more on medical error, see Allhoff (2019); Makary and Daniel (2016); and Kohn, Corrigan, and Donaldson (2000). Medical racism, both conscious and unconscious, causes much harm to minority communities. Recently, medical error due to racial bias has been emphasized (Schulman et al. 1999; Hoberman 2012; Staton et al. 2007).
3. See also Carter et al. (2015).
4. It can also be made consistent by reading both concepts as objective, but this leaves us without much epistemic access to cases of overuse and medical bases. For instance, if it is in fact the case that calcium and vitamin D supplements are not working as well as expected, then all such treatments count as overuse, despite the medical community's ignorance. This is not intuitive. Instead, we seem to be pursuing the idea that there is some gap between knowledge and practice that should be closed. This gap can present at a personal and community level: a physician might know calcium supplements do not work well and yet still prescribe them or there might be findings of this nature and yet the community has not taken steps to ensure all its members follow best known practices. There are further issues, like how we would begin to know the extent of overuse, since it depends on having perfect knowledge.
5. More will be said on this topic in the titular section of the chapter. I thank an anonymous reviewer and the editors of the KIEJ for pushing me to clarify this.
6. This is incredibly hard to find recent data on. Computed tomography scan usage certainly rose into 2007, but the rates are unclear afterwards (Larson et al. 2011). Recent studies are piecemeal and often department specific, but it appears that usage has leveled off or decreased recently (Niles et al. 2017). Regardless, the goals of anti-overtesting policies are to affect individual practice in some way, so presumably this can be assumed.
7. In what follows, I will focus largely on black Americans. It is important to acknowledge that minority experience can vary widely based on appearance, culture, and ethnicity, and so some of what is true about medical racism for black Americans will not be true for other minority groups. I do not have the space to defend each generalization from black American experience to other minority groups, so the reader is justified in rejecting any such generalizations. I am confident that if the argument is successful for black Americans, then generalizing to other minorities will only be a reason *a fortiori*.
8. For more on how health inequities are an extension of racial power dynamics to this day, see Airhihenbowan and Liburd (2006).
9. See Byrd and Clayton (2001), Byrd and Clayton (2000), Montagu (1963), Lewis (1990), and Drake (1990).
10. They also showed it is affected by gender, but I will focus on race here. One point to be made, however, is that the effect of intersectionality is clearly evident. Being both black *and* female is worse than being only black or only female in terms of clinical treatment and outcome.
11. These biases also can be passed down via the elder attending physicians and precepting. Certain forms of training, infrastructure changes, feedback, and education might correct for this.
12. Principled racism is the explicit belief that one race is better than another. Contrast this with harboring negative racial stereotypes, which can coexist with genuine affirmations of racial equality.
13. This might have relevant disanalogies. One is about susceptibility, the other about exceptionalism. Furthermore, claims about black athletes are demonstrable, whereas claims about pain require trust in the reporter. The analogy

here is not necessarily affected by these differences—instead, I wish to draw attention to the willingness to believe falsities about black bodies in general, even in the face of evidence (reported or demonstrable).

14. Some have indicated that this might be due to race being treated as entirely biological in the medical literature, or nearly so. See Doll, Snyder, and Ford (2018).

15. These are not the only factors that affect health outcome inequities. Social disadvantage, class stratification, high health-care needs without corresponding availability of care, systemic racism in other sectors (e.g., environmental racism of dumping pollutants and trash), and so on all have major impacts on health inequities. For more discussion on these and other possible drivers of health inequities, see King (2007). For more on racial segregation as a fundamental source of racial disparities in health, see Williams and Collins (2001). For more on how power plays a role in most of these inequities, see Airhihenbuwa and Liburd (2006).

16. Some of these other beliefs include thicker skin and blood that coagulates more quickly, for instance. The point is less that any one of these explanations explains the phenomena, but that whatever explanation succeeds, it will be one that includes false biological beliefs. Alternatives to these false biological belief systems are largely unsupported (e.g., that medical personnel are consistently interpersonally racist about these matters and prescribing too few pain medications to black patients out of malice).

    This also fits in with findings that indicate that overuse and underuse can be idiosyncratic to certain diagnoses (Reid, Rabideau, and Sood 2016). Here, it seems that heart disease and heart attacks in black people is precisely the kind of convergence of symptoms, biases, and practices that add up to systemic overuse or underuse.

17. A similar effect demonstrating racial bias over class-based issues was found in Williams (2015).

18. This extends to other spheres—for example, weathering and its effects might reduce political activism due to health reasons just when the population is likely to become increasingly interested in civic engagement, reducing the ability of weathered populations to gain political clout (Kilgore 2018; Bound, Geronimus, Rodriguez, and Waidmann 2015).

19. This denial or ignorance of experience is not limited to merely black women. Latina women, for example, were the least likely among women with chronic or gestational diabetes to be tested for high blood sugar in a post-partum visit (Declercq et al. 2013). They were also the most likely to be concerned that a medical error would occur around the time of birth and reported that they received poor treatment while hospitalized for birth at almost twice the rate of white women (although 2 percent lower than black women; Declercq et al. 2013).

20. This sort of objection is undermined by certain accounts of systems, institutions, organizations, and communities. When one joins the Ku Klux Klan in a sufficiently serious way, one becomes culpable (in a certain way) as a member of that group for that group's past wrongdoing. This goes both ways. Joining a charity group in a sufficiently serious way earns you praise (in a certain way) as a member of that group due to that group's praiseworthy actions.

21. Questions of redress are beyond the scope of this chapter. For discussion, see Boxill (2015), Robinson (2000), Horowitz (2003), Coates (2014), and de Greiff (2006a, 2006b).

22. At least black people in America, but possibly others. See note 8.

23. It is important to note that almost all diagnostic evaluations are cases of inference to the best explanation and are therefore probabilistic rather than all-or-nothing (see Johnson forthcoming). So while it might be the case that a physician's biases lead them so far astray that there would be a complete lack of a medical basis for care, it is more likely that most situations involve cases in which the physician is forced to make a decision on narrower probabilities.
24. There are other cases that can be constructed for using the same test fewer times than the actual situation requires due to decreased prior probability from the mistaken evaluation, and so on.
25. I thank an anonymous reviewer for making me think more carefully about how to conceptualize overtesting, both perceived and actual.
26. The point made here is very similar to the case study as presented in Krakauer and Truog (1997), although the issue is anxiety over harmless symptoms in actual overtesting and futile end-of-life care in their case.
27. This general example is meant to parallel the discussion of the black maternal mortality rate and the dismissal of black experiences in the medical field discussed previously.
28. Latina women were the least likely of all groups to receive such testing.
29. See note 7.
30. I discuss some of the advances I believe do not trigger these concerns in the final section.
31. Cf. Krakauer and Truog (1997).
32. There are interesting issues here regarding the moral luck of such circumstances. For more on this topic, see Allhoff (2019).
33. It might be objected that overtesting cannot mitigate undertreatment or undertesting because undertreatment and undertesting exist at the same time as the current climate of overtesting. But this does not consider that the climate of overtesting may well be mitigating some undertreatment and undertesting *right now*, and thus the removal of it would expand the reach of undertreatment and undertesting. Certainly allowing overtesting to continue will not solve all health inequities, but that is not my position. My position is that it may mitigate some of the harms of undertesting and the consequent undertreatment.
34. Not all or any net gains, merely some. It might be that there is some arrangement of testing such that harms go down slightly overall but the distribution of harms is racialized (e.g., perhaps black people in America experience fewer warranted tests than before). This strikes one as *prima facie* impermissible.
35. Medical costs are, unfortunately, very opaque in the United States' healthcare system. This presents a problem of its own, but whose solution is (in theory) straightforward: the cost of healthcare in the U.S. should be revised to be much clearer; else we are missing out on true informed consent.
36. A successful test is (roughly) a test in which there is a medical basis for the test, the test accurately detects whether the condition tested for is present, and the condition, if detected, can be well-treated.
37. This would entail our medical industry is a sham; doctors are acting paternalistically while deceiving patients (and the public) into thinking we have a say in our treatment. I take this route to be a dead-end.
38. This has a further problem: it seems that racial bias would also work against problems of informed consent. This might be alleviated by nuanced solutions such as feedback-focused reforms that I mention at the end of the chapter. For examples, see Hannan et al. (2010, 2014, 2018).
39. There are also proposals and research done on how to improve communication through cultural competency among other things, which will in turn increase the likelihood of securing informed consent. For more discussion and analysis, see Betsch et al. (2016).

40. Thanks to an anonymous reviewer and Sandra Borden for pushing me on this point.
41. Systems such as single-payer still care about efficiency; still, it would solve the *individual* financial case, which is what I focus on here. Costs to the system at large will be addressed shortly.
42. This is particularly true for Rawlsian arguments for universal health-care access (Rawls 1988). For example, consider premise three in Daniels (2017):

> Various socially controllable factors contribute to maintaining normal functioning in a population and distributing health fairly in it, including traditional public health and medical interventions, as well as the distribution of such social determinants of health as income and wealth, education, and control over life and work.

The social determinants of health mentioned would include racial aspects such as past injustices and physicians holding false beliefs due to cultural stereotyping and institutional racism (Hoberman 2012). Thus, the analysis given here would strongly support a crucial premise in Daniels's argument.

Deborah Stone takes this in a slightly different direction, arguing that something like market ideology guarantees racial inequality. For more, see Stone (2005).

43. Here I assume something like Rawls's Difference Principle (Rawls 1988). Political theory and philosophy are beyond the scope of this chapter, and those disagreeing with the Difference Principle or something like it may simply disagree with me here.
44. This leaves open the possibility of a system that only overtests minority groups as a solution. I take this to be an ineffective solution for two reasons: (1) it seems impossible to implement the solution without having to address the very problems causing the problem in the first place and (2) the shift to race-conscious solutions is more likely to fall in favor of the solutions studied by Hannan et al. (2010, 2018) mentioned at the end of the chapter with much less resistance and greater effect.
45. *A forteriori*, if one is convinced of some sort of reparations framework, it is entirely possible that the utilitarian calculus weighs against overtesting and yet we *still* ought to keep it due to the origin of the problem (racism) and the parties being harmed and benefitting from the system.
46. American imaging is priced to be several times more than identical procedures in other countries (International Federation of Health Plans 2010).
47. For examples, see Berwick and Hackbarth (2012).
48. Thanks to T.J. Broy for this objection.
49. Some of the waste noted in the updates by Daniel Morgan and company might also qualify.
50. Thanks to an anonymous reviewer who pointed me to this sort of solution.

Works Cited

Abaluck, Jason, Leila Agha, Chris Kabrhel, Ali Raja, and Arjun Venkatesh. 2016. "The Determinants of Productivity in Medical Testing: Intensity and Allocation of Care." *The American Economics Review* 106 (12): 3730–3764.

Airhihenbuwa, Collins, Chandra Ford, and Juliet Iwelnmor. 2013. "Why Culture Matters in Health Interventions: Lessons From HIV/AIDS Stigma and NCDs." *Health Education and Behavior* 41 (1): 78–84.

Airhihenbuwa, Collins, and Leandris Liburd. 2006. "Eliminating Health Dispari-
ties in the African American Population: The Interface of Culture, Gender, and
Power." *Health Education and Behavior* 33 (4): 488–501.
Allhoff, Fritz. 2019. "Medical Error and Moral Luck." *Kennedy Institute of Eth-
ics Journal*. Forthcoming.
Alspector-Kelly, Marc. 2019. *Against Knowledge Closure*. Cambridge University
Press.
Anderson, Karen, Carmen Green, and Richard Payne. 2009. "Racial and Ethnic
Disparities in Pain: Causes and Consequences of Unequal Care." *Journal of
Pain* 10 (12): 1187–1204.
Aristotle. 1999. *Nicomachean Ethics*. Trans. W. D. Ross. Batoche Books.
Berwick, Donald, and Andrew Hackbarth. 2012. "Eliminating Waste in US
Health Care." *Journal of the American Medical Association* 307: 1513–1516.
Betsch, Cornelia, Robert Böhm, Collins O. Airhihenbuwa, Robb Butler, Gretchen
B. Chapman, Niels Haase, Benedikt Herrmann, Tasuku Igarashi, Shinobu
Kitayama, Lars Korn, Ülla-Karin Nurm, Bernd Rohrmann, Alexander J. Roth-
man, Sharon Shavitt, John A. Updegraff, and Ayse K. Uskul. 2016. "Improving
Medical Decision Making and Health Promotion Through Culture-Sensitive
Health Communication: An Agenda for Science and Practice." *Medical Deci-
sion Making* 36 (7): 795–797.
Bishop, Tara, Alex Federman, and Salomeh Keyhani. 2010. "Physicians' Views
on Defensive Medicine: A National Survey." *Archives of Internal Medicine*
170: 1081–1083.
Boland, Benoit, Peter Wollan, and Marc Silverstein. 1996. "Yield of Laboratory
Tests for Case-Finding in the Ambulatory General Medical Examination."
American Journal of Medicine 101: 142–152.
Bonilla-Silva, Eduardo. 2017. *Racism Without Racists: Colorblind Racism and
the Persistence of Racial Inequality in the United States*, 5th ed. Rowman &
Littlefield Publishers.
Bound, John, Arline Geronimus, Javier Rodriguez, and Timothy Waidmann.
2015. "Measuring Recent Apparent Declines in Longevity: The Role of Increas-
ing Educational Attainment." *Health Affairs* 34 (12): 2167–2173.
Boxill, Bernard. 2016. "Black Reparations." *The Stanford Encyclopedia of
Philosophy* (Summer 2016 edition), edited by Edward N. Zalta. https://plato.
stanford.edu/archives/sum2016/entries/black-reparations/
Byrd, Michael, and Linda Clayton. 2000. *An American Health Dilemma: A Med-
ical History of African Americans and the Problem of Race*. Routledge.
Byrd, Michael, and Linda Clayton. 2001. "Race, Medicine, and Health-care in
the United States: A Historical Survey." *Journal of the National Medical Asso-
ciation* 93 (3): 11–34.
Carter, Stacy, Wendy Rogers, I Heath, Chris Degeling, Jenny Doust, and Amy
Barratt. 2015. "The Challenge of Overdiagnosis Begins with Its Definition."
BMJ 350: 1–5.
Centers for Disease Control. 2017. "Reproductive Health." *Centers for Disease
Control and Prevention*. https://www.cdc.gov/reproductivehealth/index.html
Cintron, Alexie, and Sean Morrison. 2006. "Pain and Ethnicity in the United
States: A Systematic Review." *Journal Palliative Medicine* 9 (6): 1454–1473.

Coates, Ta-Nehisi. June 2014. "The Case for Reparations." *The Atlantic*. Retrieved from www.theatlantic.com/magazine/archive/2014/06/the-case-for-reparations/361631/.

Comstock, Dawn, Edward Castillo, and Suzanne Lindsay. 2004. "Four-Year Review of the Use of Race and Ethnicity in Epidemiologic and Public Health Research." *American Journal of Epidemiology* 159: 611–619.

de Greiff, Pablo. 2006a. *The Handbook of Reparations*. Oxford: Oxford University Press.

de Greiff, Pablo. 2006b. "Justice and Reparations." In P. de Greiff (ed.), *The Handbook of Reparations*. (Oxford: Oxford University Press): 451–477.

Declercq, Eugene, Carol Sakala, Maureen Corry, Sandra Applebaum, and Peter Risher. 2013. *Listening to Mothers III: New Mothers Speak Out*. Childbirth Connection.

Dettling, Lisa, Joanne Hsu, Lindsay Jacobs, Kevin Moore, and Jeffrey Thompson. 2017. "Recent Trends in Wealth-Holding by Race and Ethnicity: Evidence from the Survey of Consumer Finances." *Board of Governors of the Federal Reserve System*.

Doll, Kemi, Cyndy Snyder, and Chandra Ford. 2018. "Endometrial Cancer Disparities: A Race-Conscious Critique of the Literature." *American Journal of Obstetrics & Gynecology* 218 (5): 474–482.

Douglas, S. 1926. "Difficulties and Superstitions Encountered in Practice Among the Negroes." *Southern Medical Journal*.

Drake, St. Clair. 1987. *Black Folk Here and There: An Essay in History and Anthropology*, vol. 1. Center for Afro-American Studies, University of California.

Drake, St. Clair. 1990. *Black Folk Here and There: An Essay in History and Anthropology*, vol. 2. Center for Afro-American Studies, University of California.

DuBois, William. 1899. *The Philadelphia Negro*. University of Pennsylvania Press.

FDA. 2017. "What Are the Radiation Risks from CT?" *U.S. Department of Health and Human Services*.

Feinberg, Joel. 1978. "Voluntary Euthanasia and the Inalienable Right to Life." *Philosophy and Public Affairs* 7 (2): 93–123.

Freeman, Harold, and Richard Payne. 2000. "Racial Injustice in Health-care." *New England Journal of Medicine* 342 (14): 1045–1047.

Gamble, Vanessa. 1993. "A Legacy of Distrust: African Americans and Medical Research." *American Journal of Preventative Medicine* 9: 35–38.

Gamble, Vanessa. 1997. "Under the Shadow of Tuskegee: African Americans and Health Care." *American Journal of Public Health* 87: 1773–1778.

Gamble, Vanessa, and Deborah Stone. 2006. "U.S. Policy on Health Inequities: The Interplay of Politics and Research." *Journal of Health Politics, Policy, and Law* 31 (1): 93–126.

Gee, Gilbert, and Chandra Ford. 2011. "Structural Racism and Health Inequities: Old Issues, New Directions." *Du Bois Review Social Science Research on Race* 8 (1): 115–132.

Geronimus, Arline. 1987. "On Teenage Childbearing and Neonatal Mortality in the United States." *Population and Development Review* 13 (2): 245.

Geronimus, Arline. 1992. "The Weathering Hypothesis and the Health of African-American Women and Infants: Evidence and Speculations." *Ethnicity and Disease* 2 (3): 207–221.

Geronimus, Arline, Margaret Hicken, Danya Keene, and John Bound. 2006. "'Weathering' and Age Patterns of Allostatic Load Scores Among Blacks and Whites in the United States." *American Journal of Public Health* 96 (5): 826–833.

Greenberg, Jerome, and Jonas Green. 2014. "Overtesting: Why More Is Not Better." *The American Journal of Medicine* 127 (5): 362–363.

Hannan, Edward, Michael Racz, Jeffrey Gold, Kimberly Cozzens, Nicholas Stamato, Tia Powell, Mary Hibberd, and Gary Walford. 2010. "Adherence of Catheterization Laboratory Cardiologists to American College of Cardiology/American Heart Association Guidelines for Percutaneous Coronary Interventions and Coronary Artery Bypass Graft Surgery: What Happens in Actual Practice?" *Circulation* 121: 267–275.

Hannan, Edward, Zaza Samadashvili, Kimberly Cozzens, Peter Berger, Joanna Chikwe, Alice Jacobs, Gary Walford, Frederick Ling, Ferdinand Venditti, Jeffrey Gold, and Spencer King III. 2018. "Appropriate Use Criteria for Percutaneous Cornoary Interventions: Impact on Appropriateness Ratings." *Journal of American College of Cardiology: Cardiovascular Interventions* 11: 473–478.

Hannan, Edward, Zaza Samadashvili, Kimberly Cozzens, Gary Walford, Alice Jacobs, David Holmes Jr., Nicholas Stamato, Ferdinand Venditti, Jeffrey Gold, Samin Sharma, and Spencer King III. 2014. "Assessment of the New Appropriate Use Criteria for Diagnostic Catheterization in the Detection of Cornoary Artery Disease Following Noninvasive Stress Testing." *International Journal of Cardiology* 170 (3): 371–375.

Hendee, William, Gary Becker, James Borgstede, Jennifer Bosma, William Casarella, Beth Erickson, Douglas Maynard, James Thrall, and Paul Wallner. 2010. "Addressing Overutilization in Medical Imaging." *Radiology* 257 (1): 240–245.

Hoberman, John. 1997. *Darwin's Athletes: How Sport Has Damaged Black America and Preserved the Myth of Race.* Houghton Mifflin Company.

Hoberman, John. 2012. *Black & Blue.* University of California Press.

Hoffman, Kelly, Sophie Trawalter, Jordan Axt, and Norman Oliver. 2016. "Racial Bias in Pain Assessment and Treatment Recommendations, and False Beliefs About Biological Differences Between Blacks and Whites." *Proceedings of the National Academy of Sciences of the United States of America* 113 (16): 4296–4301.

Horowitz, David. 2003. *Uncivil Wars: The Controversy over Reparations for Slavery.* Encounter Books.

Ikemoto, Lisa. 2012. "Abortion, Contraception, and the ACA: The Realignment of Women's Health." *Howard Law Journal* 55 (3): 731–769.

Institute of Medicine. March 2001. *Crossing the Quality Chasm: A New Health System for the 21st Century.* Washington, DC: National Academies Press. http://www.nationalacademies.org/hmd/~/media/Files/Report%20Files/2001/Crossing-the-Quality-Chasm/Quality%20Chasm%202001%20%20report%20brief.pd.

International Federation of Health Plans. 2010. "Comparative Price Report: Medical and Hospital Fees by Country." Retrieved from http://ifhp.com/documents/IFHP_Price _Report2010ComparativePriceReport29112010.pdf.

Jennings, A., and M. Sheldon. 1985. "Review of the Health of Children in One-Parent Families." *The Journal of the Royal College of General Practitioners* 35 (279): 478–483.

Jha, Ashish, Elliott Fisher, Zhonghe Li, John Orav, and Arnold Epstein. 2005. "Racial Trends in the Use of Major Procedures Among the Elderly." *The New England Journal of Medicine* 353: 683–691.

Johnson, David Kyle. Forthcoming. "Inference to the Best Explanation and Avoiding Diagnostic Error." In F. Allhoff and S. Borden (eds.), *Ethics and Error in Medicine*. Routledge University Press.

Jones, James. 1993. *Bad Blood*. New York: Free Press.

Kaplan, Judith, and Trude Bennett. 2003. "Use of Race and Ethnicity in Biomedical Publication." *Journal of the American Medical Association* 289 (20): 2709–2716.

Kapp, Marshall B. 1997. "Medical Error Versus Malpractice." *DePaul Journal of Health Care Law* 1 (4): 751–772. Retrieved from https://via.library.depaul.edu/jhcl/vol1/iss4/4.

King, Patricia. 1992. "The Dangers of Difference." *The Hastings Center Report* 22 (6): 35–38.

King, Patricia. 2007. "Race, Equity, Health Policy, and the African American." In L. Prograis and E. Pellegrino (eds.), *African American Bioethics: Culture, Race and Identity*. Washington DC: Georgetown University Press: 67–92.

Kohn, Linda, Janet Corrigan, and Molla Donaldson. 2000. *To Err Is Human: Building a Safer Health System*. National Academies Press.

Krakauer, Eric, and Robert Truog. 1997. "Mistrust, Racism, and End-of-Life Treatment." *The Hastings Center Report* 27 (3): 23–25.

Kramer, Michael, and Carol Hogue. 2009. "What Causes Racial Disparities in Very Preterm Birth? A Biosocial Perspective." *Epidemiologic Reviews* 31 (1): 84–98.

Larson, David, Lara Johnson, Beverly Schnell, Shelia Salisbury, and Howard Forman. 2011. "National Trends in CT Use in the Emergency Department: 1995–2007." *Radiology* 258 (1): 164–173.

Lewis Bernard. 1990. *Race and Slavery in the Middle East: An Historical Enquiry*. Oxford University Press.

Makary, Martin, and Michael Daniel. 2016. "Medical Error—The Third Leading Cause of Death in the US." *British Medical Journal* 353.

Massey, Douglas, and Robert Sampson. 2009. "Introduction: Moynihan Redux: Legacies." *The Moynihan Report Revisited: Lessons and Reflections After Four Decades, The Annals of The American Academy of Political and Social Science* 621: 17.

McBride, David. 2018. *Caring for Equality: A History of African American Health and Healthcare*. Rowman & Littlefield Publishers.

McLanahan, Sara, and Gary Sandefur. 1994. *Growing Up with a Single Parent: What Hurts, What Helps*. Harvard University Press.

Mello, Michelle, Amitabh Chandra, Atul Gawande, and David Studdert. 2010. "National Costs of the Medical Liability System." *Health Affairs* 29 (9).

Montagu, Ashley. 1963. *Race, Science and Humanity*. Van Nostrand Reinhold Co.

Morgan, Daniel, Shannon Brownlee, Aaron Leppin, Nancy Kressin, Sanket Dhruva, Les Levin, Bruce Landon, Mark Zezza, Harald Schmidt, Vikas Saini, and Adam Elshaug. 2015. "Setting a Research Agenda for Medical Overuse." *BMJ* 351: h4534.

Morgan, Daniel, Sanket Dhruva, Eric Coon, Scott Wright, and Deborah Korenstein. 2017. "2017 Update on Medical Overuse: A Systematic Review." *Journal of the American Medical Association Internal Medicine* 178 (1): 110–115.

Morgan, Daniel, Sanket Dhruva, Eric Coon, Scott Wright, and Deborah Korenstein. 2018. "2018 Update on Medical Overuse." *Journal of the American Medical Association Internal Medicine* 179 (2): 240–246.

Morgan, Daniel, Sanket Dhruva, Scott Wright, and Deborah Korenstein. 2016. "2016 Update on Medical Overuse: A Systematic Review." *Journal of the American Medical Association Internal Medicine* 176 (11): 1687–1692.

Morning, Ann. (2011) *The Nature of Race: How Scientists Think and Teach About Human Difference*. University of California Press.

Niles, Lauren, Monika Goyal, Gia Badolato, James Chamberlain, and Joanna Cohen. 2017. "US Emergency Department Trends in Imaging for Pediatric Nontraumatic Abdominal Pain." *Pediatrics* 140 (4): 1–6.

Nuland, Sherwin. 2011. *Doctors: The Biography of Medicine*. Vintage Books.

Osborne, Newton, and Marvin Feit. 1992. "The Use of Race in Medical Research." *Journal of the American Medical Association* 267 (2): 275–279.

Radzick, Linda. 2015. "Reconciliation." *Stanford Encyclopedia of Philosophy*.

Rawls, John. 1988. *A Theory of Justice*, revised ed. Cambridge, MA: Belknap Press.

Reid, Rachel, Brendan Rabideau, and Neeraj Sood. 2016. "Low-Value Health Care Services in a Commercially Insured Population." *Journal of the American Medical Association Internal Medicine* 176 (10): 1567–1571.

Rescher, Nicholas. 1969. "The Allocation of Exotic Medical Lifesaving Therapy." *Ethics* 79 (3): 173–186.

Robinson, Randall. 2000. *The Debt: What America Owes to Blacks*. Penguin.

Roeder, Amy. 2019. "America Is Failing Its Black Mothers." *Harvard Public Health*. Winter issue. https://www.hsph.harvard.edu/magazine/magazine_article/america-is-failing-its-black-mothers/

Rosenberg, Charles. 1987. *The Care of Strangers: The Rise of America's Hospital System*. Basic Books, Inc.

Schoendorf, Kenneth, Carol Hogue, Joel Kleinman, and Diane Rowley. 1992. "Mortality Among Infants of Black as Compared with White College-Educated Parents." *The New England Journal of Medicine* 326: 1522–1526.

Schulman, Kevin, Jesse Berlin, William Harless, Jon Kerner, Shyrl Sistrunk, Bernard Gersh, Ross Dube, Christopher Taleghani, Jennifer Burke, Sankey Williams, John Eisenberg, and William Ayers. 1999. "The Effect of Race and Sex on Physicians' Recommendations for Cardiac Catheterization." *The New England Journal of Medicine* 340: 618–636.

Shapiro, M.F., and S. Greenfield. 1987. "The Complete Blood Count and Leukocyte Differential Count: An Approach to Their Rational Application." *Annals of Internal Medicine* 106: 65–74.

Smedley, Brian, Alan Nelson, and Adrienne Stith. 2003. *Unequal Treatment: Confronting Racial and Ethnic Disparities in Health-care*. National Academies Press.

Smith, Richard. 1991. "Where Is the Wisdom . . .?" *BMJ* 303: 798–799.

Starfield, Barbara. 2004. "Promoting Equity in Health Through Research and Understanding." *Developing World Bioethics* 4 (1): 76–95.

Staton, Lisa, Mukta Panda, Ian Chen, Inginia Genao, James Kurz, Mark Pasanen, Alex Mechaber, Madhusudan Menon, Jane O'Rorke, JoAnn Wood,

Eric Rosenberg, Charles Faeslis, Tim Carey, Diane Calleson, and Sam Cykert. 2007. "When Race Matters: Disagreement in Pain Perception Between Patients and Their Physicians in Primary Care." *Journal of the National Medical Association* 99 (5): 532–538.

Stelfox, H., S. Palmisani, C. Scurlock, E. Orav, and D. Bates. 2006. "The '*To Err Is Human*' Report and the Patient Safety Literature." *Quality and Safety in Health Care* 15 (3): 174–178.

Stone, Deborah. 2005. "How Market Ideology Guarantees Racial Inequality." In J. Morone and Lawrence Jacobs (eds.), *Healthy, Wealthy, and Fair: Health Care and the Good Society*. Oxford University Press: 65–90.

Stone, Lisa, Nina Wallerstein, Analilia Garcia, and Meredith Winkler. 2014. "The Promise of Community-Based Participatory Research for Health Equity: A Conceptual Model for Bridging Evidence with Policy." *American Journal of Public Health* 104 (9): 1615–1623.

Thomasian, John. 2014. *Cracking the Code on Health-care Costs*. Miller Center.

U.S. Department of Health and Human Services. 2018. *National Impact Assessment of the Centers for Medicare & Medicaid Services (CMS) Quality Measures Report*. Centers for Medicare & Medicaid Services. Retrieved from www.cms.gov/Medicare/Quality-Initiatives-Patient-Assessment-Instruments/QualityMeasures/Downloads/2018-Impact-Assessment-Report.pdf.

Villarosa, Linda. 2018. "Why America's Black Mothers and Babies Are in a Life-or-Death Crisis." April 11. *The New York Times*. https://www.nytimes.com/2018/04/11/magazine/black-mothers-babies-death-maternal-mortality.html.

Williams, David, and Chiquita Collins. 2001. "Racial Residential Segregation: A Fundamental Cause of Racial Disparities in Health." *Public Health Reports* 116 (5): 404–416.

Williams, David, and Ronald Wyatt. 2015. "Racial Bias in Health Care and Health: Challenges and Opportunities." *Journal of the American Medical Association* 314 (6): 555–556.

Williams, Melissa, and Jennifer Eberhardt. 2008. "Biological Conceptions of Race and the Motivation to Cross Racial Boundaries." *Journal of Personality and Social Psychology* 94 (6): 1033–1047.

9   The Epistemology of
Medical Error in an
Intersectional World

Devora Shapiro

Situating the Analysis of Medical Error

Identifying medical error, including its incidence and causes, seems a laudable endeavor to pursue. After all, medical error is an unnecessary harm, and we have an obligation to avoid harm when we can. Medical errors happen when medicine fails to provide treatment consistent with an adequate standard of care. So we all, patients and providers alike, should be concerned with avoiding such errors and improving patient outcomes. But though we may all have an interest in preventing medical error, where we look for medical error, and how we count it, may differ depending on the interests that fuel our search. And when we consider the ways in which individuals' place in the world, their region or nation, and their position in their own community and culture can influence what we take to be the appropriate standard of care, at all, the scope of difficulty in identifying "medical error" takes an interesting turn.

In this chapter I explicate and evaluate the concept of medical error. Unlike standard philosophical approaches to analyzing medical phenomena in the abstract, I instead address medical error specifically within the context of an embodied social world. I illustrate how, as a deeply contextual concept, medical error is inextricably tied to the social conditions—and concrete, powerful interests—of the particulars in which it is found. I begin with an analysis that demonstrates the relational quality of medical error, as a functional, outcome-oriented concept, evaluating the origin and context of the term's emergence, and connecting it to a similarly contextual concept, "standard of care." I move on to note the concerning implications of medical error identification and measurement when viewed through an intersectional standpoint. To do so, I discuss what intersectional approaches can help reveal about our contemporary social world of medicine and public health. Intersectional approaches, as I will explain, focus on how intersections of social identity can unmask social structures that negatively impact groups and individuals. It appears, as I will suggest, that disparities in social goods (e.g., social standing, education, wealth) complicate our identification of medical error, itself, and compound concerns of equity and access to medical goods for those who have diminished expectations for health.

Medical Error: What Is It, What Is It for, and Who Is It for?

We often think of "ethics" as concerning issues of right and wrong, good or bad, and as guiding answers to normative questions such as "what should I do?" or "what must be done?" Such a focus in ethics is reasonable; however, it is not exhaustive. Approaches to ethical concerns manifesting in a social world can often take alternative forms, particularly when evaluating the ethical implications of social institutions such as schools, the law, or medical systems, and when evaluating such institutions as impacting not only individuals, but groups of individuals, whose social identities and statuses may promote or constrain their experiences and their actions.

"Medicine" can be considered as an abstract good, whose goal is to promote health and prevent disease. "Medical practice," however, may be less abstract, and may take on increasingly particular characteristics, drawn from the particular society in which we find it. In fact, the more that medical practice becomes part and parcel of a particular medical institution, in a particular legal environment, within a specific social and political world, the more we infuse the good of "medicine" with a particular application in medical practice (Broadbent 2019). And the more our medical practice becomes situated and embedded in a complex, particular social world that includes inequalities linked to social standing and social identities (such as race, sex, ethnicity, etc.), the more we must evaluate the structure and reality of medical practice for its ethical implications. One such embedded concept in contemporary American medical practice is "medical error" (Berlinger 2008).

Though what is meant by our term "medical error" may on its face seem reasonably straightforward, at its core it represents a deeply contextual and complicated concept (Grober and Bohnen 2005). For one, are medical errors *actions* that can be attributed to a medical practice, or only a physician? If an adverse event results from the *inaction* of a medical office or managed care company, or the legitimate lack of knowledge of particular state-licensed medical professionals (nurses, nurse practitioners) who are treating patients when licensed medical doctors are unavailable, is this a medical error? That is, if an error occurs, but there is no legally responsible physician present to shoulder the blame, does it make a sound?[1]

The landscape of medical error is, itself, complicated, convoluted, and variously defined and identified (Grober and Bohnen 2005). Before evaluating how the social world impacts how we might know that a medical error has occurred, or that a particular event should be understood as "medical error," it will be necessary to narrow the field—or at least describe the field—in which we might look for medical error, at all. Many venues and industries have entered into the foray of medical error enterprise. These include: the legal system, insurance industries (malpractice, hospital, patient, etc.), physician associations, nursing organizations, health-care business organizations, and state-sponsored agencies concerned with quality assessment and resource allocation (Grober and Bohnen 2005). Each of these industries and venues identifies, defines, and measures medical error in disparate ways and, potentially, for disparate, different ends, goals, or interests (Grober and Bohnen 2005; Elder, Pallerla, and Regan 2006).

Our current popular discussion of medical error as a concept in the United States, specifically, finds its origin in the report produced by the Institute of Medicine (IOM), the non-profit organization funded by various governmental grants and institutions. Produced at the turn of the twenty-first century, this report spurred the explosion of an industry of quality control in health care, with the United States Congress allocating $50 million to the Agency for Healthcare Research and Quality (AHRQ) for the purpose of medical error reduction (U.S. Department of Health and Human Services 2018). At the time the IOM variously reported between $17billion and 29 billion in total costs related to errors in hospitals, alone, and between 44,000 and 98,000 deaths in hospitals as a result of medical error (IOM 2000). Such dramatic reporting of the incidence, severity, and cost of medical errors was sufficient to prompt an increase of interest from all sectors of society, and follow-up studies were engaged. In the flurry of activity that ensued, however, no standard measure of "medical error" was settled upon, and no proper scope was defined (Harrington 2005). Since that time numerous researchers in a variety of fields have taken up the project of identifying and mitigating medical error, and in doing so have potentially proliferated—rather than consolidated—the concept.

Some researchers, noting the inherent problems stemming from vagueness and ambiguity, have systematically approached the definitional effort for clarifying the concept of "medical error." Grober and Bohnen offer a summary of many such efforts, categorizing medical error definitions as either "outcome-dependent" or "process-dependent" (Grober and Bohnen 2005, 40). Process-dependent definitions of medical error[2] focus on explaining deficient processes that more often give rise to medical error, with an aim toward improving such processes, and reducing negative outcomes. In contrast, outcome-dependent definitions are those that focus on "patients experiencing adverse outcomes or injury as a consequence of medical care," that are often adopted in the context of patient safety research (Grober and Bohnen 2005, 40). Such definitions have variously identified their objects of study under the terms "noxious events," "potentially compensable event," "adverse event," "preventable adverse event," "negligent adverse event," and "adverse patient out-come" (Grober and Bohnen 2005, 40).

Each of these various terms identifies an undesirable outcome experienced by a patient. However it is notable that each of these terms also captures slightly different objects in its net. To begin, a "potentially compensable event" would be a subset of undesirable outcomes for a particular patient, and is a term specifically developed and employed within the context of insurance interests. It derives from the well-known 1978 California Medical Insurance Feasibility Study, and, as the name suggests, was undertaken for the purpose of identifying the "type, frequency, and severity of those disabilities *for which compensation might be paid*" (Mills et al. 1978, 360).[3] The original 1978 study was expressly pursued in order to manage the limited availability of liability insurance and its "skyrocketing premium costs" (Mills et al. 1978, 360). Based on the interests of the study, only those adverse outcomes that might have resulted in compensation to a harmed patient would be included. These would include what some refer to as "never events,"[4] such as surgery to the wrong part of the body, or artificial insemination with the wrong donor sperm. While such dramatic and easily identifiable errors are indisputably bad, such kinds of outcomes do not account for all of what we generally understand as a "medical error." Further, only those events that occurred in a hospital were included in the study; though the authors note that their purpose in the study was to "obtain adequate information about patient disabilities resulting from health care management" (Mills et al. 1978, 360), they supposed that for their purposes—for the purposes of evaluating the overall costs of potentially compensable events—they needed only to include the frequency of such events in hospitals.

While hospitals surely are sites of health-care management, there are presently many other kinds of health-care management sites, that differ importantly in their legally set standards, and in the state and industry regulations regarding staffing, treatment criteria, patient insurance statuses, and so on. These distinctions are important for two reasons: first, we might imagine that the dramatic kinds of compensable never events that might occur in hospital surgeries would not occur in managed care outpatient clinics, and second a compensable event is directly defined by the laws of the land. For an adverse event to be compensable, that event must demonstrate failure to meet a legally required standard or a violation of a legally enforceable rule or regulation. Since such rules and regulations largely govern hospitals and medical doctors, adverse outcomes in standalone outpatient clinics that are focused on delivering basic community health have far fewer restrictions—and thus opportunities for legal violation. Further, their staffing requirements are significantly more diffuse, allowing professionals outside of licensed medical doctors to perform basic patient care. When a failure in a clinic occurs, patients will find it difficult to locate an entity that is legally responsible for the error, or a law that has been broken. This reduces the likelihood of an error leading to a compensable event.

Finally, with regard to placing attention on "compensable" events as the focus for error, there are many errors that might occur in a medical setting that, *if* one had herculean motivation, endless time and financial resources, and access to particularly skilled and creative legal counsel, then one *might* succeed in demonstrating a health-care company responsible for in a civil court. But few harmed patients meet such conditions, and very few, in fact, bring legal suits to court (Mello et al. 2007, 837).[5]

The evaluation of medical error in the literature is strongly focused on medical error in the hospital setting. In 2011, Bishop, Ryan, and Casalino estimated that there are over 30 times as many outpatient visits as inpatient, and reported that during the five-year period spanning 2006–2011 the AHRQ funded in-patient studies of medical error at a rate 10 times that of outpatient studies (Bishop, Ryan, and Casalino 2011). This strong focus on medical error in the hospital setting originates with the noted studies' interest in curbing costs for insurers and extends to cost management efforts driven by hospitals, as well as by the shareholders who hold an interest in these increasingly privately owned facilities (Mello et al. 2007). Mello et al. note that the overwhelming focus on medical error and related cost control concerns focuses on hospitals' inpatient costs, and therefore limit themselves to considering those costs that are paid by hospitals and medical insurers. As Mello et al. point out, however, additional costs to individual patients and families include "lost income, lost household production, future medical expenses, noneconomic losses, and other components" (Mello et al. 2007, 838). Moreover, "although patients are often injured by medical negligence, only a tiny proportion has their injury costs reimbursed by health-care providers and their insurance companies" (Mello et al. 2007, 838), and only 50 percent of the estimated 2–3 percent of injured patients who actually file legal claims even receive compensation (Mello et al. 2007, 838). With a focus on "potentially compensable events" as the scope for medical error, the impact of errors on patients, therefore, will be lost.

Accordingly, attempts have been made to identify alternative measures of error in medicine. Other categories that have been used as a proxy for medical error include the category "adverse event." This unqualified category, however, has been accused of being overly broad; AHRQ provides one definition of "adverse event" that suggests an adverse event includes "an injury caused by medical management (rather than the disease process) that resulted in either prolonged hospital stay or disability at discharge" (U.S. Department of Health and Human Services 2019). But this category would be so broad as to include unexpected bleeding or wound infection—both of which are likely to occur some of the time, even with standard precautions and appropriate patient care. Most studies therefore limit the scope of the category to "preventable" adverse events (of which "negligence" is a subset). AHRQ, for example, understands an adverse event to be preventable "if it was avoidable by any means currently available unless that means was not considered standard care" (Thomas and Troyen 2000, 741).

Determining whether an adverse event is preventable is highly contextual, however, because of its connection to "standard care." Standard care in the United States will vary greatly: from standard care in communities existing within disastrous or disaster-stricken infrastructure, political unrest, environmental crises, and so on, on the one hand, to standard care in wealthy communities or at health-care sites that treat only well-insured or self-pay patients, on the other. Surely we would not suppose that the most attentive and successful doctor in a remote community situated in the Congo, for example, would be able to (or expected to) provide the same treatments to patients, or hold to the same standard care, or "standard of care," as she would in the exceedingly affluent community of Potomac, Maryland. Nonetheless, studies focused on medical error as definitionally tied to "standard of care" generally do not address—or even note—such issues.

In the foundational and well-known Harvard Medical Practice Study concerned with adverse events and negligence in hospital settings (Brennan et al. 1991), they connect their outcome-dependent concept of "preventable adverse events" with "medical negligence," supposing those adverse events that are attributable to negligence could have been avoided and are also legally significant. They define adverse events, therefore, as those events leading to either prolonged hospital stay or to injury due to the management of care, and further specify negligence as "care that fell below the standard expected of physicians in their community" (Brennan et al. 1991, 370). Though their results were intended to inform discussions of malpractice and litigation, this use of standard of care language further extends the context dependency of the medical error conversation, and extends the connection to more deeply entrenched social and politically laden contingencies including economic status, geographic location, racial identity, and education level.

"Standard of care" as a concept has been present in medicine, informally, for over a century, according to (Moffett and Moore 2011). They offer a chronological approach to understanding the concept, and cite a lack of physician awareness of the connection between medical practice, on the one hand, and the legal implications of standard of care for medical *mal*practice, on the other. Standard of care, they explain, is a mutable and evolving concept that, like medical error, is contextually dependent: it depends on the circumstances of the patient encounter, the patient's medical history, the physician's interpretation of a root medical cause, and the physician's choice of treatment, all things considered. Legal negligence standards generally focus on "minimum competence," and being determined to have performed "competently" will insulate a physician from liability for basic judgment errors, diagnostic mistakes, and generally undesirable results (Moffett and Moore 2011, 110). Though specialty-specific clinical guidelines determine what physicians look to for baseline standard of care guidelines, courts evaluating legal liability for malpractice focus instead on establishing minimum competence for the physician, within the context of their present environment.

The environment that informs both minimal competency judgments and clinical guidelines, however, includes physician licensing boards and interactions with one's professional community, not to mention the multitude of non-clinical influences that may directly or indirectly inform a clinician's interpretation of relevant guidelines. Hajjaj et al. discuss the breadth and depth of what they identify as non-clinical influences on clinical decision making (2010, 178). They define clinical decision making as "the process of making an informed judgment about the treatment necessary for . . . patients," and they describe this process as involving "an interaction of application of clinical and biomedical knowledge, problem-solving, weighing of probabilities and various outcomes, and balancing risk-benefit" (Hajjaj et al. 2010, 178). They further suggest that the key task of physician clinical-decision making is to "balance personal experience and prevalent knowledge" (Hajjaj et al. 2010, 178). Examples included here are: patient socio-economic status; patient's race; patient's age, gender and "personal" characteristics; "patient's adherence to treatment or inappropriate behavior that may influence adherence"; and outside influences of family members and faith communities, etc. (Hajjaj et al. 2010, 179).

Hajjaj et al. note the relevance of such non-clinical factors on decision making by referencing the very real influence of socio-economic factors on management decisions in the U.S. specifically (2010, 178). They note that doctors may change treatment strategies of aggressiveness of treatment in response to patient's financial resources, and because of the assumption that socio-economically disadvantaged patients are reported, as a group, to be less compliant than non-disadvantaged patients. Physicians make similar assumptions about black patients' adherence to treatment regimens, and their adherence to "do not resuscitate" (DNR) orders is more likely when treating black patients (Hajjaj et al. 2010, 180). Differences in treatment decisions linked to the racial identifier "black," for example, have been documented in treatment for: depression; renal cell carcinoma; and HIV treatment (Hajjaj et al. 2010, 180). And there are examples for each of the categories of non-clinical factors in clinical decision making that are associated with physician-related characteristics, as well as features of the health-care practice where the patient's care is being managed and delivered.

As a result, "standard of care," like "medical error," can be described and defined for multiple purposes and in multiple contexts. Kinney clarifies that standard of care definitions can be constructed from within medical practice—by doctors and clinical researchers, or from without, by federal regulators, health-care management organizations with financial interests, and so on (Kinney 2004, 574). These definitions include "medical (or clinical) practice guidelines" that she defines as "systematically developed statements to assist practitioners in their decision making in specific clinical settings" (Kinney 2004).[6] This definition is characterized by Kinney as arising from "within" medical practice, whereas the remaining definitions she reviews are constructed as quality measures from "without" medical practice, by health regulators. If standard of care, particularly from the perspective of physicians within medical practice, is dependent on clinical setting, professional judgment, and resource availability, and includes non-clinical factors for decision making (as it unavoidably will), then those treatment decisions (and whether they conform to "standard of care") will legitimately be justifiable with regard to all of these factors. And all of these factors are demonstrably socially laden: they are tied up with, constructed with, contingent upon, and infused by the social.

What does this mean for medical error? Medical error, as we have now seen, is closely tied to interests invested in minimizing adverse events that prolong hospital stays, increase treatment costs, or that are likely to put hospitals at risk of lawsuit. Included as a factor in all of these calculations are statistical data comprised of such things as racial make-up of health-care consumers, compliance expectations based on socioeconomic ascriptions including wealth, age, race, and ethnicity, access to medical resources based on geographic location, and so on. "Standard of care" guidelines, in many forms, are similarly influenced by such factors, and constitute an element of the evaluations of medical negligence that are included in the health-care industry's efficiency and/or quality concept of "medical error." The guidelines are also significant in establishing that an "adverse event" would have been "preventable."

"Medical error," as such, is always treated as a subset of adverse events and "bad outcomes" (death) that are due to negligence or a failure to maintain a minimally competent standard of care for their legally understood comparison class. Further, medical error is a category closely connected to the larger swath of "preventable" adverse events. Already, it is clear that medical error is context-dependent. The full scope of such a realization is deeply ethically concerning, however, when paired with a theoretical standpoint that can identify, articulate, and bring into the foreground the concerns arising from this context-dependency.

Medical Error: Why Do We Care?

Tomas is a 12-year-old boy being treated for Stage III, Nodular Sclerosing Hodgkins Lymphoma, in November of 1991. At this time, Tomas is given a good prognosis, and his doctor feels he will likely recover fully and permanently, after six months of chemotherapy and two months of radiation. He is receiving his care at a community hospital in a major metropolitan area and receives his rotating courses of four chemotherapeutic drugs every two weeks. His immediate family of two parents, two younger siblings, and his grandmother are all legal immigrants without larger ties to any relatives in the United States, and both of his parents are full-time hourly wage workers. They are native Spanish speakers. Tomas does not have full coverage, or private insurance, and his treatment is instead covered through various public insurance programs.

Tomas experiences standard side effects from his treatments, including severe nausea and vomiting. This includes vomiting every 10–15 minutes, beginning two–three hours following treatment, and continuing uninterrupted for up to an additional 16 hours, after which time the vomiting slows. He is regularly given Compazine and Benadryl—a very low cost, standard treatment at the time in 1991, amounting to just a few dollars per treatment. This anti-emetic treatment, however, appears ineffective in curbing Tomas's vomiting. With each successive treatment he becomes increasingly weak, and his recovery time longer. Tomas, after two months of treatment, is no longer able to attend school, due in part to the severity of his nausea, vomiting, and related issues: esophageal ulcers, possible pneumonia caused from aspiration, fatigue, and malnourishment. His family has lost significant wages due to Tomas's care, and his extended time away from school.

Eventually he is admitted to hospital for his treatments, as his state deteriorates. Though Tomas's cancer is shrinking, he is increasingly frail and in danger of significant additional complications that could prove life-threatening or cause permanent damage and disability.

Jessica, 15 years old, is also being treated by the same physician, in a nearby private research hospital, and for the same disease. However Jessica's parents are both salaried government workers, with excellent insurance. When Jessica undergoes her first treatment, she is also given Benadryl and Compazine, to no effect. Like Tomas, her reactions are significant, and her parents ask their physician for alternatives to help with the nausea and vomiting. Her doctor is enthusiastic to introduce Zofran,[7] a newly approved anti-emetic that has demonstrated remarkable effects in patients undergoing the kinds of chemotherapy that Jessica has been assigned. At her next treatment she receives Zofran, and the results are dramatic: she vomits only twice over the 24 hours following her treatment, resumes eating within two days, and returns to school after a long weekend.

Jessica and Tomas meet at a community event for pediatric cancer patients and share stories of their experiences with one another. As Jessica realizes the difference between the treatment she is now receiving, as compared to Tomas's treatment, she asks her physician why Tomas can't receive Zofran, too. Her doctor explains that Tomas does not have insurance that will cover the treatment, and that without insurance to cover the expense his family could not possibly afford it.[8]

Intersectionality and Medical Error

In 1991, the drug Ondansetron, better known by its trade name "Zofran," was approved for use in the United States (Cancer Network 2006). At the time, it was cost-prohibitive for patients without insurance to receive Zofran (and even those *with* insurance coverage were often placed on the "fail-first" regimen). Initial studies in the United Kingdom had demonstrated remarkable improvements, particularly in cancer patients undergoing chemotherapy, and these improvements were specifically in response to one of the most significant adverse effects of chemotherapy: nausea and vomiting. In 1991 it was reported that after treatment with Zofran "complete control of emesis was achieved in 42–87% of patients, and complete plus major control of emesis (0–2 emetic episodes) was achieved in 65–98% of children" (Stevens 1991, S20). By 1992, studies in the US reported "82–100% (0–24 hours) vomiting free patients" (Tanneberger et al. 1992, 326).

These were impressive results and significantly improved not only quality of life for patients, but both reduced time in hospital and overall morbidity. Though early studies noted the increased cost of treatment with Zofran (of about 6 percent; Tanneberger et al. 1992, 326), by 1999 the *Journal of Clinical Oncology* published a retrospective assessment detailing the antiemetic costs of treatment with Zofran including "drug costs, nursing time, pharmacy time, physician's time, supplies, and facility 'hotel costs'" for the six months before the availability of Zofran as compared to the six months after Zofran became available (Stewart et al. 1999, 344). The study found a significant savings in cost per patient per month, largely attributed to a reduction in hospital bed days and increased effectiveness in case management (Stewart et al. 1999, 344). Still, in 2006, when the FDA approved the release of generic Ondansetron, it was the twentieth *most* expensive brand-name drug used in US hospitals (Cancer Network 2006).

But what does the example of Zofran, and the cases of Tomas and Jessica, mean for medical error? As demonstrated in the first section, the term "medical error" is largely an outcome-based concept, generally associated with identifying preventable adverse events, particularly those occurring in the context of inpatient hospital care. Those events that are generally identified are events that carry with them the potential to generate payouts to patients as compensation for harm, and/or that have the potential to increase costs to insurers, for unnecessary follow-up patient care costs and extended hospital stays. Medical error, as established previously as well, is a concept of interest primarily to insurers, hospitals, and medical providers interested in reducing expenditures, protecting against legal liability for adverse outcomes, and, at times, concerned with increasing profit margins. Since merely half of the two–three percent of patients who are harmed by a preventable adverse event ever receive compensation for their losses, patients have little to gain directly from increased tracking of medical error, as it stands now.

What the cases of Tomas and Jessica help to add is an entry point to viewing the larger—and deeply significant—ethical issue that an interrogation of the concept "medical error" helps reveal: that there is something not quite right about the reasons we are given for caring about medical error, and that suspected "something" has to do with medical error serving interests that may diverge or be in conflict with patients' interests—particularly those who are members of vulnerable or disadvantaged populations. But standard, single-variable approaches to evaluating this diffuse and difficult-to-grasp worry are not particularly helpful. For example, approaches to evaluating patients who experience harm in the form of "adverse events" or "bad outcomes" as a result of medical treatment might more often belong to a particular racial group. But noting that adverse events are associated with disadvantaged racial identities does nothing to inform us as to why such association exists, or to how simultaneous membership in different social positions increases or mitigates risk for harm.

"Intersectionality" refers to the now well-known theory first articulated by legal theorist and professor, Kimberlé Crenshaw, in 1989. Intersectional theory is an outgrowth of the Black feminist thought of the 1970s and 1980s, and challenges standard approaches to evaluating social and political problems. Rather than identifying group characteristics as single-variable, unitary wholes, intersectional theory conceptualizes identity as multidimensional, thus not confining it to a single-axis analysis that distorts and cannot capture, for example, Black women's (and potentially other oppressed minorities') experiences (Crenshaw 1989). She uses the example of Black women to demonstrate that the traditional, "additive" approach to identity fails to capture the complexity of Black women's experiences in the U.S. What she means by this is that merely collecting data on "women" and on "Blacks" and "adding" these together, will fail to give us insight into the intersecting nature of the unique experience as a "Black woman." Instead, the category of "women" will be skewed to White women's experiences, and the category "Black," to Black men's experiences. Combining these two categories fails to represent the experience of the erased: the Black woman in late twentieth-century America (Crenshaw 1991).

Over two decades later, Bowleg contextualizes intersectional theory within contemporary social science research stating: "Intersectionality is a theoretical framework for understanding how multiple social identities such as race, gender, sexual orientation, SES, and disability intersect at the micro level of individual experience to reflect interlocking systems of privilege and oppression (i.e., racism, sexism, heterosexism, classism) at the macro social-structural level" (Bowleg et al. 2012, 1267). She emphasizes the particularly strong fit between this theory and the project of those engaging in public health research, citing the common ends of both endeavors as focused on social justice. Intersectional theory has increasingly gained attention as a promising framework for evaluating and analyzing marginalization in the social sciences and health research, and as Glass et al. recently explain, intersectionality can "formalize the notion that adverse health outcomes [owe] to having a marginalized social position, identity, or characteristic" (Glass et al. 2017, 516). Said another way, intersectional analyses offer us the ability to recognize and make visible the experiences—and in this case, poor health experiences—of individuals and groups of individuals living at the intersections of multiple axes of disadvantage and disenfranchisement. An intersectional analysis further offers a framework that can expose the underlying, interlocking social systems and institutions that create and perpetuate the possibility of such an existence.

Intersectionality has been used effectively in a variety of areas of public and population health, including in conjunction with quantitative studies. Glass et al. demonstrate one example of this theory applied as an intersectional approach to generate hypotheses regarding the expected increase of the effects of alcohol consumption within impoverished communities, on men and women, and with regard to race, gender, and ethnicity. They had hypothesized that the effects of identifying with multiple layers of less socially privileged positions would yield multiplicative, rather than additive, negative outcomes. In their case the outcomes were informative and confirmed intersectionally supported hypotheses. More to the point, however, their study demonstrated the value of a successful application of intersectional theory: it allowed them to pinpoint the central factors most significant to experiences of harm and the intersectional identities most likely to experience harm, and it allowed for the narrowing in on particular systems that supported and perpetuated this harm (Glass et al. 2017).

Applied within the context of a discussion of medical error, intersectional theory offers a unique ability to refocus the lens through which we evaluate the use, purpose, and effects of such a concept, as embedded in the deeply social world it purports to inform and improve. From an intersectional perspective, our goal is twofold: (1) to acknowledge the positionality of different persons and groups of people, shaped and informed in connection with their socially significant identities, and as importantly valuable and unique nodes of experience worth considering. Our further goal is (2) to help make visible—to reveal—and to aid in identifying and interrogating the structures that encourage or reinforce conditions for injustice: in this case health disparities and social inequalities associated with class, race, and other group-based social positions.

Let us return, then, to the cases of Tomas and Jessica. I have claimed that intersectionality will help "reveal" something that other theories will miss or obscure. How do the cases of Tomas and Jessica remain obscured in the absence of intersectionality? What is it that standard analyses of "medical error" cannot grasp? How does this case even represent an instance of medical error?

To review, each child is being treated within the range of the accepted standard of care for Hodgkin's Lymphoma, and by an apparently competent doctor. And yet they receive different treatment (the anti-emetics are not the same), while receiving treatment in the same town, and by the same doctor. Jessica responds well to the treatment she receives, and Tomas responds poorly to his treatment. Though Tomas's cancer is shrinking, he is not well; he loses considerable weight, demonstrates the effects of malnourishment, develops ulcers in his esophagus, shows clear signs of both depression and fatigue, has increasingly extended stays in the hospital, and misses school. That is, Tomas demonstrates that he is medically less well than might be achieved by available medication, displays deleterious psychosocial impact, and has been impeded by his inability to access education, which would aid him in reintegrating into the post-treatment life that his prognosis suggests he is expected to secure. Further Tomas's family is significantly impacted in ways that extend beyond Tomas, alone, and in ways that affect his siblings by compromising their ability to secure food, shelter, general health, access to education, and an overall groundwork to productive futures.

Our definitions of medical error included: "potentially compensable event," "preventable adverse event," "negligent adverse event," and "adverse patient outcome." AHRQ, the current central regulatory government agency, sums this up by defining medical error as "an act of commission (doing something wrong) or omission (failing to do the right thing) leading to an undesirable outcome or significant potential for such an outcome" (U.S. Department of Health and Human Services 2019). They specifically define preventable adverse events as "those that occurred due to error or failure to apply an accepted strategy for prevention" and they define the subset of those events that were due to negligence as "those that occurred due to care that falls below the standards expected of clinicians in the community."

So what about Tomas? The physician chooses to omit a possible treatment, introducing numerous preventable adverse events, due to care that falls below that physician's own standard of care for other patients, and on the basis of the physician's personal judgment. It is this last bit, however, that weakens Tomas's case from being considered "potentially compensable," and it is precisely for this reason that an intersectional approach can be fruitful.

An intersectional lens will interrogate elements in its view that may be socially relevant to the decisions made in the treatment of Tomas:

Tomas is on public insurance, Hispanic, and part of a family of immigrants who are native Spanish speakers. Both of Tomas's parents have heavily accented English, and his parents are working jobs that do not require a high level of education. Given these non-clinical factors, the physician believes the family does not have sufficient resources to afford the alternative medication. Often an intersectional analysis will identify such socially significant categories of analysis as race, class, and gender; here I extend those and focus instead on the similarly socially significant categories of ethnicity and immigration status, rather than race, per se, and include specific categories such as employment type and insurance status as a manifestation of class.

Though the doctor is aware of a readily available remedy, he does not offer it due to the lack of resources he envisions Tomas's family has available. Jessica however, appears to be a white, middle-class daughter of well educated, presumably citizen-from-birth parents, who has excellent private insurance and likely additional resources available should they become necessary. The doctor offers the available remedy, and Jessica responds very well. There is no reason to believe that Tomas would not respond similarly (studies available at that time suggest that nearly all treated children responded remarkably well). Tomas's adverse outcomes, therefore, are likely to be medically preventable ones. The drug is withheld from Tomas due to a lack of financial resources.

While it might appear that a standard, single-variable analysis of this case would suffice, and that lack of insurance adequately explains—and potentially justifies—the scenario, this situation is not so simple. The doctor made clinical judgments in treatment based on non-clinical features of his patient that may reflect nonclinical features of himself and of the medical setting, including acculturated biases specific to his experience as a doctor in an urban, metropolitan area. An intersectional analysis interrogates how these multiple axes of Tomas's identity intersect to distinguish his experience not simply as a poor patient, or as an immigrant patient, or as a Hispanic patient, but as a patient uniquely situated at the intersection of these socially significant identities. Further, once the positionality of Tomas has been identified and made intelligible, an intersectional analysis can conceptualize the structures (e.g., racism and classism) that stand in relief to these identities. These structures and social systems, or institutions, provide the possibility and continued support for the negative experiences connected to Tomas's disadvantaged identity. The quality of the care delivered to Tomas was markedly inferior to what it could have been. An intersectional analysis will look for the systemic issues that make the physician's rationalized choices seem reasonable.

As it happens, there is convincing evidence that the quality of care delivered to comparable patients, even in the same hospital, will vary by insurance type (Spencer et al. 2013). Though doctors take an oath to treat all patients equally, racial identity and insurance status accurately predicts different treatment; a patient's race and ethnicity pervades throughout their movement in the health-care system, impacts their access to resources, and impacts their interactions with health-care providers, and ultimately their treatment and treatment outcomes (Tello 2017; Egede 2006).

One might object that the standard of care—a contextually informed clinical guideline—allows for some variation according to a physician's clinical judgment. But should we suppose then, that we will allow as legitimate, differences in treatment when the deciding difference in clinical judgment is informed by insurance coverage rates and non-clinical and medically irrelevant features of patients? Such a supposition seems dubious, to say the least.

Still, we might respond that in instances of scarcity we must allocate resources inequitably at times. If the resources needed to treat Tomas were truly "scarce," one might argue that a physician has no choice but to treat with whatever means are available (Morreim 1989). However in this case, the resource (Zofran) is not scarce—in fact it is in large supply. It's just not available for those who can't afford it.

Had the medication been requested for a non-medical purpose, or had the medication been unproven in its superior effectiveness, perhaps this refusal to treat with Zofran might have reasonably been understood to be within the standard of care. But Zofran was already proven to be successful and safe in the target population, would have significantly reduced the likelihood of adverse events, and the omission of treatment with Zofran is the direct cause of the increased risk for harm, hospital stay, and potential disability in the patient. On all but one measure, the withholding of treatment with Zofran meets the qualification of "medical error"; this one outlying measure is a potentially compensable event. Since Tomas's treatment outcomes are so varied, and the causally significant factors in his current state of sickness so diffuse, they do not constitute a case that is in any way likely to support a malpractice claim. But what does this tell us?

When viewed through an intersectional lens this case reveals a considerable amount of thought-provoking content related to medical error and the underlying system in which it is an active and meaningful concept. What is revealed is that (1) the medical error-as-compensable-event, though purportedly concerned with quality control and patient harm, fails to be framed in a way that can capture or mitigate the common harms that the poor, poorly insured, or socially less respected patients experience; (2) medical error as a preventable adverse event *does* successfully capture the harm that is done to socio-economically vulnerable patients such as Tomas, but the system that supports medical error *does not acknowledge this*, instead reinforcing the belief that insurance coverage and individual wealth is a legitimate decider, alone, for determining treatment; (3) that the system in which medical error is utilized—the rhetoric of quality control and patient safety—reinforces inequalities between patients and contributes to the reinforcing of inequality beyond the medical setting (through the long-term harms that sub-par treatment produces in affected patients); and (4) that the concept of medical error does not directly serve patients (though it presumably has helped in many ways); it is instead a concept first and foremost created and implemented in service of larger, powerful, capital-rich industries, including the "quality health-care" industry, itself.

Conclusion: Intersectionality and What It Can Reveal About Medical Error

The lack of consistency regarding standards and definitions of medical error across studies and industries is not surprising. After all, why *would* they all agree, when their interests are so divergent? Take health-care management and business, for example. The interests and stated purpose of corporations *qua* corporations is to generate profit for shareholders. In the business of health care, businesses intend to profit, and shareholders invest in such businesses with the understanding that they will receive benefit—monetary benefit, from such endeavors (Poplin 2017). This means that the monetary costs of delivering services must be outweighed by the monetary benefits received by the company.[9]

All of this suggests one central and fundamental point: our claim to know that a medical error has occurred is a contextual claim: it depends on who we are, where we are, and where our interests lie. The epistemic issue of medical error—of knowing when an error has occurred—bleeds into the social and, therefore, the ethical. The contextual nature of medical error is not only abstractly based in the various industries that have an interest in medical error, it is also embedded in the social particularities of the site of origin.

Medical errors occur in a variety of socio-economic places, and they manifest in patients—people who live in different places, circumstances, and times, and who are experienced by their health care providers through the social lenses and background histories that such providers bring with them. Our evaluation of whether a medical error has occurred, at all, may at times be influenced by socio-economic factors affecting physician expectations, resource availability, and the real or imagined expectations for a given patient's access to future medical care. But the one constant that becomes clear through an intersectionally focused analysis of medical error is that equality and equity in health care are not central tenets of current medical practice; that justice for those who are harmed by the systems that support and deliver health care in our contemporary American society can miss the mark of justice, and errs in its delivery of medicine.

Notes

1. For more on blame and the proper culture of justice, see Chapter 3: "A Just Culture Approach to Medical Error" by Garrett and McNolty and Chapter 4: "Rehabilitating Blame" by Reis-Dennis.
2. Most notably represented by James Reason's "Swiss-cheese" model of medical error.
3. Italics mine.
4. Additional examples include: patient death or disability associated with a fall, electric shock, or a medication error (Berlinger 2008).
5. Moral luck in the context of medical error complicates this issue as well. If a medical procedure is done incorrectly but, luckily, leads to a positive result (such as amputating the wrong limb only to learn it was cancerous) would mean that the event is not a compensable one, despite having all of the other properties of a medical error. For more on this, see Chapter 2: "Medical Error and Moral Luck" by Allhoff.
6. Kinney notes that these definitions are based on the 1990 IOM report.
7. Even Jessica only receives Zofran after the "fail first" requirement has been met.
8. The particulars of this fictional case are woven from various accounts during the period from patients and providers, and from within the relevant specialties.
9. Additional concerns about increased mortality due to cost reduction practices at hospitals keen on staying "competitive" have also been raised (Mukamel et al. 2002).

Works Cited

Berlinger, Nancy. 2008. "Medical Error." In Mary Crowley (ed.), *From Birth to Death and Bench to Clinic: The Hastings Center Bioethics Briefing Book for Journalists, Policymakers, and Campaigns*. Garrison, NY: The Hastings Center: 97–100.

Bishop, Tara, Andrew Ryan, and Lawrence Casalino. 2011. "Paid Malpractice Claims for Adverse Events in Inpatient and Outpatient Settings." *JAMA* 305 (23): 2427–2431. doi:10.1001/jama.2011.813

Bowleg, Lisa. 2012. "The Problem with the Phrase Women and Minorities: Intersectionality—An Important Theoretical Framework for Public Health." *American Journal of Public Health* 102 (7): 1267–1273. doi:10.2105/AJPH.2012.300750

Brennan, Troyen, et al. 1991. "Incidence of Adverse Events and Negligence in Hospitalized Patients. Results of the Harvard Medical Practice Study I." *New England Journal of Medicine* 324: 370–376. doi: 10.1056/NEJM199102073240604

Broadbent, Alex. 2019. "What is Medicine? Why It's So Important to Answer This Question." *Medical Xpress*. Retrieved from https://medicalxpress.com/news/2019-01-medicine-important.html

Cancer Network. 2006. "FDA Approves the First Generic Versions of Ondansetron." *Journal of Oncology* 15 (12). Retrieved from www.cancernetwork.com/nausea-and-vomiting/fda-approves-first-generic-versions-ondansetron

Crenshaw, Kimberle. 1989. "Demarginalizing the Intersection of Race and Sex: A Black Feminist Critique of Antidiscrimination Doctrine, Feminist Theory and Antiracist Politics." *University of Chicago Legal Forum*: 1, (8).

Crenshaw, Kimberle. 1991. "Mapping the Margins: Intersectionality, Identity Politics, and Violence against Women of Color." *Stanford Law Review* 43 (6): 1241–1299.

Dovey, Susan, D. Meyers, R. Phillips, L. Green, G. Fryer, J. Galliher, J. Kappus, and P. Grob. 2002. "A Preliminary Taxonomy of Medical Errors in Family Practice." *Quality & Safety in Health Care* 11 (3): 233–238.

Donaldson, Molla. 2008. "An Overview of To Err is Human: Re-emphasizing the Message of Patient Safety." *Patient Safety and Quality: An Evidence-Based Handbook for Nurses.* Agency for Healthcare Research and Quality (US): Chapter 3.

Egede, Leonard. 2006. "Race, Ethnicity, Culture, and Disparities in Health Care." *Journal of General Internal Medicine* 21 (6): 667–669. doi:10.1111/j.1525-1497.2006.0512.x

Elder, Nancy, Harini Pallerla, and Saundra Regan. 2006. "What Do Family Physicians Consider an Error? A Comparison of Definitions and Physician Perception." *BMC Family Practice* 7: 73. doi:10.1186/1471-2296-7-73

Femi, Hajjaj, Sam Salek, M. Basra, and Andrew Finlay. 2010. "Non-Clinical Influences on Clinical Decision-Making: A Major Challenge to Evidence-Based Practice." *Journal of the Royal Society of Medicine* 103 (5): 178–187. doi:10.1258/jrsm.2010.100104

Glass, Joseph, Paul Rathouz, Maurice Gattis, Young Joo, Jennifer Nelson, and Emily Williams. 2017. "Intersections of Poverty, Race/Ethnicity, and Sex: Alcohol Consumption and Adverse Outcomes in the United States." *Social Psychiatry and Psychiatric Epidemiology* 52 (5): 515–524. doi:10.1007/s00127-017-1362-4

Grober, Ethan, and John Bohnen. 2005. "Defining Medical Error." *Canadian Journal of Surgery. Journal* 48 (1): 39–44.

Harrington, Maxine. 2005. "Revisiting Medical Error: Five Years After the IOM Report, Have Reporting Systems Made a Measurable Difference." *Health Matrix* 15: 329–382.

Institute of Medicine. 2000. *To Err is Human: Building a Safer Health System.* Washington, DC: The National Academies Press. https://doi.org/10.17226/9728.

Kephart, George, and Yukiko Asada. 2001. "Need-Based Resource Allocation: Different Need Indicators, Different Results?" *BMC Health Services Research* 9 (122): 21. doi:10.1186/1472-6963-9-122

Kinney, Eleanor. 2004. "The Origins and Promise of Medical Standards of Care." *Virtual Mentor* 6 (12): 574–576. doi:10.1001/virtualmentor.2004.6.12.mhst1-0412

Mello, Michelle, David Studdert, Eric Thomas, Catherine Yoon, and Troyen Brennan. 2007. "Who Pays for Medical Errors? An Analysis of Adverse Event Costs, the Medical Liability System, and Incentives for Patient Safety Improvement." *Journal of Empirical Leal Studies* 4 (4): 835–869. https://doi.org/10.1111/j.1740-1461.2007.00108.x

Mills, Don. 1978. "Medical Insurance Feasibility Study. A Technical Summary." *Western Journal of Medicine* 128 (4): 360–365.

Moffett, Peter, and Gregory Moore. 2011. "The Standard of Care: Legal History and Definitions: The Bad and Good News." *Western Journal of Emergency Medicine* 12 (1): 109–112.

Morreim, Haavi. 1989. "Stratified Scarcity: Redefining the Standard of Care." *Law, Medicine and Health Care* 17 (4): 356–367.

Mukamel, Dana, Jack Zwanziger, and Anil Bamezai. 2002. "Hospital Competition, Resource Allocation and Quality of Care." *BMC Health Services Research* 2 (1): 10. doi:10.1186/1472-6963-2-10

Poplin, Caroline. 2017. "Why Medicine is Not Manufacturing." *New England Journal of Medicine Catalyst*. Retrieved from https://catalyst.nejm.org/medicine-not-manufacturing-business/

Spencer, Christine, Darrell Gaskin, and Eric Roberts. 2013. "The Quality of Care Delivered to Patients Within the Same Hospital Varies By Insurance Type." *Health Affairs* 32 (10): 1731–1839.

Stevens, R. 1991. "The Role of Ondansetron in Paediatric Patients: A Review of Three Studies." *European Journal of Cancer* 27 (S1): S20–22.

Stewart, David, Simone Dahrouge, Doug Coyle, and William Evans. 1999. "Costs of Treating and Preventing Nausea and Vomiting in Patients Receiving Chemotherapy." *Journal of Clinical Oncology* 17 (1): 344–344.

Tanneberger, S., G. Lelli, A. Martoni, E. Piana, and F. Pannuti. 1992. "The Antiemetic Efficacy and the Cost-Benefit Ratio of Ondansetron Calculated with a New Approach to Health Technology Assessment (Real Cost-Benefit Index)." *Journal of Chemotherapy* 4 (5): 326–331.

Tello, Monique. "Racism, Discrimination, and Healthcare." *Harvard Health Blog*. January 16, 2017. Retrieved from www.health.harvard.edu/blog/racism-discrimination-health-care-providers-patients-2017011611015.

Thomas, Eric, and Troyen Brennan. 2000. "Incidence and Types of Preventable Adverse Events in Elderly Patients: Population Based Review of Medical Records" *BMJ* 320: 741.

U.S. Department of Health and Human Services. Agency for Healthcare Research and Quality. 2018. "Advancing Patient Safety." Retrieved from www.ahrq.gov/professionals/quality-patient-safety/patient-safety-resources/resources/advancing-patient-safety/index.html.

U.S. Department of Health and Human Services. Agency for Healthcare Research and Quality. 2019. "Adverse Events, Near Misses, and Errors." *PSNet*. Retrieved from https://psnet.ahrq.gov/primers/primer/34/Adverse-Events-Near-Misses-and-Errors.

10 The Harm of Ableism
Medical Error and Epistemic Injustice[1]

Joel Michael Reynolds and David Peña-Guzmán

Introduction

Improper diagnosis and treatment due to medical error lead to tens of thousands of deaths every year (Makary and Daniel 2016). While there is a significant body of research analyzing the nature, causes, and effects of medical error as well as the effectiveness of various error-reduction strategies (IOM 2000), the medical error literature has historically undertheorized a specific kind of error—namely, epistemic error—that is brought about by epistemic schemas linked to group- or identity-based biases based upon categories such as race, sex, gender, sexuality, and disability. In this chapter, we turn to the field of social epistemology with the double aim of filling this gap in the literature as well as better understanding the role that epistemic schemas play in the production of medical errors that disproportionately affect patients from marginalized social groups.

Our argument moves in three stages. First, we sketch dominant taxonomies of medical error, define what we mean by "epistemic schema" and "epistemic error," and situate our project in the context of the larger literature on epistemic injustice. Second, we look at the socially uneven distribution of epistemic error by using ableism as a case study. Ableism, which we here define as an epistemic schema, plays a pernicious role in patient–provider communication (PPC). It distorts communication between non-disabled physicians and disabled patients, subjecting the latter to various forms of epistemic injustice and exposing them to a higher risk of medical error and, consequently, harm. Our analysis of this case study will demonstrate that even though the possibility of medical error impacts everyone, it does not impact everyone *equally*. Socially vulnerable patients, such as disabled patients, are more likely to be affected by it. Finally, we contend that medical errors due to epistemic schemas rooted in prejudice, such as ableism, are issues of justice that must be addressed at all levels of health-care practice. We offer this analysis in the hope of clarifying the role epistemic schemas play in the production of medical errors and reducing the number of lives hurt or lost in their wake.

Kinds of Medical Error

Medical errors take many forms. To better understand them and to assist in efforts to reduce their frequency, researchers have developed various taxonomies of medical error, most of which are based on their causes or effects. For example, taxonomies that carve the joints of medical error along the lines of effect often classify errors as *fatal, life threatening, serious,* or *significant.* Meanwhile, those that track differences in origin produce rather different tables of elements. Taking this approach, for instance, Aronson (2009) classifies medical errors as *knowledge-based, rule-based, action-based,* or *memory-based.*[2]

Taxonomies are powerful resources that help us conceptualize phenomena in specific ways and frame how we think about issues. Like all conceptual resources, however, taxonomies come with limitations. Taxonomies of medical error that focus on effects, for example, can be misleading because not all medical errors have observable consequences. "Many errors," as Weingart, Wilson, Gibberd, and Harrison note, "do not produce injury; they are caught in time, the patient is resilient, or luck is good" (2000, 390). Similarly, taxonomies based on origin can misconstrue or entirely miss errors that are multi-factorial or whose source of origin is either unknown or hard to discern.

In this chapter, we focus on the specific kind of error that Aronson (2009) describes as "knowledge-based." Knowledge-based medical errors result, in one way or another, from deficient knowledge on the part of providers. As Aronson defines them, these errors involve "any type of knowledge, general, specific, or expert."

> It is *general knowledge* that penicillin can cause allergic reactions; knowing that your patient is allergic to penicillin is *specific knowledge*; knowing that co-fluampicil contains penicillin is *expert knowledge*. Ignorance of any of these facts could lead to a knowledge-based error.
>
> (2009, 603)

For Aronson, a central way doctors can inadvertently harm their patients is by failing to know or otherwise being ignorant about things that they ought to know at the moment they ought to know them. This could be due to a lack of true beliefs about X or due to the possession of false beliefs about X. In the example Aronson gives, one might not know that a patient is allergic to penicillin or one might falsely believe that a patient isn't allergic to it. In the literature on medical error, knowledge-based failings such as these are typically referred to as "epistemic errors."

Even though epistemic errors are frequently referenced in this literature, they are often equated with what we call "factical errors," which are errors that stem from the lack or the misapplication of information.

Factical errors occur, for example, when not all the medically relevant information provided by a patient is made available to all the medical experts said patient interacts with at different stages of care, when information is missing from key medical spaces at key medical moments (as when a drug container does not specify that a drug must be diluted), or when providers are ignorant of new research, methods, or protocols. We call these errors "factical" because they pertain to the possession or non-possession of relevant facts and beliefs and not, as is the case with "schematic errors," to cognitive and perceptual habits.

The unstated assumption in much of the extant literature on medical error seems to be that if experts knew all the relevant facts, then they would not make errors. We disagree with this assumption, for not all epistemic errors are factical in nature. Surely, medical errors can occur based on *what providers know*, but one of our chief claims in this chapter is that medical errors also depend on *how providers know*. It is a mistake, therefore, to equate epistemic errors with factical errors since these categories are related but not co-extensive; the latter is a subset of the former. All factical errors, in other words, are epistemic; but not all epistemic errors are factical. To improve medical practices and institutions, we must attend to the plurality of medical error types and recognize that different types of errors have different causes and effects. Epistemic errors in particular require us to look not only at the information that is available to medical providers at various moments, but also at the broader social character of medicine because the production, operationalization, and dissemination of medical knowledge is a social and relational process that goes beyond the brute application of facts. When it comes to the epistemology of medicine, factical errors are only the tip of the medical iceburg.

Schematic Errors: Beyond Medical Facts

Over the last few decades, social epistemology has emerged as a burgeoning field of philosophical inquiry. On the whole, the field is based on the premise that knowledge is fundamentally social, which is to say, produced, shared, interpreted, and transmitted through complex human practices, interactions, and institutions. This insight, which grew primarily out of feminist scholarship on the relationship between knowledge and power, can help us make sense of those medical errors that cannot be traced to purely factical concerns and that involve *how*, rather than *what*, providers know. We call these errors "schematic" rather than "factical" because they are outgrowths of *epistemic schemas* that shape the larger processes, judgments, and pool of hermeneutic resources upon which providers draw. Epistemic schemas are thereby central to how medical providers position themselves relative to their patients and, as we explore later in this chapter, this can have especially significant ramifications for patients who are perceived to be unlike a provider in different regards, especially patients who come from historically marginalized social groups.

The concept of a schema has been widely and variably used in linguistics, cognitive psychology, the philosophy of mind, and even the philosophy of science. In this context, we understand epistemic schemas simultaneously as "manifold cognitive structures exerting influence over memory encoding and retrieval" (Ghosh and Gilboa 2014) and structures which make it possible for epistemic agents to arrive at "shared meanings or frames of reference" (Dotson 2012; cf. Bartunek and Moch 1987). Epistemic schemas, then, are constellations of implicit and explicit values, norms, biases, impulses, desires, fantasies, and assumptions that condition what counts as knowledge, who counts as a knower, and how knowledge claims are interpreted, assessed, and adjudicated within a given epistemic community.[3] At once perceptual, cognitive, and hermeneutical, they are structures that shape how epistemic agents participate in the life of a community by making, sharing, interpreting, and communicating knowledge claims. And because they influence how we experience, reflect upon, and communicate information about the world we share with others, these schemas are more than simple biases or habits. Yet, like biases and habits, epistemic schemas are often implicit rather than explicit, meaning that typically most of us are unaware of the pull they exert over our thoughts, actions, and ways of knowing and the various ways in which we have been socialized into them.

Our use of the concept of an "epistemic schema" is thus related to concepts such as "body schema" and "gender schemas" that denote how networks of information are interpreted through a dynamic process of filtering and framing (Bem 1981; Johnson 1987). By definition, schemas are information-filtering mechanisms that downgrade the import of some information whilst amplifying and prioritizing the significance of other information. But they aren't passive sieves that merely let (some) information pass. They are also meaning-making processes that present information in a certain light, that frame the information they themselves filter in sense-conferring ways. This is why we ought to think of epistemic schemas as meaning-making mechanisms that have a significant influence on how people think about themselves (personal identity dynamics) and their place in larger social formations (in-group/out-group dynamics).

Epistemic schemas can grow out of religious, philosophical, and even scientific worldviews, but the ones that interest us here are tied to social markers of identity, such as race, ethnicity, gender, sex, sexuality, class, and disability, among others. Racism, for instance, is a social, material, and political reality that profoundly affects the lives of racial minorities and shapes the larger society as a whole. It can also function as an epistemic schema in our sense of the term because it also affects how differently racialized agents *think about* and communicate with one another. Racism, understood as an epistemic schema, structures how one knows, what one knows, which voices and bodies of knowledge one includes or excludes and how, and, more broadly, the ways one engages in the world as a knower, as an organism who gathers, processes, judges, and communicates *about* its experiences to itself and others. Although schemas such as racism and sexism do not offer an ordered interpretation of *all* one's experiences, they can determine—and, in some cases, wildly over-determine—how epistemic agents interact with one another as knowers, which is to say, how they interpret the meaning, validity, and force of one another's claims. That is to say, although they may appear to be domain specific, their impact easily bleeds into all sorts of knowing activities. And, while not all epistemic schemas are rooted in prejudices of these sorts, those that are, typically lead to epistemic injustice.

One reason epistemic schemas, and especially those rooted in prejudice, are so powerful and recalcitrant is because they reinforce epistemic ignorance, which is to say, modes of knowing that *depend* upon ignorance concerning others and the world in such a manner as to maintain the privileges of the knower.[4] Historically, philosophers have understood ignorance quite simply as the absence of knowledge. Recent work in epistemology, much of which heavily draws upon past feminist and anti-racist work, suggests instead that ignorance may be better defined as "the other side of knowledge" (Mills 2010; see Alcoff 2007, 18ff) because there are cases when someone's ignorance is predicated upon, and a boon for, extant social injustices. Put simply, what one is ignorant of is no simple matter and does not absolve one from culpability. On the contrary, ignorance is shot through with ethical, social, and political choices that carry profound effects. Epistemic ignorance, this literature demonstrates, is a driver of epistemic injustice; it leads to harms against marginalized groups and individuals in their capacity as knowers. That is to say, fundamentally prejudicial epistemic schemas such as those of racism, sexism, and ableism are problems not just because of the way they lead epistemic agents to know, but also because of the way they lead agents *not* to know. Ignorance can be just as unjust, if not more so, than unjust forms of knowing.

In these cases, then, it would be inaccurate to describe ignorance as an innocent lack of knowledge and more accurate to talk about it as the controlled effect of a system of power that actively seeks to keep certain things *un-known*. As Linda Alcoff notes, "the study and analysis of [epistemic] ignorance poses some special epistemological questions beyond the expected sociological and educational ones, questions having to do with how we understand the intersection between cognitive norms, structural privilege, and situated identities" (Alcoff 2007, 39). In what follows, we explore the role epistemic schemas play in fostering epistemic ignorance through the case of ableism. We demonstrate that ableism, understood as an epistemic schema, leads to medical error by fostering epistemic ignorance rooted in privilege and prejudice on the part of health-care providers, and we use research on PPC with respect to patients with disabilities to illustrate our point.

Case Study: Ableism

While the philosophical literature on social epistemology has made significant strides in exposing how systems of oppression, such as racism and sexism (Song et al. 2014), mold people's experience of medical care, this literature has paid comparatively little attention to ableism, aside from the notable exceptions we discuss in detail here. In this section, our principal objective is to show that ableism affects the quality of care that people with disabilities receive by exposing them to a higher-than-average risk of medical error and, consequently, medical harm. Given that (a) people with disabilities make up the largest legally protected minority group of health-care users and given that (b) the types of epistemic ignorance associated with the schema of ableism and the epistemic injustices that result from it lead to people with disabilities being impacted by medical error disproportionately, this is a serious lacuna.

One of the chief ways that ableism brings about this regrettable state of affairs is by undermining effective patient–provider communication (PPC), which is to say, by generating communication failures between disabled patients and their typically non-disabled providers.[5] An important caveat is in order here: Because empirical research on ableism and PPC is scarce, much of our analysis will be speculative in nature. Hence, in articulating some of the mechanisms by means of which ableism warps PPC, we take ourselves to be hypothesizing, rather than proving, a potential causal connection between these terms, and we take ourselves to be calling for further empirical research that might confirm or deny our hypothesis. More than anything, we offer this analysis in the hope of providing a research program for other medical humanists, clinical researchers, and social scientists to pursue in greater detail.

One of the reasons there is such little research on the subject of ableism, PPC, and medical error is because of the lack of dialog between two bodies of research: the medical literature on PPC and the fields of disability studies and philosophy of disability.[6] On the one hand, the medical literature on PPC is extensive, but comparatively little of it deals specifically with disability. That which does, however, typically doesn't deal with ableism understood as an epistemic schema that affects both *what* and *how* providers "know" disability and interact with people with disabilities as epistemic agents. On the other hand, since at least the 1980s, experts spanning the humanities and social sciences who work in disability studies have shown that ableism harms people with disabilities in a number of ways (see, e.g., Shakespeare 2014; Wong 2009). For example, it harms them economically (e.g., by contributing to discrimination in employment and housing opportunities), socially (e.g., by contributing to their exclusion from public spaces and social interaction), and politically (e.g., by contributing to their denial of sound political representation and equal rights). Yet, what these experts have not documented in an equally nuanced manner is how the harm of ableism manifests itself in relation to medical error. When medical experts investigate misdiagnosis patterns, failures in PPC, and the causes of low patient satisfaction, among other things, they rarely investigate it along the lines of disability and specifically with respect to ableism understood as an epistemic schema. The result is a gap in the literature that demands rectification. This chapter is a first step in tackling this lacuna by demonstrating the central and general role of epistemic schemas in poor PPC leading to medical errors and, second, by arguing more specifically that ableism is a significant contributor to poor PPC with patients with disabilities.

Poor PPC Leads to Preventable Medical Error

Since at least the 1980s, it has been well established in the medical communication literature that PPC plays a key role in determining health outcomes (Stewart and Roter 1989; Kaplan, Greenfield, and Ware 1989; Stewart 1995). A vast body of clinical and social-scientific research shows that effective communication between patients and providers leads to *better* health outcomes (Street, Makoul, Arora, and Epstein 2009)[7] and that, conversely, poor communication harms patients, increasing the likelihood of medical error. Indeed, studies of semi-structured interviews between patients and providers (Sutcliffe, Lewton, and Rosenthal 2004) and of medical malpractice lawsuits (Beckman, Markakis, Suchman, and Frankel 1994; Vincent, Young, and Phillips 1994; Hickson et al. 2002; Huntington and Kuhn 2003) overwhelmingly suggest that, while not the only variable in play, breakdowns in PPC lie at the heart of the problem of error in medicine.

Communication failure—which includes any situation in which what Alvarez and Coiera (2006) dub "the communication space" of medicine is diminished, obfuscated, or obstructed—leads to medical error in at least two ways. First, whenever an encounter between patient and provider is not conducive to mutual understanding, patients are less likely to be forthcoming about their symptoms and concerns. This may be because they do not feel comfortable enough to share them with their physician or because they don't understand what might count as medically relevant information and what might not. Either way, communicational failure reduces the amount and quality of diagnostically relevant information that a medical expert receives from the patient. Even in cases where patients have a condition for which an objective diagnostic test exists, diminished communication can threaten the diagnostic moment. As anyone with clinical experience will attest, not all salient information can be gleaned from diagnostic tests, and even information that can be gleaned from them cannot always be properly interpreted in the absence of patient input (Wanzer, Booth-Butterfield, and Gruber 2004; Stewart et al. 2000).

Second, poor PPC can destroy the trust that patients need to have in providers in order for the clinical encounter to run smoothly. Although many people think of the experience of going to the doctor as a one-off event that exists largely in isolation, this is rarely the case. Much of the time medical care is a protracted process that requires multiple visits to the clinic, interaction with testing laboratories, and even more encounters between the patient and what at times appears to be an interminable flow of medical knowers (nurse practitioners, residents, physician assistants, etc.). For this entire process to work, patients and providers must build a framework of trust that enables them to recognize each other as partners in a mutually reciprocal relationship. Unfortunately, poor PPC erodes this trust by making patients feel unheard and under-valued, as if the very experts on whom they depend do not see them as persons to be cared for but as names on a list to be crossed off (Neumann et al. 2009, 342). A trusting relationship between patient and provider determines the extent to which patients listen to what doctors say, whether or not they adhere to medication protocols, and even whether or not they seek out care when non-emergency medical incidents arise again in the future. Trust, in short, has a substantial effect on the quality of care and on overall health outcomes. Repairing that trust after it has been broken is no easy task (Berlinger 2005). The feelings of desperation, isolation, and frustration experienced by patients who report poor PPC eat away at the mutual trust that is the bedrock of medical practice.

Although medical error can change people's experience of the healthcare system for the worse and corrode their trust in this system, it also kills morale among health-care providers, which research shows further compromises quality of care (Kohn 2001). And, most importantly, it harms patients in tangible, and sometimes horrendous, ways. The medical error literature is replete with illustrations of the catastrophic effects medical errors can have on patients, which range from intense physical and psychological suffering (on account of, say, having the wrong leg amputated) to severe chronic illness or death (on account of, say, being systematically misdiagnosed) (IOM 2000).

Ableism as an Epistemic Schema

Within both social epistemology and medical error research, the concept of ableism is rarely utilized to understand the types of epistemic injustices and harms pertinent to people with disabilities. This claim is true both with respect to studies examining epistemic injustice in relation to mental illness (Crichton, Carel, and Kidd 2017; Sanati and Kyratsous 2015; Kurs and Grinshpoon 2018; Dohmen 2016) and those that discuss a wider range of disability experiences (Reiheld 2010; Ho 2011; Li 2016; Buchman, Ho, and Goldberg 2017; Tremain 2017; Scully 2018). Even in the philosophy of disability, the concept of ableism sometimes plays a secondary analytic role. For example, in *The Minority Body* Elizabeth Barnes defines ableism not in terms of an epistemic schema, but as "social prejudice and stigma directed against the disabled in virtue of the fact that they are disabled" (2016, 5).[8] More often than not, she deploys the term as a way to understand counterfactual claims about the badness of disability in a world without ableism (2016, see esp. 59, 66, 92, and 163). While ableism certainly involves prejudice and stigma, we hope to show it involves much more than that.

Especially insofar as our knowledge about people invariably involves assessments of and knowledge about their abilities, ableism, we argue in this section, can regularly impact how we interact with others as epistemic agents. In other words, because ability expectations are central to the conception of any given individual, ableism serves to determine *in essential ways* how and what people know and don't know about their own experiences and that of others. It is in light of the breadth and depth of ableism's impact that we suggest research on epistemic justice, medical error, and their connection would be improved through a greater focus on ableism and the ways in which it functions as an epistemic schema.

With respect to its role as an epistemic schema, we will use the term *ableism* to mean the assumption that forms of embodiment considered "abnormal" are necessarily experienced both differently and negatively in comparison to forms of embodiment considered "normal." Ableism functions as a framework for preemptively knowing about the abilities and ability expectations of bodies based upon their perceived disability status, including even *what it is like* to have a particular body and mind. Ableism leads providers to *other* patients with disabilities.[9] Like racism and sexism, the concept of ableism involves both descriptive and normative aspects. Ableism is a way of understanding the quality, meaning, value, and differences of human life through the lens of abilities and ability expectations shaped via socially dominant conceptions of normality. While the idea of normality is historically and culturally variable, in modern medical contexts it takes on a far more specific meaning (Cryle and Stephens 2017; Davis 2013).[10] Modern medicine invariably makes assumptions about "normal" bodily shape, size, motion, and function. It also perforce makes specific assumptions based upon statistical analyses of bodily metrics, ranging from those that determine everything from "normal" blood pressure to "normal" levels of anxiety.

Part of what is so pernicious about the way ableism functions inside of medical institutions and across various domains of medical practice is the way that it forecloses upon the vast range of meanings of disability as a fact of human life as well as the vast range of discrete disability experiences. The term "disability" is notoriously hard to define, serving to cover everything from Albinism to cystic fibrosis to autism to deafness to short stature to ADHD. Ableism flattens out these differences in deeply problematic ways.

Consider that since the origins of the field of disability studies in the 1980s, a core distinction has been made between medical and social models of disability. On the medical model, disability is a personal tragedy or hardship resulting from a congenital abnormality, environmental accident, or result of old age. In other words, disability is a bad thing that befalls one. On social models of disability (sometimes erroneously referred to as *the* social model), a core distinction is made between "disability" and "impairment." One is impaired insofar as one's body is different in ways that impact one's ability to function in the world as compared to most people. One is disabled, however, insofar as one is negatively impacted by the treatment of others on account of one's impairment, including impacts due to larger societal norms and institutions. What is crucial about social models of disability is the way they point to the social, cultural, political, and historical factors that shape how one is treated, including how one is treated by medical experts on account of one's particular body and mind.[11]

Ableism persists in medical contexts especially through the dominance of the medical model of disability inside of medical education, ranging from pre-med to residency to continuing education and spanning across all manner of medical institutes and centers (Iezzoni and O'Day 2006; Iezzoni 2006; Reynolds 2018). Insofar as medical providers assume that a disabled patient is automatically a person dealing with a personal tragedy or hardship, they operate with an epistemic schema that results in them pre-judging and mis-judging their patients. The epistemic schema of ableism leads providers to not only misunderstand the lived experience of their disabled patients, but also to think that they *know* what being disabled is like.[12]

Ableism thus leads to epistemic ignorance about disability in multiple respects and to epistemic injustices as a result. As we will discuss in greater detail in the next section, it leads providers to dismiss and remain ignorant of the qualitatively distinct differences between different kinds of disabilities, to exhibit overconfidence concerning claims about disability experience in general as well as specific types of disability, and to distrust, discredit, or otherwise dismiss people with disabilities as experts about their own experiences and that of their communities. The negative effects of the epistemic schema of ableism are manifold. To better understand the effects of this epistemic schema, we will now turn to lay out the four principal mechanisms by means of which ableism undermines PPC.

Ableism's Impact on PPC: Four Mechanisms

Let us begin by observing that we already know that PPC failures are more common when it comes to people with disabilities (Blackstone

2015; Nordness and Beukelman 2017) and that patients with disabilities suffer more misdiagnoses than non-disabled patients. For example, people with intellectual and developmental disabilities are systematically misdiagnosed (Mastroianni and Miaskoff 1997). Well into at least the 1990s, people with moderate hearing loss were misdiagnosed as "mentally retarded" (Berke 2007). Today, people with cerebral palsy "are at three times the risk of experiencing adverse events as compared with adults without preexisting communication vulnerabilities" (Hemsley and Balandin 2014; Nordness and Beukelman 2017). Meanwhile, physical impairments are regularly underdiagnosed in people with intellectual disabilities (Kiani and Miller 2010), as are cognitive impairments in people with spinal cord injury (Tolonen et al. 2007). All this we know. What we need to investigate further is *how* these failures in communication and misdiagnoses come into being and interact with one another. What causes these breakdowns in PPC and produces such an asymmetrical distribution of the possibility of error along the lines of disability? We argued earlier that the answer turns on the dominant schema through which people without disabilities "see" and "know" disability, which is to say, the schema of ableism. Ableism brings about these disastrous effects by means of at least four mechanisms.

The first is what Fricker (2007) calls *testimonial injustice.* This is a form of epistemic injustice wherein a speaker's testimony is unfairly downgraded in credibility thanks to a prejudice on the hearer's part. Put otherwise, testimonial injustice occurs when a social agent does not take someone else's testimony as credible *because of the social identity of the testifier.* This kind of injustice treats its targets as agents incapable of contributing to a community's shared knowledge resources, an injustice which is associated with treating them as lacking the very capacity to reason—a feature typically (although problematically) held to be central to the attribution of personhood (Fricker 2007, 44; Scully 2018, 111). The social epistemology literature has produced a number of illustrations of testimonial injustice, such as the (historical) case of the black slave whose testimony was not seen as authoritative in American courts unless "validated" by the testimony of a white man or the case of the female rape victim whose testimony is not believed by the males in her life simply because those men impute onto women a credibility deficit concerning sexual violence.

Testimonial injustice occurs in medical spaces when, for example, a doctor holds a group-based belief that black people have higher pain thresholds than those who are not black (Hoffman, Trawalter, Axt, and Oliver 2016). In doing so, they commit a testimonial injustice against their black patients by discounting the validity of their testimony concerning the extent and quality of pain they are experiencing. Similarly, a disabled person with a mobility impairment suffers from an arbitrary credibility deficit when medical knowers, for example, discount their testimony concerning the specific reason they entered the clinic ("I've got a recurring rash I think is due to an allergic reaction"), focusing instead on their impairment and tying diagnosis solely to it ("it's probably from rubbing up against your wheelchair"). That example is not an innocent instance of misunderstanding because the person with a disability is being "seen" through the schema of ableism. On that schema, being disabled means being *worse off* by virtue of one's disability, and so even information that is not clearly related to an impairment (a spinal cord issue) can easily become a *reason* for potentially any medical issue (including a rash). By not treating the person as a full-fledged epistemic agent, but instead interpreting them through an ableist lens, their testimony ("I've got a recurring rash I think is due to an allergic reaction") is down-graded in credibility. As this happens more frequently, mistrust on the part of the patient increases. Testimonial injustice, then, is not simply a phenomenon that occurs interpersonally. Insofar as it results from epistemic schemas that track historically oppressed groups and that depends upon prejudicial knowledge and forms of knowing, patterns of testimonial injustice can be systemic and pervasive. These patterns can become historically entrenched within the social, political, cultural, and even economic norms of a community.[13]

According to Jackie Leach Scully, medical experts often ascribe "a global epistemic incapacity to people affected by impairment" because they assume that any disability, whether cognitive or physical, manifests itself as an incapacity to engage in meaningful dialog with non-disabled agents (Scully 2018). In one of the few, but growing number of studies of epistemic injustice in health care, Carel and Kidd (2014) contend that medical professionals frequently and presumptively attribute "characteristics like cognitive unreliability and emotional instability" to people with disabilities in ways that "downgrade the credibility of [the] testimonies [of people with disabilities]."

This is confirmed by research in disability studies and the philosophy of disability. For example, in *The Meaning of Illness: A Phenomenological Account of the Different Perspectives of Physician and Patient*, S. Kay Toombs describes her experience of going to the doctor in a wheelchair and with her husband (Toombs 1992; see also 1987). She reports that people would talk to her husband as if she wasn't there, assuming that being in a wheelchair meant she was non-verbal. This feeling of not having one's word be heard by those in positions of power is quite widespread among people with disabilities, which indicates that ableism brings about the regular disregard of the knowledge claims (testimony) and lived experiences (phenomenology) of people with disability. Smith (2009) claims that people from all over the disability spectrum report a feeling of invisibility in medical spaces. "Those with a disability," he writes,

> are significantly more likely than persons without a disability to perceive that the physician does not listen to them, does not explain

treatment so that they understand, does not treat them with respect, does not spend enough time with them, and does not involve them in treatment decisions.

(206, cf. 213–14)

And the invisibility is not just social (i.e., feeling that medical experts do not recognize one's presence in a shared environment), but also testimonial (i.e., feeling that these experts simply do not take one's word as meaningful or consequential even when they elicit it directly). A good example of this is a recent study that concluded that medical experts overwhelmingly *do not* believe the testimony of people with chronic fatigue syndrome (Blease, Carel, and Geraghty 2017). This problem takes on a particularly acute form when it comes to people with communicative disabilities (Hemsley and Balandin 2014).

A second mechanism through which ableism bankrupts PPC is what Cassam (2017) calls *epistemic overconfidence*.[14] We have seen that ableism produces credibility deficits for people with disabilities, which results in an imbalance between social agents on the basis of disability status. This imbalance is compounded by another factor that is not unique to disability, but that has unique implications for it given the way that disability is often seen solely via a medical lens, which is the credibility excess medical experts enjoy as a matter of course.[15] We habitually extend long lines of epistemic credit to medical experts, especially physicians; we assume that they must know what they are talking about even in cases where the evidence points to the contrary. In some sense, of course, it makes sense that we would give medical experts a credibility excess in medical settings since the reason we go to see a doctor is precisely because we assume that the doctor's knowledge of health and illness far outstrips our own.

The problem is that doctors often internalize this epistemic privilege riding on the back of their expert status to such a degree that it can mutate into epistemic overconfidence. This term refers to an excess of self-assurance about what one knows and how far their knowledge extends. Epistemic overconfidence impedes the ability of doctors to exercise the kinds of epistemic self-monitoring we expect of them and that is expected of them by their own profession. It can lead to medical error by making experts less likely to question first intuitions, to request further diagnostic tests, to entertain alternative hypotheses, to consider referring patients to other specialists, to get a second opinion, to reflect more critically about social conditions and determinates of health, and so on—all of which can culminate in a misdiagnosis and can serve to undermine trust with a patient. In short, it produces in experts an active ignorance that blocks them from recognizing the limits of their own knowledge and its impact on care.

For example, it has been reported that epilepsy is regularly misdiagnosed among people with intellectual disabilities because doctors cannot tell the difference between epileptic events and non-epileptic self-stimulatory events (Chapman et al. 2011). Yet, the problem is not necessarily that doctors *don't know* how tell the difference per se. The problem is that they often *don't know that they don't know* how to tell the difference and jump straight to a diagnosis when they should be getting a second opinion, discussing things further with the patient, more substantively educating themselves about epilepsy as well as about various expressions of certain sorts of intellectual disability, or referring the patient to a more qualified expert.

As Cassam (2017) formulates it, epistemic overconfidence can affect all patients independently of disability status. But we argue that ableism amplifies it in particular ways. Consider the so-called "disability paradox." This term refers to the fact that non-disabled people rate the quality of life of people with disabilities significantly lower than people with disabilities do. As Albrecht and Devlieger formulate the paradox: "why do many people with serious and persistent disabilities report that they experience a good or excellent quality of life when to most external observers these individuals seem to live an undesirable daily existence?" (1999, 977). One would expect that among non-disabled people, health-care providers would buck this trend since presumably their expert knowledge of medicine translates to a better understanding of impairment than the average person. But the exact opposite turns out to be true. Medical experts have an inaccurate perception of the quality of life of disabled people and systematically rate the quality of life *lower* than the average non-disabled person does (Basnett 2001).[16] What's more, because of their expert status, medical practitioners are unlikely to call into question their own assumptions, which are continuously reinforced by the medical model of disability in which they have been reared and to which in most cases they remain committed. Research concerning the disability paradox suggests that doctors often walk into a consultation with fixed and fundamentally flawed assumptions about disability.

Bioethicist Anita Ho argues that this disability-specific overconfidence on the part of experts puts disabled patients in a dangerous Catch-22 situation in which (i) they may put themselves at risk if they do not trust their doctors (given that trust correlates with positive outcomes) and, somewhat paradoxically, (ii) they may put themselves at even higher risk if they *do* trust them (since trusting an epistemically overconfident expert can lead to harm). "Trust may increase epistemic oppression and perpetuate the vulnerability of people with impairments" (Ho 2011). A doctor who believes that he or she is the leading authority on disability even when a disabled person is in the room may put this patient in harm's way, even if unintentionally. Ho continues:

> While more empirical evidence is necessary to ascertain the multiple determinants of patients' dissatisfaction, numerous studies show

that [health care providers] continue to hold negative attitudes and assumptions toward impairments and the quality of life of people living with these impairments. Reported negative attitudes raise questions of whether these patients can take professionals' proclaimed good will for granted.

(2011, 113)

When the good will of the medical expert can no longer be taken for granted, all bets are off for people with disabilities. How could one, in good faith, ask disabled patients to put their trust, perhaps even their lives, in the hands of a provider who believes that their quality of life is poor anyways *and* who is so confident about this belief that they see no point in even putting it up for debate? This has serious ramifications not just for particular providers, but for medicine as a whole. As Grasswick (2018) has argued, when an institution such as medicine has historically failed members of a specific community, the latter have good reasons to mistrust the institution as a whole even if they don't necessarily mistrust the particular individuals who represent it.

To be clear, it may be true that a provider has more medical information about a particular impairment and rightfully considers themselves to be an expert in that sense—but medical information is wholly insufficient to understand the *lived experience* of a person with a particular impairment, an experience saturated with social, cultural, political, and historical complexities typically untouched by even the best and most capacious forms of medical education. It is the transferal of confidence in medical knowledge concerning impairments to confidence in knowledge concerning the *meaningfulness* of living with a given impairment that helps produce epistemic overconfidence.

A third mechanism operative in medical spaces is *epistemic erasure*. Epistemic erasure functions by removing entire categories or swaths of hermeneutical resources from a communicative space where they would otherwise reside because the speaker's perceived social identity is erroneously thought to render those subjects categorically inapplicable.[17] In the case of disabled patients, epistemic erasure vitiates communication by removing entire subjects of possible medical interest from conversation and thereby foreclosing from the outset certain avenues of dialog that might not have been foreclosed in the absence of disability.

Consider sexual health. One of the ways in which ableism operates is by turning people with disabilities into objects of pity, which is often accomplished through the de-sexualization of disabled bodies.[18] In light of this de-sexualization, many abled-bodied individuals express surprise or even shock upon learning that disabled people have typical sex drives and lead fully active sex lives. Health-care providers are not exempt from this way of thinking and, like the rest of the population, tend to de-sexualize people with disabilities (Wieseler forthcoming).

This prejudice is likely to rear its ugly head in the personal lives of providers, including in the choices they make about who counts for them as a possible object of romantic or sexual interest and who doesn't. But this prejudice will also rear its head in their professional lives as it may cause them *not to* pose certain questions, such as questions concerning sexual health, to their disabled patients even if said questions are typically routine. As Shakespeare, Iezzoni, and Groce (2009) note, "by assuming that people with disabilities are not sexually active, physicians may exclude them from health information or screening that non-disabled people receive as a matter of course—for example, for sexually transmitted diseases, cervical cancer, or HIV." Of course, the de-sexualization of disabled bodies is offensive. But it is medically dangerous, too. The route from epistemic erasure to medical error is both *direct* and *indirect.* Directly, we can say that epistemic erasure does not *lead* to medical error but is itself an expression of it. Indirectly, it leads to medical error in the same way testimonial injustice does—that is to say, by limiting the information patients are called upon to provide as well as that which they feel comfortable in providing, and, consequently, the sorts of diagnoses providers are in a position to make.[19]

People with disabilities often report being treated by abled-bodied individuals as objects of a violent and voracious curiosity, as "freaks" to be looked at and gazed upon (Garland-Thomson 1996). This is because ableism teaches non-disabled people to "reduce" people with disabilities to their disabilities, thereby objectifying them. In the perceptual field of one under the sway of ableism, a person with epilepsy registers simply as an epileptic object, a blind person as a walking cane on the precipice of danger, and a person in a wheelchair as one "confined" and "bound" to ever-limited self- or other-pushing. As van de Ven, Post, de Witte, and van den Heuvel (2005) point out, sometimes the only way to explain able-bodied people's behavior in the presence of disability is to assume that, somehow, "they only see the disability and not the person behind it." Disability, which is to say, ableist assumptions about disability, crowds their perceptual field so thoroughly that they are incapable of *not* looking at it, *not* talking about it, *not* being distracted by it. The tricky part, here, of course, is that it is not the disability that is responsible for producing this effect, but the way in which the disability is perceived and interpreted by the abled-bodied individual. It is an effect of ableism as a way of knowing about the world and others. The problem lies in the gaze—and epistemic schemas—of the able-bodied.

Like all of us, medical experts are a product of their environment. Yet, medical experts are also part of an institution with a long and dark history concerning disability. Historically, medicine has played a central role in the construction of disability as both spectacle and tragedy, as something to be gawked at and pitied. This explains, in part, why the disability community tends to distrust the medical establishment and its historically teratological understanding of disability.[20] And while dominant social narratives of the inevitability of social progress incline us to believe that we have transcended this dark history, the ongoing experiences of people with disabilities suggest otherwise. They suggest that medical providers too often continue to treat disability as something to be poked and prodded, as a fascinating object to be stared at and squinted at.

The fourth mechanism by which ableism leads to medical error depends on this unique dynamic whereby disability becomes so visible, indeed hyper-visible, that it derails PPC from the real locus of medical concern. We call this *epistemic derailing*. Epistemic derailing occurs when the qualities and features assumed to track a speaker's perceived identity overdetermine hermeneutic space, preemptively shutting down more relevant hermeneutic resources and pathways. We here use the term "epistemic derailing" to pick out one of effects of the medical and able-bodied gaze: it erroneously narrows the communicative space between a disabled patient and a provider.[21] It can prevent medical experts from truly listening to what the patient has to say. By making providers assume from the start that the patient is in front of them *because* of their disability (i.e., the phenomenon that crowds the expert's field of perception), ableism derails the conversation and places an undue epistemic burden on the patient to constantly redirect the doctor's gaze back to what matters from a medical standpoint: their actual symptoms.

Let us briefly look at a case of epistemic derailing that is not directly connected to paradigmatic cases of disability: the treatment of HIV-positive people. HIV-positive patients often find that doctors cannot seem to get past the fact that that they are HIV-positive and assume that whatever complaints they make are due to their status. This is why depression is severely under-diagnosed in people living with HIV (Rodkjaer, Laursen, Balle, and Sodemann 2010)—doctors, held epistemically captive by the concept of HIV, may assume that patients are simply sad about having contracted HIV. Here, the over-attentiveness to HIV status interacts with other background assumptions, such as beliefs about how sad and meaningless life with HIV must be, to create a magnetic field that pulls PPC in a specific direction and that, ultimately, leads to medical error and medical harm.[22]

In summary, patients with disability experience this derailing effect of ableism in terms of an over-inquisitiveness on the part of providers about their disability status and a cascade of assumptions about patients with disabilities that are untethered from any concrete facts or judgments based upon the patient's actual experience. This levies a hefty "epistemic tax" on people with disabilities, who suddenly shoulder the onus of educating a non-disabled person, in this case a medical provider, about disability (Kattari, Olzman, and Hanna 2018). It also undermines the dialog between patient and provider because the patient now understands that his or her disability takes so much space in the provider's imaginary that the latter will devote most of her or his epistemic resources to it and perhaps it alone.[23] Both of these forms of testimonial injustice/oppression can lead to what Dotson calls "testimonial smothering," wherein "the speaker perceives one's immediate audience as unwilling or unable to gain the appropriate uptake of proffered testimony" and thus self-censors (Dotson 2011). Dotson continues to explain: "testimonial smothering, ultimately, is the truncating of one's own testimony in order to insure that the testimony contains only content for which one's audience demonstrates testimonial competence. Testimonial smothering exists in testimonial exchanges that are charged with complex social and epistemic concerns" (244). In the contexts under discussion, a patient with disabilities may purposely limit the information they provide because they know that, if included, additional information will not be heard and may even exacerbate the epistemic and communicative issues at play.

Motivated to combat this phenomenon, Shakespeare, Iezzoni, and Groce (2009) draw an important distinction between "need to know" and "want to know" questions. The first category refers to questions that providers should ask; the second, to those they *tend* to ask out of ignorance and curiosity whenever disability enters the scene. The dark side of "want to know" questions is that, aside from re-enacting medicine's historical treatment of people with disabilities as freaks and monsters, they cast a shadow on "need to know" questions. When providers cannot see anything but the disability, they cannot think of anything but the disability; and when this happens, they cannot come up with the questions whose answers they really "need to know." These questions drop out of focus and, before providers realize it, their hyper-attentiveness to the patient's disability snowballs into a situation in which patients and providers may be technically exchanging words but aren't communicating in ways that will promote positive health outcomes.

Ableism and Contributory Injustice

The four aforementioned mechanisms—testimonial injustice, epistemic overconfidence, epistemic erasure, and epistemic derailing—are all functions of the ableist schema that mediates how providers think about, and relate to, their disabled patients. But what is it about providers, or the medical establishment more generally, that cultivates this ableism? We submit that at the root of these mechanisms is the medical community's lack of engagement with critical, non-medical modes of knowledge concerning disability, including and especially with respect to knowledge created by disability communities themselves as well as bodies of work which draw directly on such knowledge, as literature in disability studies and philosophy of disability regularly does. In other words, a root cause of ableism in medicine is *medicine's own understanding of disability* as an objective lack rather than as a diverse set of phenomena that are thoroughly socially mediated. This reliance constitutes a form of what Dotson calls "contributory injustice," which turns on the willful exclusion of a certain set of hermeneutical resources from the worldview of a socially privileged agent. "Contributory injustice is caused by an epistemic agent's situated ignorance, in the form of willful hermeneutical ignorance, in maintaining and utilizing structurally prejudiced hermeneutical resources that result in epistemic harm to the epistemic agency of a knower" (Dotson 2012, 31).

Contributory injustice results from histories of epistemic exclusion and entrenched relations of power. As Dotson explains:

> [Miranda] Fricker [in her book *Epistemic Injustice*] seems to assume that there is but one set of collective hermeneutical resources that we are all equally dependent upon. I do not share this assumption. We do not all depend on the same hermeneutical resources. Such an assumption fails to take into account alternative epistemologies, counter mythologies, and hidden transcripts that exist in hermeneutically marginalized communities among themselves . . . the agent plays a role in contributory injustice by willfully refusing to recognize or acquire requisite alternative hermeneutical resources. [Gaile] Pohlhaus calls this refusal willful hermeneutical ignorance.
>
> (2012: 31–32)

Put differently, contributory epistemic injustice results from what Dotson (2014) and Leach Scully (2018) call *epistemic exclusions*. As Scully puts it:

> Epistemic exclusion is the notion that social position and power align with certain forms of epistemic power, that is, power over the ways in which knowledge is accumulated within, acknowledged by, and disseminated through communities, with the result that some kinds of knowledge can be kept out of mainstream sight.
>
> (107)

Contributory injustice is thus one form of epistemic exclusion, though not all epistemic exclusions are harmful or unjust. For example, a white provider who has completed her medical education may see no reason to learn about the history of medical practice, much less the way that that history today affects the differential treatments of patients along lines of racialization. She may assume that her education, especially if it comes from a privileged institute of higher education, is *enough*. She may assume that her life experience has taught her all she needs to know about social relations. Why would the provider need to draw upon hermeneutic resources from communities of color to learn about racism and its history and contemporary role in medicine? Or, analogously, sexism?

Or cissexism? Or ableism? By not attending to such bodies of knowledge, a provider commits contributory injustice. Perhaps the simplest way to think about contributory injustice is in terms of which bodies of knowledge register to people in positions of privilege as legitimate or illegitimate, and which simply fail to register at all. Contributory injustice is about the ways in which relations of oppression can be produced and exacerbated by the implicit choices we make about which hermeneutic resources matter and which do not.

As Dotson notes, one assumption of the theory of contributory injustice—and, in this regard, she differs from Fricker—is that there is no such thing as "the" pool of hermeneutic resources because not all members of a political community (say, the United States) interact with the world using the same stockpile of hermeneutic resources. Rather, different communities develop different modes of thinking about the world (or a particular slice of it) that may or may not coincide with the mode of thinking that happens to be dominant. Hence, when we witness instances of epistemic injustice, it is possible that the problem isn't that a socially privileged agent unjustly doubts someone's testimony or that the community is at a loss for the kinds of hermeneutical resources the testifier needs to shed light on an important aspect of her experience. In these cases the problem is that while there *are* hermeneutic resources that tackle the specific problem at hand, the socially privileged agents aren't familiar with them because they have no interest in learning about them since doing so is likely to challenge their own epistemic schemas. They may in fact have a vested interest in *not* learning about them insofar as that ignorance maintains their privileges and attendant experiences in the world.

An illustration will make this clearer. Gender-affirmation surgery (GAS) is often discussed in the medical and bioethical literatures as controversial because medical experts disagree about whether it counts as "therapy" or "enhancement" (Hongladarom 2012). But this way of thinking about GAS leaves trans individuals in a terrible double bind. On the one hand, if trans communities accept the therapeutic interpretation, then they must also accept the secondary claim that GAS is essentially a corrective, a "fix" for the condition that the DSM V calls "gender dysphoria." This, in turn, implies that to be trans *is* to have a "mental disorder." As Emma Inch (2016) rightly observes, this medicalization of trans identities fuels transphobia and contributes to the ongoing marginalization of trans subjects. On the other hand, if trans communities opt for the enhancement interpretation of GAS as a way of resisting the adverse effects of medicalization, they can be left in a medically vulnerable situation since, under contemporary medical-legal frameworks, trans people often need a diagnosis to change their names in legal documents and to offer a socially intelligible explanation of their situation to friends and family members. In many places, a diagnosis is required for GAS itself.

A medical diagnosis, in addition to exercising a social control function in modern societies, can help individuals gain access to care and treatment. Gender-reassignment surgery and hormone treatments are very expensive, and the fear is that neither publicly funded health providers, nor private medical insurance schemes will pay for treatments that are not prescribed with the intention of relieving a diagnosed condition. Some trans people ultimately view the label of disorder as the price that must be paid for access to treatment. For some, medical treatment truly is a matter of life or death, and they fear the removal of it from diagnostic manuals could have devastating consequences. Members of the WHO Working Group acknowledge this quandary and insist that diagnostic manuals like the ICD "find a balance between the competing issues of stigma versus access to care" (Inch 2016, 199).

The double bind between medical stigmatization and access to medical services is real and painful, but it may not be inevitable. This bind is only an inevitable effect of the specific hermeneutic resources the medical community mobilizes when it thinks about GAS and trans identity, which is what makes it a good example of contributory injustice. As soon as the hermeneutic resources of the medical establishment are used to frame discussions of GAS (Is it enhancement? Is it therapy?), it becomes difficult to think about this complex phenomenon in any other way.

But the trans community—especially trans scholars working in the field of trans studies—has generated an entire body of knowledge that affords radically different understandings of what it means be trans. The trans community, in other words, has generated its own hermeneutic resources (concepts, questions, methods, problematics, ways of framing, etc.) to think about trans identity in ways that evade the therapy/enhancement double bind. If the therapy/enhancement double bind continues confining trans people, this is because the medical establishment continues to approach GAS using hermeneutic resources that are outmoded, ill-suited, prejudicial, and ultimately harmful—resources that have been historically produced without the direct input of the trans community itself. From the standpoint of social epistemology, the medical establishment commits contributory injustice against trans individuals by privileging a set of hermeneutic resources that are prejudiced but do not register as such and by ignoring alternate resources, including those directly from the trans community.

The same can be said in relation to the disability community. Because the medical establishment on the whole embraces the medical model of disability, it relies on hermeneutic resources that were not designed with disabled people in mind and that are often directly at odds with how disability communities understand the meaning of disability and with how disabled people experience their own lives. The four mechanisms of epistemic injustice we have outlined here result from an active ignorance on the part of providers about how disabled people understand themselves and their own experiences, not to mention how the medical model harms people with disability. In a world in which multiple alternative models of disability exist and where the medical community has the power to access them, engage them, and incorporate them into its institutional structure, failure to do so constitutes contributory injustice because it reflects a decision on the part of the medical community that the harms its hermeneutic resources inflict on disabled patients do not matter as much as the comfort it itself takes in the continued use of these resources.

Medical Error in a Historical and Social Context

We have argued that testimonial injustice, epistemic overconfidence, epistemic erasure, and epistemic derailing undercut PPC and expose people with disabilities to an unjustifiably high risk of medical error and medical harm. Of course, medical errors that terminate in suffering are always harmful insofar as they cut against the grain of the two most fundamental interests of patients irrespective of disability status: their interest in getting better and their interest in not getting worse. While error is obviously good for no one, we argue that medical errors are *particularly* harmful when they happen to people with disabilities and other marginalized identities because they tend to not only have first-order physical effects (e.g., suffering), but also second-order symbolic effects. Furthermore, they are particularly harmful at a first-order level insofar as they contribute to the disproportionate distribution of error against an already marginalized group.

This symbolic harm, however, can be interpreted in a different way. When a disabled patient suffers a first-order medical harm at the hands of experts because of the ableism that permeates the institution of medicine, this harm takes place not just in a historical context in which the history of medicine is implicated, but also in a social context in which the collective imaginary already conflates disability with pain and suffering. What Reynolds (2017) calls "the ableist conflation" is the persistent conflation of experiences of disability with experiences of pain, suffering, and disadvantage. That is why the most common reaction to disability is an uncritical rush to pity and an assumption of low quality-of-life. By equating disability with suffering in this way, non-disabled individuals construct in their minds an identity for people with disabilities that denies the latter agency and the possibility of a rich, meaningful life. While it is possible for the non-disabled to suffer, the ableist conflation leads non-disabled people to think it is impossible for the disabled *not* to suffer, restricting both the facts and imagined possibilities of a life. This conflation produces a pernicious "master narrative" (Lindemann 2001, 157ff) that defines what it means to be disabled from the vantage point of the non-disabled.

We have also argued that schematic epistemic errors deserve more attention in the medical error literature. While epistemic errors are frequently referenced in this literature, most of the time they are reduced to what we call "factical errors," which are errors resulting from lack of information. But we showed that medical errors can occur not only because of *what* providers know, but also because of *how* they know. Schematic epistemological errors pertain to "ways of knowing" that involve entire constellations of values, norms, biases, impulses, desires, fantasies, and assumptions of which we are sometimes unaware but that nevertheless shape our activities of knowing in any given milieu. It is these schematic epistemological errors, we hypothesized, that are largely responsible for the unequal distribution of medical errors.

Finally, we would like to close by suggesting that schematic epistemic errors deserve special attention in the medical error literature because of their *recalcitrant* nature. Schematic epistemic errors not only involve the ins and outs of a hyper-complex health-care system, but also the ways in which epistemic agents interact with this system, with one another, and with the broader local, national, and international environments of which this system is only one component. Epistemic errors can persist despite improvements in medical education and the efforts of individual providers and teams aimed specifically at reducing medical error. In short, they are obdurate because they are not explicit, easily localizable, or particularly supple. On the contrary, they are distributed, implicit, and resistant to change. Often, they are the result of long-acquired habits of thinking and knowing that sediment and ossify with the passage of time—and these habits easily reflect entrenched hierarchies of social power that reinforce difficulties faced by patients from vulnerable populations. For this reason, individuals often lack the will, not to mention the ability, to uproot them. Calls to mobilize against them can even be met with collective resistance. Schematic errors, in particular, can serve to undermine care even when providers are actively working to address factical-based errors and actively working to provide equal care across populations.

Schematic errors present a special problem for patients with disabilities given the fraught historical relationship between disability and medicine. Medicine has surely contributed to improving the lives of some people with disabilities, but it has also defined disability and treated people with disabilities in ways that harm them. Medical errors due to ableism literally add insult to injury insofar as they crystallize the medical institution's historical disregard for and disparagement of the lives of people with disabilities (Nielsen 2012).

Preventable medical errors due to ableism only fuel this conflation and further re-entrench an identity that has been constructed (with the historical aid of medicine) *for* people with disabilities, *without* them—the inverse of one of the most important maxims of the disability rights movement: *nothing about us without us*. And this forms a vicious circle. Ableism leads to medical error. Error leads to first-order harm. First-order harm makes people with disabilities suffer. This suffering, when perceived by others under the aegis of ableism, reinforces the ableist conflation upon which ableism rests and contributes to second-order symbolic harms and damaging master narratives.

At some point, persistent medical error ceases to be a purely medical problem connected to a doctor's fiduciary and ethical duties to their patient and becomes a political problem tied to the question of justice. We can think through the connection between error and justice using a Rawlsian framework. Although Rawls's understanding of justice is traditionally framed in terms of the fair distribution of goods, such as material resources and political rights, this could easily be expanded to include the fair distribution of potential harms. Of course, no social institution can immunize itself against the possibility of accident. But all institutions should strive to ensure that the possibility of accident is not so unfairly distributed among its population that certain sub-sections of it bear all, or even most, of the brunt of it. When such an imbalance occurs, we can infer that there are deep structural problems that need to be addressed in the interest of justice, especially if we also have compelling reasons to believe that the accidents in question could be prevented with due diligence. If our analysis above is correct and the possibility of medical error is indeed not evenly distributed among all social groups in medical spaces, justice would demand that we strive to uproot the cause or causes of this asymmetrical distribution. One such cause is ableism.

Acknowledgements

Each author contributed equally to the conception, research, writing, and editing of this chapter. For helpful feedback on earlier drafts, we thank Sandra Borden, Fritz Allhoff, Derek Anderson, as well as two anonymous reviewers.

Notes

1. Reynolds, Joel Michael and David Peña-Guzmán. "The Harm of Ableism: Medical Error and Epistemic Injustice." *Kennedy Institute of Ethics Journal* 29: 3 (2019), 205–242. © 2019 Johns Hopkins University Press. Adapted and reprinted with permission of Johns Hopkins University Press.
2. Aronson presents his taxonomy specifically in relation to medication errors, but it is clear that it suitably extends to medical errors more generally.
3. For us, epistemic schemas include both epistemic elements (such as beliefs and intentions) as well as elements that traditional theories of knowledge may not consider properly epistemic (such as values, norms, and implicit biases). Schemas are conglomerations of beliefs, intentions, values, norms, and biases through which epistemic agents arrive at an ordered interpretation of their experience or of important aspects of it.

4. While here we describe the relationship between epistemic schemas and epistemic ignorance as causal (i.e., schemas cause ignorance), in reality the relationship is dialectical. Schemas and ignorance are mutually reinforcing insofar as schemas generate various types of epistemic ignorance, which in turn reinforces the schemas by shielding them from conscious reflection and, therefore, the possibility of criticism. They are both causes and effects of one another.

5. We do not mean to suggest that ableism negatively impacts *only* people with disabilities. Though we cannot defend the point here, insofar as what counts as being "able-bodied" and "normal" intersects with assumptions about race, gender, sex, sexuality, and the like, it can have a negative impact on people who are not disabled or who do not have impairments (we here mean both "disability" and "impairment" in the sense of social models of disability). We are, however, assuming that those *most* negatively affected by the epistemic schema of ableism in a medical context are disabled people.

6. The Society for Disability Studies defines "disability studies" as an interdisciplinary field born in the second half of the twentieth century that "encourages perspectives that place disability in social, cultural, and political contexts" (SDS 2017). There is disagreement within disability studies scholarship and disability activism across the globe concerning whether "persons with disabilities," "disabled persons," or some other such term should be used. In recognition of the underlying pluralism about ways of conceiving of the relationship between disability and personhood that these voices and ensuing disagreements represent as a whole, we will use both terms interchangeably.

7. Street, Makoul, Arora, and Epstein (2009) posit seven pathways through which communication can lead to better health: "increased access to care, greater patient knowledge and shared understanding, higher quality medical decisions, enhanced therapeutic alliances, increased social support, patient agency and empowerment, and better management of emotions."

8. To be fair, it is entirely possible that by using the terms "prejudice" and "stigma" to describe ableism, Barnes was in fact thinking of something along the lines of an epistemic schema. Our only point is to show that otherwise insightful and important analyses of disability have not engaged the concept of ableism, especially with respect to its role as an epistemic schema, as fruitfully and as in depth as they might.

9. On the concept *othering*, see (Shapiro 2008; Roberts and Schiavenato 2017).

10. For a fantastic study on the concept of normality and its connections to the "natural" and the "normative," see Gail Weiss's "The normal, the natural, and the normative: A Merleau-Pontian legacy to feminist theory, critical race theory, and disability studies" (2015).

11. One might counter that our analysis does not attend sufficiently to the differences between intellectual and physical disability. Although our examples are indeed taken more often than not from examples of physical disability, and although we agree that there are crucial and often substantive differences between intellectual and physical disability with respect to the topics at hand, we nevertheless maintain that our more general analysis is a boon to analyses of medical error and people with disabilities of both types (or of both). It should also be noted that the concept of "impairment," as well the social models of disability more generally, have come under significant criticism from disability theorists and philosophers of disability. These debates, though important, are orthogonal to our concerns here.

12. There are many drivers of ableism in medicine. One of them, which we do not have space to discuss here, has to do with how disability becomes a

synecdoche for human vulnerability as such, which ignores the fact that vulnerability comes in many forms. Scully (2013), for instance, distinguishes between "contingent" and "intrinsic" vulnerabilities. Rogers, Mackenzie, and Dodds (2012) similarly distinguish between "inherent," "situational," and "pathogenic" vulnerabilities. Following Scully (2013), we hold that many dependencies, and the vulnerabilities that come with them, are not "incompatible with full autonomy" (204). There are no vulnerabilities inherently and uniquely connected with disability (or, rather, impairment) as such. Vulnerabilities emerge as a product of the relationship between an individual and his or her environment. As historians of disability and disability studies scholars more generally have shown, many of the vulnerabilities disabled people face result from environments designed to not support or which are actively hostile to them, whether due to inaccessible built environments, ableist ideologies, underdeveloped assistive technologies, or medicalized understandings of disability, impairment, and vulnerability, etc.

13. Our thanks to one of the anonymous reviewers for nudging us to reflect upon this point. With respect to sexist and racist epistemic injustices, Medina (2013) offers an illuminating analysis. With respect to testimonial injustices experienced by people with chronic illness, see Kidd and Carel's (2018) analysis of what they call "pathocentric epistemic injustices."

14. Karen Jones's (2012) "The Politics of Intellectual Self-Trust" also discusses this phenomenon in a general way. Our thanks to Derek Anderson for pointing us to this reference and those in the next footnote.

15. Among other sources that discuss credibility excess, see (Medina 2011, 2013; Davis 2016; Yap 2017).

16. According to Ho, in the case of people with chronic conditions, this pessimistic judgment "can inadvertently thwart physicians' motivation to treat a patient's other conditions aggressively on the assumption that the patient's overall quality of life is poor anyway" (Ho 2009, 192). Scully also notes that while the disability paradox needs to be taken seriously as an indicator of the prevalence of ableism, that impairments come along with about an average quality of life "is not always the case, especially not for more recently disabled people whose impairment constitutes a significant loss and who are still struggling to adapt to their changed circumstances" (Scully 2018, 109–110).

17. With regards to both *epistemic erasure* and what we discuss shortly later as *epistemic derailing*, we take ourselves to be exploring forms of (or, depending upon precisely how they are construed in a given context, at least closely related phenomena to) what Pohlhaus (2012) calls "willful hermeneutical ignorance." To be clear, by coining these terms, we do not take ourselves to be the first to point to these issues—on the contrary, we are using these phrases to point to experiences that we take to be well attested in disability studies writ large (as our citations throughout indicate).

18. In 2016, *InterAlia: A Journal of Queer Studies* published a two-part special issue on the subject. In the introduction to the special issue, "Let's Talk About (Crip) Sex," Tomasz Sikora and Dominika Ferens note that the various contributions are important reminders of disabled people's struggle for sexual recognition. Endless narratives depict people with disabilities as either a-sexual or non-sexual, indeed as barely having sexual organs in the first place. According to Sikora and Ferens, this contributes to the oppression and marginalization of the disability community.

19. Epistemic erasure—among other types of epistemic injustice we discuss in this chapter—takes on a different form and can have different effects with respect to invisible disabilities. Due to space, we are limiting our discussion

here primarily to visible disabilities and hope that further research in this vein will explore questions relating to invisible disabilities.

20. In *Exile and Pride: Disability, Queerness, and Liberation*, Eli Clare observes that medicine played a key role in the "medicalization" of disability in the early twentieth century and that one of the first tools used by medical experts to turn disabled bodies into objects of interest was the language of teratology, "the centuries old study of monsters" (Clare 2009, 97).

21. Throughout this chapter, we have assumed that the medical provider in question is able-bodied. This is, of course, an assumption that leaves out disabled providers. It is sadly beyond the scope of this chapter to address the specific types of challenges disabled providers might face with respect to PPC, ableism, and epistemic injustice more generally. (See, for example, Meeks 2019.) Insofar as disabled providers experience ableism along the lines we discuss here, we hope that this chapter may, mutatis mutandis, afford some insights.

22. People who are HIV-positive are not the only ones who feel this pull in the context of PPC. Overweight patients do too. Often, when patients who are overweight, obese, or, as some prefer to be called, fat, show up to the clinic, they are confronted with a labyrinthine setting in which all paths lead to the same destination: "It is because of your weight." As in the case of ableism, fatism narrows the provider's field of vision and causes them to fail to make inferences that they otherwise would have likely made. This would explain why conditions such as mood disorders (Da Silva, Da Silva, Azorin, and Belzeaux 2015) and sleep disorders (Mears, Mears, and Chelly 2007) are underdiagnosed among overweight patients.

23. To be clear, epistemic erasure is closely related to epistemic derailing. Keeping to our primary example, the former is when a topic of medical relevance disappears from the doctor's perceptual field and really is *invisible*. The provider might express surprise at the patient who insists on talking about this. By contrast, epistemic derailing is a subtle deviation in the conversation where one topic slowly pulls the conversation in its direction even though the conversation begins, or should reasonably go, somewhere else. Derailing is a question of *hyper-visibility*. Each, then, are like the inverse of one another. Put more simply, erasure occurs when the epistemic schema of ableism puts patients in a situation where their impairment has the effect of hiding something from a provider that is relevant and derailing occurs when their impairment becomes so bright, as it were, that nothing else can be seen.

Works Cited

Albrecht, Gary L., and Patrick J. Devlieger. 1999. "The Disability Paradox: High Quality of Life Against All Odds." *Social Science & Medicine* 48: 977–988.

Alcoff, Linda. 2007. "Epistemologies of Ignorance: Three Types." In Shannon Sullivan and Nancy Tuana (eds.), *Race and Epistemologies of Ignorance.* Albany, NY: SUNY Press.

Alvarez, George, and Enrico Coiera. 2006. "Interdisciplinary Communication: An Uncharted Source of Medical Error?" *Journal of Critical Care* 21 (3): 236–242.

Aronson, Jeffrey K. 2009. "Medication Errors: Definitions and Classification." *British Journal of Clinical Pharmacology* 67 (6): 599–604. doi: 10.1111/j.1365-2125.2009.03415.x.

Barnes, Elizabeth. 2016. *The Minority Body.* New York, NY: Oxford University Press.

Bartunek, Jean, and Michael Moch. 1987. "First-Order, Second-Order, and Third-Order Change and Organization Development Interventions: A Cognitive Approach." *The Journal of Applied Behavioral Science* 23 (4): 483. doi: 10.1177/002188638702300404.

Basnett, Ian. 2001. "Health Care Professionals and Their Attitudes Toward Decisions Affecting Disabled People." In Kathryn Seelman Gary Albrecht and Michael Bury (eds.), *Handbook of Disability Studies.* Thousand Oaks, CA: Sage Publishers: 450–467.

Beckman, Howard B., Kathryn M. Markakis, Anthony L. Suchman, and Richard M. Frankel. 1994. "The Doctor—Patient Relationship and Malpractice. Lessons from Plaintiff Depositions." *Archives of Internal Medicine* 154 (12): 1365–1370. doi: 10.1001/archinte.1994.00420120093010.

Bem, Sandra Lipsitz. 1981. "Gender Schema Theory: A Cognitive Account of Sex Typing." *Psychological Review* 88 (4): 354–364. doi: 10.1037/0033-295X.88.4.354.

Berke, Jamie. 2007. "Deaf, Not Retarded: When Misdiagnoses Are Made, Everyone Pays." *About.com.* Retrieved from http://deafness.about.com/cs/featurearticles/a/retarded_2.ht.

Berlinger, Nancy. 2005. *After Harm: Medical Error and the Ethics of Forgiveness.* Baltimore: Johns Hopkins University Press.

Blackstone, Sarah W. 2015. "Issues and Challenges in Advancing Effective Patient – Provider Communication." In David Beukelman. Sarah W. Blackstone, and Kathryn Yorkston (eds.), *Patient Provider Communication.* San Diego, CA: Plural Publishing: 9–35.

Blease, Charlotte, Havi Carel, and Keith Geraghty. 2017. "Epistemic Injustice in Healthcare Encounters: Evidence from Chronic Fatigue Syndrome." *Journal of Medical Ethics* 43 (8): 549. doi: 10.1136/medethics-2016-103691.

Buchman, Daniel Z., Anita Ho, and Daniel S. Goldberg. 2017. "Investigating Trust, Expertise, and Epistemic Injustice in Chronic Pain." *Journal of Bioethical Inquiry* 14 (1): 31–42. doi: 10.1007/s11673-016-9761-x.

Carel, Havi, and Ian James Kidd. 2014. "Epistemic Injustice in Healthcare: A Philosophical Analysis." *Medicine, Health Care and Philosophy* 17 (4): 529–540. doi: 10.1007/s11019-014-9560-2.

Cassam, Quassim. 2017. "Diagnostic Error, Overconfidence and Self-Knowledge." *Palgrave Communications* 3: 17025. doi: 10.1057/palcomms.2017.25.

Chapman, Melanie, Pam Iddon, Kathy Atkinson, Colin Brodie, Duncan Mitchell, Garry Parvin, and Steve Willis. 2011. "The Misdiagnosis of Epilepsy in People with Intellectual Disabilities: A Systematic Review." *Seizure: European Journal of Epilepsy* 20: 101–106. doi: 10.1016/j.seizure.2010.10.030.

Clare, Eli. 2009. *Exile & Pride: Disability, Queerness and Liberation.* Cambridge, MA: South End Press.

Crichton, Paul, Havi Carel, and Ian James Kidd. 2017. "Epistemic Injustice in Psychiatry." *British Journal of Psychiatry* 41 (2): 65–70.

Cryle, Peter, and Elizabeth Stephens. 2017. *Normality: A Critical Genealogy.* Chicago and London: The University of Chicago Press.

Da Silva, Virginie Borgès, Roxane Borgès Da Silva, Jean Michel Azorin, and Raoul Belzeaux. 2015. "Mood Disorders Are Highly Prevalent but Underdiagnosed among Patients Seeking Bariatric Surgery." *Obesity Surgery* 25 (3): 543–544. doi: 10.1007/s11695-014-1557-7.

Davis, Emmalon. 2016. "Typecasts, Tokens, and Spokespersons: A Case for Credibility Excess as Testimonial Injustice." *Hypatia* 31 (3).

Davis, Lennard J. 2013. *The End of Normal: Identity in a Biocultural Era.* Ann Arbor: University of Michigan Press.

Dohmen, Josh. 2016. "A Little of Her Language." *Res Philosophica* 93 (4): 669–691.

Dotson, Kristie. 2011. "Tracking Epistemic Violence, Tracking Practices of Silencing." *Hypatia* 26 (2): 236–257. doi: 10.1111/j.1527-2001.2011.01177.x.

Dotson, Kristie. 2012. "A Cautionary Tale. On Limiting Epistemic Oppression." *Frontiers: A Journal of Women Studies* 33 (1): 24–47. doi: 10.5250/fronjwomestud.33.1.0024.

Dotson, Kristie. 2014. "Conceptualizing Epistemic Oppression." *Social Epistemology: A Journal of Knowledge, Culture, and Policy* 28 (2): 115–138.

Fricker, Miranda. 2007. *Epistemic Injustice: Power and the Ethics of Knowing.* Oxford and New York: Oxford University Press.

Garland-Thomson, Rosemarie. 1996. *Freakery: Cultural Spectacles of the Extraordinary Body.* New York: New York University Press.

Ghosh, Vanessa E., and Asaf Gilboa. 2014. "What Is a Memory Schema? A Historical Perspective on Current Neuroscience Literature." *Neuropsychologia* 53: 104–114. https://doi.org/10.1016/j.neuropsychologia.2013.11.010.

Grasswick, Heidi. 2018. "Understanding Epistemic Trust Injustices and Their Harms." *Royal Institute of Philosophy Supplement* 84: 69–91.

Hemsley, Bronwyn, and Susan Balandin. 2014. "A Metasynthesis of Patient—Provider Communication in Hospital for Patients with Severe Communication Disabilities: Informing New Translational Research." *AAC: Augmentative & Alternative Communication* 30 (4): 329–343. doi: 10.3109/07434618.2014.955614.

Hickson, Gerald B., Charles F. Federspiel, James W. Pichert, Cynthia S. Miller, Jean Gauld-Jaeger, and Preston Bost. 2002. "Patient Complaints and Malpractice Risk." *JAMA* 287 (22): 2951–2957. doi: 10.1001/jama.287.22.2951.

Ho, Anita. 2009. " 'They Just Don't Get It!' When Family Disagrees with Expert Opinion." *Journal of Medical Ethics* (8): 497. doi: 10.1136/jme.2008.028555.

Ho, Anita. 2011. "Trusting Experts and Epistemic Humility in Disability." *IJFAB: International Journal of Feminist Approaches to Bioethics* 4 (2): 102. doi: 10.2979/intjfemappbio.4.2.102.

Hoffman, Kelly M., Sophie Trawalter, Jordan R. Axt, and M. Norman Oliver. 2016. "Racial Bias in Pain Assessment and Treatment Recommendations, and False Beliefs About Biological Differences Between Blacks and Whites." *Proceedings of the National Academy of Sciences of the United States of America* 113 (16): 4296. doi: 10.1073/pnas.1516047113.

Hongladarom, Soraj. 2012. "Sex Change Surgery: Therapy or Enhancement?" *Asian Bioethics Review* 4 (4): 283–292.

Huntington, Beth, and Nettie Kuhn. 2003. "Communication Gaffes: A Root Cause of Malpractice Claims." *Baylor University Medical Center Proceedings* 16 (2): 157–161. doi: 10.1080/08998280.2003.11927898.

Iezzoni, Lisa I. 2006. "Make No Assumptions: Communication Between Persons with Disabilities and Clinicians." *Assistive Technology* 18 (2): 212.

Iezzoni, Lisa I., and Bonnie O'Day. 2006. *More Tan Ramps: A Guide to Improving Health Care Quality and Access for People with Disabilities.* Oxford and New York: Oxford University Press.

Inch, Emma. 2016. "Changing Minds: The Psycho—Pathologization of Trans People." *International Journal of Mental Health* 45 (3): 193–204. doi: 10.1080/00207411.2016.1204822.

IOM. 2000. *To Err Is Human: Building a Safer Health System.* Washington, DC: Institute of Medicine.

Johnson, Mark. 1987. *The Body in the Mind: The Bodily Basis of Meaning, Imagination, and Reason.* Chicago: University of Chicago Press.

Jones, Karen. 2012. "The Politics of Intellectual Self-Trust." *Social Epistemology* 26 (2): 237–251.

Kaplan, Sherrie H., Sheldon Greenfield, and John E. Ware. 1989. "Assessing the Effects of Physician—Patient Interactions on the Outcomes of Chronic Disease." *Medical Care* 27 (3): S110—S127.

Kattari, Shanna K., Miranda Olzman, and Michele D. Hanna. 2018. '"You Look Fine!' Ableist Experiences by People with Invisible Disabilities."*Affilia* 33 (4): 477–492. doi: 10.1177/0886109918778073.

Kiani, Reza, and Helen Miller. 2010. "Sensory Impairment and Intellectual Disability." *Advances in Psychiatric Treatment* 16 (3): 228–235. doi: 10.1192/apt. bp.108.005736.

Kidd, Ian James, and Havi Carel. 2018. "Healthcare Practice, Epistemic Injustice, and Naturalism." *Royal Institute of Philosophy Supplements* 84: 211–233.

Kohn, Linda T. 2001. "The Institute of Medicine Report on Medical Error: Overview and Implications for Pharmacy." *American Journal of Health-System Pharmacy* 58 (1): 63–66.

Kurs, Rena, and Alexander Grinshpoon. 2018. "Vulnerability of Individuals with Mental Disorders to Epistemic Injustice in Both Clinical and Social Domains." *Ethics & Behavior* 28 (4): 336–346. doi: 10.1080/10508422.2017.1365302.

Li, Yi. 2016. "Testimonial Injustice without Prejudice: Considering Cases of Cognitive or Psychological Impairment." *Journal of Social Philosophy* 47 (4): 457–469. doi: 10.1111/josp.12175.

Lindemann, Hilde. 2001. *Damaged Identities, Narrative Repair.* Ithaca: Cornell University Press.

Makary, Martin A., and Michael Daniel. 2016. "Medical Error—The Third Leading Cause of Death in the US." *BMJ* 353: i2139. doi: 10.1136/ bmj.i2139.

Mastroianni, Peggy R., and Carol R. Miaskoff. 1997. "Coverage of Psychiatric Disorders under the Americans with Disabilities Act." *Villanova Law Review* (2): 723.

Mears, Dana C., Simon C. Mears, and Jacques E. Chelly. 2007. "Two-Incision Hip Replacement in the Morbidly Obese Patient." *Seminars in Arthroplasty* 18: 272–279. doi: 10.1053/j.sart.2007.09.011.

Medina, José. 2011. "The Relevance of Credibility Excess in a Proportional View of Epistemic Injustice: Differential Epistemic Authority and the Social Imaginary." *Social Epistemology* 25 (1): 15–35.

Medina, José. 2013. *The Epistemology of Resistance: Gender and Racial Oppression, Epistemic Injustice, and Resistant Imaginations.* Oxford and New York: Oxford University Press.

Meeks, Lisa. 2019. "Coalition for Disability Access in Health Science Education." Accessed June 22. Retrieved from www.hsmcoalition.org/articles.

Mills, Charles W. 2010. *Radical Theory, Caribbean Reality: Race, Class and Social Domination.* Kingston, Jamaica: University of the West Indies Press.

Neumann, Melanie, Jozien Bensing, Stewart Mercer, Nicole Ernstmann, Oliver Ommen, and Holger Pfaff. 2009. "Analyzing the 'Nature' and 'Specific Effectiveness' of Clinical Empathy: A Theoretical Overview and Contribution towards a Theory-based Research Agenda." *Patient Education and Counseling* 74 (3): 339–346.

Nielsen, Kim E. 2012. *A Disability History of the United States.* Boston: Beacon Press.

Nordness, Amy S., and David R. Beukelman. 2017. "Supporting Patient Provider Communication Across Medical Settings." *Topics in Language Disorders* 37 (4): 334–347. doi: 10.1097/TLD.0000000000000133.

Pohlhaus, Gaile. 2012. "Relational Knowing and Epistemic Injustice: Toward a Theory of Willful Hermeneutical Ignorance." *Hypatia* 27 (4): 715–735. doi: 10.1111/j.1527-2001.2011.01222.x.

Reiheld, Alison. 2010. "Patient Complains of . . . : How Medicalization Mediates Power and Justice." *International Journal of Feminist Approaches to Bioethics* 3 (1): 72–98. doi: 10.2979/FAB.2010.3.1.72.

Reynolds, Joel Michael. 2017. " 'I'd Rather Be Dead Than Disabled'—The Ableist Conflation and the Meanings of Disability." *Review of Communication* 17 (3): 149–163. doi: 10.1080/15358593.2017.1331255.

Reynolds, Joel Michael. 2018. "Three Things Clinicians Should Know About Disability." *AMA Journal of Ethics* 20 (12): E1181–E1187. doi: 10.1001/amajethics.2018.1181.

Roberts, Mary Lee A., and Martin Schiavenato. 2017. "Othering in The Nursing Context: A Concept Analysis." *Nursing Open* 4 (3). doi: 10.1002/nop2.82.

Rodkjaer, Lotte, T. Laursen, N. Balle, and M. Sodemann. 2010. "Depression in Patients with HIV Is Under-Diagnosed: A Cross-sectional Study in Denmark." *HIV Medicine* 11 (1): 46–53.

Rogers, Wendy, Catriona Mackenzie, and Susan Dodds. 2012. "Why Bioethics Needs a Concept of Vulnerability." *International Journal of Feminist Approaches to Bioethics* 5 (2): 11–38. doi: 10.3138/ijfab.5.2.11

Sanati, Abdi, and Michalis Kyratsous. 2015. "Epistemic Injustice in Assessment of Delusions." *Journal of Evaluation in Clinical Practice* 21 (3): 479–485. doi: 10.1111/jep.12347.

Scully, Jackie Leach. 2016. "Disability and Vulnerability: On Bodies, Dependence, and Power." In Catriona Mackenzie, Wendy Rogers and Susan Dodds (eds.), *Vulnerability: New Essays in Ethics and Feminist Philosophy.* New York, NY: Oxford University Press: 204–221.

Scully, Jackie Leach. 2018. "From 'She Would Say That, Wouldn't She?' to 'Does She Take Sugar?' Epistemic Injustice and Disability." *IJFAB* 11 (1): 106–124. doi: 10.3138/ijfab.11.1.106.

SDS. 2017. "Mission and History." Society for Disability Studies, Accessed April 10. Retrieved from https://disstudies.org/index.php/about-sds/mission-and-history/.

Shakespeare, Tom. 2014. *Disability Rights And Wrongs Revisited*, 2nd ed. London and New York: Routledge.

Shakespeare, Tom, Lisa I. Iezzoni, and Nora E. Groce. 2009. "Disability and the Training of Health Professionals." *The Lancet* 374 (9704): 1815–1816. doi: 10.1016/S0140-6736(09)62050-X.

Shapiro, Johanna. 2008. "Walking a Mile in Their Patients' Shoes: Empathy and Othering in Medical Students' Education." *Philosophy, Ethics, and Humanities in Medicine* 3 (1): 10. doi: 10.1186/1747-5341-3-10.

Sikora, Tomasz, and Dominika Ferens. 2016. "Introduction: Let's Talk about (Crip) Sex." *Inter Alia: A Journal of Queer Studies* 11: i–ix.

Smith, Diane L. 2009. "Disparities in Patient—Physician Communication for Persons with a Disability from the 2006 Medical Expenditure Panel Survey (MEPS)." *Disability and Health Journal* 2: 206–215. doi: 10.1016/j.dhjo.2009.06.002.

Song, Lixin, Mark A. Weaver, Ronald C. Chen, et al. 2014. "Associations Between Patient—Provider Communication and Socio-Cultural Factors in Prostate Cancer Patients: A Cross-Sectional Evaluation of Racial Differences." *Patient Education and Counseling* 97 (3): 339–346. doi: 10.1016/j.pec.2014.08.019.

Stewart, Moira A. 1995. "Effective Physician—Patient Communication and Health Outcomes: A Review." *Canadian Medical Association Journal* 152 (9): 1423–1433.

Stewart, Moira A., Judith B. Brown, Allan Donner, Ian R. McWhinney, Julian Oates, Wayne Weston, and John Jordan. 2000. "The Impact of Patient-Centered Care on Outcomes." *The Journal of Family Practice* 49 (9): 796–804.

Stewart, Moira A., and Debra Roter. 1989. *Communicating with Medical Patients*. Thousand Oaks, CA: Sage Publications, Inc.

Street, Richard, Gregory Makoul, Neeraj Arora, and Ronald Epstein. 2009. "How Does Communication Heal? Pathways Linking Clinician—Patient Communication to Health Outcomes." *Patient Education and Counseling* 74 (3): 295–301.

Sutcliffe, Kathleen M., Elizabeth Lewton, and Marilynn M. Rosenthal. 2004. "Communication Failures: An Insidious Contributor to Medical Mishaps." *Academic Medicine* 79 (2): 186–194.

Tolonen, Anu, Jukka Turkka, Oili Salonen, Eija Ahoniemi, and Hannu Alaranta. 2007. "Traumatic Brain Injury Is Under-Diagnosed in Patients with Spinal Cord Injury." *Journal of Rehabilitation Medicine (Stiftelsen Rehabiliteringsinformation)* 39 (8): 622–626.

Toombs, S. Kay. 1987. "The Meaning of Illness: A Phenomenological Approach to the Patient—Physician Relationship." *Journal of Medicine and Philosophy* 12 (3): 219–240.

Toombs, S. Kay. 1992. *The Meaning of Illness: The Phenomenological Account of the Different Perspectives of Physician and Patient*. Dordrecht: Springer. Book Review.

Tremain, Shelley. 2017. "Knowing Disability, Differently." In Jose Medina, Gaile Pohlhaus Jr., and Ian James Kidd (eds.), *Routledge Handbook of Epistemic Injustice*. New York: Routledge: 175–184.

van de Ven, Leontine, Marcel Post, Luc de Witte, and Wim van den Heuvel. 2005. "It Takes Two to Tango: The Integration of People with Disabilities into Society." *Disability & Society* 20 (3): 311–329. doi: 10.1080/09687590500060778.

Vincent, C., M. Young, and A. Phillips. 1994. "Why Do People Sue Doctors? A Study of Patients and Relatives Taking Legal Action." *Lancet* 343 (8913): 1609–1613.

Wanzer, Melissa Bekelja, Melissa Booth-Butterfield, and Kelly Gruber. 2004. "Perceptions of Health Care Providers' Communication: Relationships Between Patient-Centered Communication and Satisfaction." *Health Communication* 16 (3): 363–383.

Webb, James, Edward R Amend, Paul Beljan, et al. 2005. *Misdiagnosis and Dual Diagnoses of Gifted Children and Adults; ADHD, Bipolar, OCD, Asperger's, Depression, and Other Disorders.* Tucson, AZ: Great Potential Press.

Weingart, Saul N., Ross McL. Wilson, Robert W. Gibberd, and Bernadette Harrison. 2000. "Epidemiology of Medical Error." *Western Journal of Medicine* 172 (6): 390–393.

Weiss, Gail. 2015. "The Normal, the Natural, and the Normative: A Merleau-Pontian Legacy to Feminist Theory, Critical Race Theory, and Disability Studies." *Continental Philosophy Review* 48 (1): 77–93. doi: 10.1007/s11007-014-9316-y.

Wieseler, Christine. Forthcoming. "The Desexualization of Disabled People as Existential Harm and the Importance of Temporal Ambiguity." In Susan Bredlau and Talia Welsh (eds.), *Normality, Abnormality, and Pathology in Merleau-Ponty.* Ithica, NY: State University of New York Press.

Wong, Sophia Isako. 2009. "Duties of Justice to Citizens with Cognitive Disabilities." *Metaphilosophy* 40 (3–4): 382–401. doi: 10.1111/j.1467-9973.2009.01604.x.

Yap, Audrey S. 2017. "Credibility Excess and the Social Imaginary in Cases of Sexual Assault." *Feminist Philosophy Quarterly* 3 (4): Article 1.

11 Error and Determinations of Decision-Making Capacity in Mentally Ill Patients

Kelsey Gipe

Introduction

Medical error is characteristically thought of in terms of mistakes made during procedures or in prescribing and dispensing medications. However, there is an earlier point in the process of care when equally impactful and morally troubling errors may be made: during determinations of a patient's capacity to give informed consent, particularly in cases of mental illness. Psychological illness does not necessarily preclude a patient from possessing the capacity necessary to give genuine informed consent, but it has the serious potential to do so.[1] Recently, a physically healthy 24-year-old Belgian woman named Emily was granted medical assistance to end her life due to unbearable psychological suffering as the result of persistent and severe depression (O'Gara 2015; 24 & Ready to Die 2015). Many agree that we should provide medical aid in dying (e.g., physician-assisted suicide, active voluntary euthanasia, withdrawal of care necessary to sustain life) to terminally ill patients who find themselves in excruciating and intractable pain (e.g., Dworkin et al. 1997; Brock 1992; Dworkin 1994). But cases like Emily's raise some difficult ethical questions. If individuals may opt for physician-assisted dying due to unremitting psychological pain in the absence of terminal biophysical illness, this leaves us with some troubling epistemic uncertainty; the particular uncertainty that motivates the current project is that surrounding how to determine capacity for medical decision making in the face of illness that is itself fundamentally and inextricably bound up with the patient's mentation.

Potential for error is more troubling the more is at stake, so requests for medical aid in dying provide a good starting point for highlighting and teasing apart the ethical challenges accompanying determinations of decision-making capacity in mentally ill patients. I will in this chapter focus not only on cases in which medical aid in dying is requested by a mentally ill patient, but in which there is the added moral complexity of such a request being made in the absence of terminal biophysical illness and/or when the patient's death is far from imminent. Figuring out how to determine whether all of the criteria for decision-making capacity are met by particular patients in a rigorous and standardized way is a daunting challenge (and one which physicians in, e.g., the Netherlands, seem to be struggling with). However, it is imperative we get it right, given the immense and irrevocable import of a decision to seek medical aid in dying.[2] If we err on the side of assuming patient capacity, we risk providing medical aid in dying to patients who may not have made such a choice rationally. If we err on the side of assuming patient incapacity, we risk withholding medical aid in dying from patients who are suffering greatly and who, with capacity, request death in order to escape severe and refractory suffering.

To make progress in understanding and working to solve this problem, I will first explicate the framework for capacity determinations I will be relying on here and briefly run through the current landscape of medical aid in dying, particularly in the United States. I will then build a rational entailment from moral endorsement of palliative sedation therapy to treat severe and refractory psychological suffering at the end of life to endorsement of palliative sedation therapy to severe and refractory psychological suffering when death is far from imminent. I will then consider as a paradigm case Julian Savulescu's example of an anorexic who wishes to opt for voluntary palliated starvation (VPS) (Savulescu 2014). I will argue that an anorexic patient might judge a world in which she must eat—given the pain of her illness and little to no prospect of a cure in her specific case—as worse than death, and thus rationally opt for VPS as a means to death. In such a case, she would be opting for death on the basis of refractory and severe suffering. This would be importantly different from opting for VPS as a means to persist in a state of starving herself, with death as a mere side-effect. In the former case, the patient is evaluating the suffering that accompanies her mental illness and choosing on that basis. In the latter, the patient's illness leads her to fixate on avoiding weight restoration, even in the face of death from starvation. If a request for medical aid in dying by an anorexic patient were directly motivated by a fear of weight restoration, this would be a request that issues from the illness itself and thus precludes the patient from making a rational choice. In contrast, in a case like the one outlined above—where the patient's illness has been judged refractory and she opts for medical aid in dying on the basis of a desire to avoid a future of suffering and slow death from anorexia—it may be possible for the patient to make a rational choice to die.

However, it would be challenging to apply such a distinction to real-world cases. In reality, the motivations of patients may be mixed. Furthermore, a patient's genuine motivations may be opaque to us and sometimes even to the patient herself. This uncertainty leads to situations ripe for error in making determinations of decision-making capacity. Further, compounding elements of a mentally ill patient's situation (such as social isolation) also have the potential to compromise decision-making capacity. In light of such concerns, I argue that a blanket assumption of incapacity—with possible room for exceptions—may be the best approach to take to capacity determinations in the sorts of cases under consideration. But this prompts and leaves open the question of whether there are cases in which a patient's psychological suffering may be severe enough to warrant granting medical aid to end her life, even in the absence of capacity.

A Framework for Capacity Determinations

I will here adopt Allen Buchanan and Dan Brock's account of decision-making capacity in medical settings. This is a "process standard" that focuses "primarily not on the content of the patient's decision but on the *process* of the reasoning that leads up to that decision" (Buchanan and Brock 1995, 50–51). A process standard of capacity, on their view, requires that two main questions be answered. First, what *level of reasoning* must the patient exhibit in order to be judged to have capacity? And, second, what *level of certainty* requiring the patient's ability to reason and understand facts relevant to her situation is required by those evaluating the patient's capacity (ibid.)? It is the second question that is the primary focus of this chapter. However, it is worth characterizing the capacities necessary to meet the level of reasoning required for decision-making capacity.

Decision-making capacity in medical settings requires certain abilities. Such abilities include "the capacity for understanding and communication and the capacity for reasoning and deliberation" (Buchanan and Brock 1995, 23). In addition to these abilities, decision-making capacity requires that the patient "have a set of values or conception of the good" (ibid.). What the capacity for understanding and communication amounts to is prima facie straightforward (at least in theoretical terms; in clinical reality, as with most things, matters may be less clear cut). The patient must be able to understand the content being relayed to her and be able to express her preferences and decisions and ask questions when necessary. Understanding requires that the patient have the cognitive abilities required to take in and process information, along with the ability to do at least some basic perspective-taking and mental time travel when it comes to envisioning what the future might be like in the face of different treatment alternatives. The capacity for reasoning and deliberation again requires certain cognitive abilities. The patient must have at least some ability to draw inferences and reason probabilistically and must be able to retain information long enough to run through a process of deliberation. Finally, the patient's possession of some (at least minimally stable and consistent) set of values or conception of the good is required for decision-making capacity because, without these, the patient would be unable to reasonably and consistently assign weights to different considerations and options in terms of goodness or desirability. For example, the relative weights assigned to four additional weeks of life in great pain would be radically different for a patient with a strong Protestant work ethic as opposed to one who greatly valued hedonic goods.

On the conception of decision-making capacity I endorse here, the standard of capacity required to make a particular choice regarding treatment is *variable*. This means that it will (ideally) vary in proportion to the seriousness of the decision being made in terms of the information required to make an adequately informed choice, level of risk accompanying that choice, expected harms, and the probability of such harms coming about. Buchanan and Brock explain the relation as follows:

> The greater the risk [of a patient's choice] relative to other alternatives—where risk is a function of the severity of the expected harm and the probability of its occurrence—the greater the level of communication, understanding, and reasoning skills required for competence to make that decision.[3]
>
> (Buchanan and Brock 1995, 55)

This means that, for instance, the level of such skills required to consent to a life-saving blood transfusion will be much lower than that required to refuse the same transfusion. Roughly put, the risk and magnitude of foreseen harm that accompanies a particular choice will be directly proportional to the level of cognitive ability required to have capacity to make that choice. On this view, the same patient may be able to consent to, for example, a routine mammogram, but unable to competently consent to a prophylactic double mastectomy. This variability has clear implications for the project at hand. After all, a decision to seek medical aid in dying is one in which there is much (perhaps everything) at stake for a patient. In light of this, the level of cognitive skill required to consent to such an intervention would generally be quite high. Further, the level of certainty required of those evaluating the patient's capacity should also be quite high in cases in which a patient is opting for medical aid in dying.

Current Landscape of Medical Aid in Dying

In the United States, physician-assisted suicide (PAS) is currently legal in only a handful of states, and active euthanasia illegal in all. How exactly PAS is regulated varies from state to state. Take, for instance, Oregon's Death With Dignity Act, on which physician-assisted suicide legislation in other states has been based. In order to receive assisted suicide, a person must have a terminal illness, a prognosis of six months or less to live, approval from at least one physician that she is has capacity to make such a decision, and approval from a psychiatrist or psychologist if her decision-making capacity is unclear (Oregon Health Authority 2018). This system precludes many of the sorts of situations that generate the difficult ethical questions arising from physician-assisted dying to relieve psychological suffering. By limiting the availability of physician-assisted suicide to those who are terminally biophysically ill and at the end of their lives, the question of whether (or when) to accommodate cases of intractable and severe psychological suffering in the absence of terminal illness by providing medical aid in dying does not even arise.

However, there is an end-of-life (EOL) intervention available throughout the United States that can be employed to relieve unremitting psychological suffering: palliative sedation therapy (PST). And, even though it currently only takes place in EOL contexts, I will argue that endorsing its moral permissibility for use at the end of life rationally entails that we endorse it for use in the absence of terminal illness and when death is far from imminent, if criteria of sufficiently severe refractory suffering and patient consent obtain. This is because—if severe suffering, refractoriness, and consent are present in both cases—it is unclear why we ought to permit a patient to opt for PST in the EOL case, but not in an earlier case identical in morally relevant respects. Thus, a commitment to the moral permissibility in EOL cases further rationally commits us to the moral permissibility of early PST.

Defining Palliative Sedation Therapy

Palliative Sedation Therapy (PST), also referred to as "palliative sedation" or "terminal sedation," is an intervention that may be employed by physicians at the end of a patient's life to relieve intractable pain by dropping the patient below the level of consciousness until she eventually passes away. PST is defined by Susan Chater and colleagues as follows:

> [D]eliberately inducing and maintaining deep sleep . . . in very specific circumstances. These are: 1) for the relief of one or more intractable symptoms when all other possible interventions have failed and the patient is perceived to be close to death, or 2) for the relief of profound anguish that is not amenable to spiritual, psychological, or other interventions, and the patient is perceived to be close to death.
> (Chater et al. 1998, 257–258)

PST may be used to treat both physical and psychological symptoms. The requirements for employing PST are that the patient be suffering from refractory physical or psychological symptoms, that death be close at hand, and that consent be obtained from the patient herself and/or her surrogate decision-maker. Refractory symptoms are those that cannot be adequately alleviated by any other means (e.g., psychotherapy, drugs, spiritual and/or familial support and so on). Patients are administered sedatives that keep them in a state of unconsciousness, and food and fluids are often withheld. PST can last from hours to weeks, but typically a patient will die within the first few days (Morita 2004, 448; Rousseau 2000, 1065–1066).

Although some object to the use of Palliative Sedation Therapy on the grounds that it is akin to euthanasia, it is widely employed and generally acknowledged to be a beneficial and morally permissible medical treatment (e.g., ten Have and Welie 2013; Taylor and McCann 2005; Chater et al. 1998). One of the main reasons that PST is legal throughout the United States, while active euthanasia remains illegal in all but a handful of states, is because PST is prima facie easily differentiated from active euthanasia in terms of the rule of double effect. Roughly put, this rule states that certain actions with bad effects may be morally permissible if those effects are foreseen but not intended, and if the action meets further conditions of goodness (of the action itself), intention (of the agent performing the action), and proportionality (of good to bad effects of the action) (Quill et al. 1997, 1786). It is easy to see how the rule of double effect might justify PST but not active euthanasia. In PST cases, the action is good in that it relieves pain. The agent (usually understood to be the relevant physician) intends to relieve the patient's pain through sedation. Death in this case is foreseen but not intended, and it is not a means to the end of pain relief, but rather a side-effect of achieving that end.[4] And, in PST cases, the good effect of pain relief is proportional to the "bad" effect of death. This is because the patient is suffering greatly, to such an extent that permanent unconsciousness is desirable. Even if the patient were not sedated, this suffering would in all likelihood continue until the patient passes away from her underlying illness. If being unconscious for the remainder of one's life is preferable to being conscious, given the degree of suffering consciousness entails, it is at least prima facie reasonable to say that one would be better off dead. If the patient's quality of life is so low that she prefers to be rendered unconscious, and if there is no reason to think the patient's suffering will eventually abate (as it would if the patient were suffering from an illness from which she would be expected to recover, or temporarily sedated in order to let her heal from some sort of trauma), then the bad effect of death would, for that patient, be proportional to the good effect of relieving the patient's suffering. In cases of *active* euthanasia, on the other hand, death is a clear means to the end of relieving suffering. Ending the patient's life is itself the method employed to alleviate suffering, rather than an anticipated side-effect of another method of pain relief.

Even if one holds that PST is morally permissible, while active euthanasia is not, it is still the case that we can have reason to administer PST to the not-imminently-dying while maintaining accordance with the rule of double effect. This is because the intention to relieve severe and intractable suffering holds regardless of whether the patient is terminally ill or not. I would argue that, if the same degree of intractable suffering is present in a patient who is not imminently dying and one who is, there is no reason to limit the administration of PST to the former. If PST is the only means of relieving such pain, then it seems equally justified in both sorts of cases. This will be so unless it is the case that death is a greater bad the earlier it occurs, such that the bad effect of death will not be proportional to the good effect of relieving suffering. The notion that death is worse if it occurs earlier in life, or that death is worse if it occurs during a certain pivotal time period in one's life, is put forward by philosophers such as Jeff McMahan, who argues that, from about age 10 onward, death is worse *for an individual* the more good life years are lost (McMahan 2002). This is an intuitive notion. After all, death after one has had the opportunity to live a long and full life seems like a much lesser evil than death in one's prime, or even before one's life has had a chance to really begin.

However, it also seems to be the case that more suffering is worse than less suffering, and so the total badness of suffering is worse the longer it lasts. If this is true, then the necessity of relieving suffering may be greater if it is anticipated that the patient will suffer greatly for many years. Eduard Verhagen and Pieter J.J. Sauer, for instance, found that in a sample of cases of neonatal euthanasia in the Netherlands under the Groningen Protocol, long life expectancy was a consideration in favor of euthanasia in over 50 percent of cases sampled. This was because "[t]he burden of other considerations is greater when the life expectancy is long in a patient who is suffering" (Verhagen and Sauer 2005, 960). Temporal length of suffering seems to be an important consideration in determining whether medical aid in dying is warranted. How are we to weigh the increased badness of death earlier in life against the increased suffering that accrues to a longer timespan?

Many of the general assumptions that undergird accounts of the badness of death do not apply to the sorts of patients who would opt for PST when not-imminently-dying. The tragedy of dying early is the loss of good life years, and so if the life years lost do not meet some minimum threshold of goodness in quality-of-life terms, it seems that death would be less bad for the person than it would be if she had life years of adequate quality to look forward to (as McMahan himself does acknowledge). If psychological suffering has made it such that a person will not be able to do the things that make human life valuable then, in such a case, an early death might not be any worse for that person than it would be if she were elderly. We might say that death is more tragic *in a sense*, but we would not have real reason to say that death would be worse *for the individual* if she is, for example, in her early 20s, given sufficient severity and persistence of suffering.

Unbearable Suffering

One requirement to receive euthanasia in accordance with the Dutch Euthanasia Act is that "the physician must be convinced that the patient's suffering is unbearable" (Pasman et al. 2009, 1). Now, it is true that whether a patient's level of well-being is bearable from her point of view will depend at least partly upon subjective evaluations on the part of the patient. However, I think it is possible to sketch in broad strokes some general features that contribute to making one's life bearable. Being able to pursue activities and projects one enjoys without being racked with pain is important to having a bearable level of well-being. On a more fundamental level, being able to function at all without being racked with pain seems to be a prerequisite for having a bearable level of well-being. Although the point at which life becomes unbearable in the face of that pain may differ from individual to individual, it will usually or always be characterized by seriously impairing the individual's ability to function. A protracted process of dying often involves having to experience the deterioration of one's mind and body until one is almost entirely dependent upon others for the necessities of daily life. It is hard to imagine wanting to lose control of one's body, have one's activities constrained by chronic pain, or rely on others to take care of daily activities, such as bathing and eating, to name just a few factors. States such as being bedridden, having to be helped with basic tasks such as using the toilet, bathing oneself, and eating, and a state of extreme dependence generally (and which, in EOL contexts, will often last indefinitely) all have the potential to seriously compromise a patient's well-being. PST may be opted for out of a desire to either alleviate the individual's suffering when she is in that state, or to alleviate her distress at the prospect of falling into that state. PST enables the patient to escape from this intolerable state at the EOL, in cases in which such suffering becomes both severe and refractory.

It is important to note here that it is not just terminal biophysical illness that can render a patient's life unbearable to her. Psychological suffering can be at least as painful as physical suffering, and so we have good reason to take psychological suffering as seriously as we take physical suffering. Furthermore, in many real-life circumstances it is near-impossible to tease the two apart. Particularly in end-of-life situations in which physical illness is often accompanied by psychological and existential distress, psychological problems, such as agitation and confusion, may be directly caused by or bound up with physical suffering, such as dyspnea (shortness of breath), or even the disorienting effects of pain medication used to treat the patient's physical suffering. Pain is complicated and may have vastly different causes and characters. Moreover, the fact that the root cause of psychological suffering may be "all in one's head" in no way renders it less painful or less genuine than something with clear biophysical correlates. This entails that the same obligations that accrue to medical providers in the face of straightforwardly biophysical pain equally apply in cases of psychological suffering.

A Rational Entailment From EOL to "Early" PST

PST involves:

1. the presence of severe and refractory patient suffering (physical or psychological)
2. chemical sedation to unconsciousness
3. requested by the patient or proxy consenter
4. taking place in an end-of-life context (and/or terminal illness)

Now suppose that genuinely refractory symptoms were present earlier in life. Chemical sedation (2) could thus be used to relieve severe refractory suffering (1) with the consent of the patient or proxy (3), but it is unclear as to why feature (4) ought to be necessary at all. That is, in the presence of genuinely refractory suffering, it is unclear what difference the patient being at the end of her life ought to make.

Consider the real-life example of the pseudonymous "Elizabeth," a Belgian woman in her late 50s who opted to begin the process for receiving medical euthanasia in 2014 (van de Perre and Daenen 2016).[5] Elizabeth has struggled with chronic anorexia since its onset at age 14. Over decades she has been in and out of psychiatric wards, sometimes for years at a time, and has tried medications and therapy with no great success. Her underlying mental illness has resulted in an inability to form romantic attachments and meaningful friendships and alienated Elizabeth from her family. Although the case as it is presented is under-described, I think it is safe to assume that Elizabeth struggles at the very least with depression as a comorbidity of her anorexia. Her life is suffused by suffering, and she finds herself practically overwhelmed by a desire to end this suffering. This desire is what led Elizabeth to request that her psychiatrist begin the euthanasia process. Suppose Elizabeth were a resident of the United States rather than Belgium. What should be done for her? If Elizabeth's pain truly is refractory and she has exhausted all treatment options, then it seems that medical professionals in the United States might ultimately be left with the choice of either allowing her suffering to continue or sedating her to the point at which she is no longer aware of her suffering. If Elizabeth were sedated and continued to receive food and fluids, then she would likely live for quite a long time, ultimately dying of some complication related to being hospitalized, which would probably take the form of an infection. If food and fluids were withheld, she would pass away sooner.

The case of Elizabeth illustrates how all the central moral considerations behind EOL PST can apply far in advance of a person's projected natural death. Elizabeth has expressed a persistent wish to die. She has autonomously consented to have her life ended with medical aid. The reason she wishes to die is that her subjective quality of life is so low as to be worse, on her own evaluation, than death. Her unremitting and severe psychological suffering is such that Elizabeth cannot derive any substantial and lasting joy or hope from life, and assuming that it has been accurately judged refractory, there is no prospect for that pain to be alleviated, apart from an unanticipated breakthrough in treatment or change in the way her brain is "wired." In light of this, it seems that it would be morally justified to use PST to end Elizabeth's suffering and the suffering of patients like her. This is evidence that our commitment to the moral permissibility of PST at the end of life rationally commits us to endorsing the moral permissibility of PST earlier in life and in the absence of terminal illness, when the conditions of very intense and unremitting refractory suffering and informed consent obtain. Going forward, I will employ as shorthand "early PST" to refer to cases of PST in which the death of the patient in question is not imminent and "EOL PST" to refer to cases of PST that take place at the end of a patient's life.[6]

Voluntary Palliated Starvation and Anorexia

Although it may seem far-fetched to imagine non-terminally ill patients who are tired of life coming to the hospital in droves and requesting to be sedated below the point of consciousness, Julian Savulescu has posited that something very similar could at least be possible (Savulescu 2014, 2015). Savulescu argues that, since it would be immoral to compel a capacitated individual who has made the reasoned decision to refrain from eating to eat, and doctors have the obligation to care for patients regardless of whether harm is self-inflicted or not, a patient who voluntarily chooses to starve herself in order to die has the right to receive palliative care, likely including PST (Savulescu 2014, 111). Voluntarily stopping eating and drinking can take place at any point of life by individuals who have decided it would be better to die for whatever (capacitated) reason. In such cases, PST would presumably take place when suffering from starvation becomes refractory. A patient who voluntarily stops eating and drinking and who receives such palliative care will thus be in the process of what Savulescu terms "Voluntary Palliated Starvation" (VPS).[7] Savulescu goes on to make the following statement, which will serve as a sort of motivating case for the remainder of this chapter:

> Some anorexics, perhaps many, are competent and psychiatric illness does not necessarily render a person incompetent. The competent wishes of people with psychiatric illness should be respected, even wishes to die, or choices that foreseeably result in death. Psychiatric illness can be a good reason to want to die, just as physical illness can be.
>
> (ibid.)

How might we make sense of Savulescu's claim that some (perhaps many) anorexic patients have capacity to consent to VPS? Might Elizabeth, for instance, have capacity to consent to VPS? And, even if it were possible for Elizabeth to consent to VPS, how would we go about determining whether she actually has capacity to make such a decision in any particular case?

It is clear that psychiatric illness does not always render a person incapacitated, and that the requests of mentally ill patients with capacity should, in general, be respected. However, anorexia may pose some unique challenges to decision-making capacity in the context of VPS. As the Mayo Clinic characterizes it, anorexia involves "an abnormally low body weight, intense fear of gaining weight and a distorted perception of body weight" (Mayo Clinic Foundation for Medical Education and Research 2018). If an anorexic person prioritizes not eating over living on the basis of her fear of gaining weight or inaccurate conception of her body as being too large, then she is choosing on the basis of a skewed perception of the world that is rooted in psychological illness, which would preclude her from being able to make a reasoned decision with capacity.

Characteristics of anorexia that may further impair capacity include "the cognitive changes associated with acute and chronic starvation; the psychological distortions and phobias that are inherent to the diagnosis; and, the deeply rooted ambivalence that most patients have towards recovery, given its inextricable link to their most feared outcome—weight restoration" (Bryden et al. 2010, 139). There is also evidence that decision making in general is impaired in people with anorexia nervosa, manifesting specifically in "a preference for immediate reward despite the long-term adverse consequences" (Adoue et al. 2015, 121). So there is at least prima facie reason to think that an anorexic patient will not have capacity to opt for VPS *as a means to persist in a state of starving herself.* It is also worth noting that, although the existence of such consensus far from settles matters in moral terms, "there is a broad consensus that involuntary treatment of patients with eating disorders is ethically and legally justifiable when the patient is at acute risk of death from the medical complications of his or her disorder" (Bryden et al. 2010, 139).

I take the motivation of anorexics who would prioritize not eating over remaining alive to show that the intention behind VPS matters when it comes to determining whether or not (a) the person making the decision does in fact have capacity to make that decision, and (b) whether a case of VPS is chosen with the aim of permanently relieving suffering (physical, psychological, or existential). The key to making sense of this is Savulescu's claim that psychiatric illness can provide just as good a reason to desire to die as biophysical illness. It is not out of the question that an anorexic patient might judge that a world in which she must eat, given the pain of her psychological illness and little to no prospect of a cure in her particular case, would be worse than death, and rationally choose VPS as a means to death. However, this is importantly different from using VPS as a means to persist in a state of starving oneself with death as a mere side effect (there is here a reversal of the sort of argument that applies the rule of double effect to distinguish between PST and euthanasia).

There is thus a difference between using voluntary starvation as a means to die when life has become unbearable and assigning *not eating itself* such a high priority that resulting death does not matter to one as much as the importance of refraining from eating. If an anorexic chooses to die rather than eat on the basis of the suffering generated by her psychological illness being unbearable to her, this might be a situation in which she could make a capacitated decision to opt for VPS. After all decision to opt for VPS. After all, anorexia is a painful illness to suffer from, especially when one is in the later stages of starvation. So, it might be the case that an anorexic could have capacity to choose to end her life rather than eat because her illness itself has rendered life intolerable to her. And, if her suffering could be proven severe and refractory, then she would possibly be a candidate for early PST under the entailment I've built in this chapter.

It is unclear how exactly to separate a rational desire to die in which the patient is motivated, such that she *accepts as a reason* the suffering of her mental illness, from a desire to die that *issues from the illness itself* in a way that precludes the patient from choosing rationally. In reality, the motivations of patients may be mixed. And a patient's genuine motivations may be opaque to us and sometimes even to the patient herself. In light of these fundamental uncertainties, there would be a significant chance of error in determining the intentions of any particular anorexic. And this uncertainty alone might provide reason to judge anorexics incapacitated in general to make such a choice. But it would be morally troubling to remove the option of receiving medical aid in dying from capacitated mentally ill patients, such as anorexics who are suffering greatly and rationally desire to die *taking as a reason* their severe and refractory psychological suffering.

Anorexia is a particularly interesting example of mental illness to consider here because VPS is essentially an accelerated version of the starvation process an anorexic will often already be undergoing as a product of her illness. Further, some data on the lived experience of anorexia indicates inner alienation from the disorder, with an "anorexic voice" present as something distinct from the rest of the self. This "anorexic voice" often begins as a helpful "friend" and coping mechanism then becomes a dominating "enemy" (Williams and Reid 2012, 2010). So, it may be simpler to distinguish between preferences of the "self" and those of the "anorexic voice" than it would be to distinguish between preferences that issue from the authentic self and those that issue from mental illness in, for example, cases of serious depression. Because depression characteristically casts a negative valence on one's thoughts and experiences in a sweeping and pervasive way, there will likely be no "depressive voice" a patient can point to as something distinct from, or at least a distinct part of, herself. Taken together, the method of starvation, coupled with the inner experience of anorexia, have the entailment that it may be more difficult to determine the patient's motivations *from the outside*, but perhaps easier for the patient to determine her own motivations *from the inside* in cases of anorexia than it would be for patients suffering from (at least some) other mental illnesses.

It seems that, although Savulescu is correct that it is not outside the realm of possibility that an anorexic patient may have capacity to consent to VPS, there are deeply troubling uncertainties on the part of the evaluator, as well as perhaps even the patient herself, as to whether the patient is choosing taking as a reason the suffering of her illness or whether the choice is issuing from the illness itself. This is because the direct method the patient is taking to die lines up with what her underlying illness compels her to do, namely self-starvation. It would be challenging to determine—both from the inside (i.e., from the patient's perspective) and from the outside (i.e., from the perspective of an evaluator)—whether stopping eating and drinking in the case of any particular anorexic patient were genuinely *voluntary*. So, at the very least, it seems that there is good reason to operate under a blanket assumption of incapacity for anorexic patients specifically when it comes to VPS as a method of medical aid in dying.

Social Alienation as a Compounding Concern

Even apart from the unique challenges that accrue to determining the capacity of an anorexic patient to consent to a form of medical aid in dying that is precipitated by complete cessation of eating, there are further concerns that ought to be taken seriously in determining the capacity of mentally ill patients in general to consent to end their lives early and in the absence of terminal illness. And, even apart from concerns such as explicit financial pressure or overt coercion which might compromise a patient's ability to make a free and reasoned choice, there are numerous non-explicit pressures which may compromise patient capacity, including ableism as a social force that discounts the lives of the mentally ill, caretaker fatigue, and social alienation.[8] While these issues are by their nature difficult to quantify, I think a reasonable story can be told as to how a patient may be led to value her life less highly than she might otherwise as a result of them.

I will here focus on and motivate one locus of concern which, by itself and combined with the inherent uncertainties that accompany capacity determinations in the face of mental illness, may give us reason to pause: social alienation. Social alienation may be a substantial component or compounding factor of psychological suffering but it is difficult to quantify and even more difficult to fix. One might be hesitant to "medicalize" something like social isolation or atomization in the form of familial estrangement, a dearth of meaningful relationships, or lack of community involvement. But such factors have an immense impact on patient's lives, one that can may ground a preference for continuing to live or not.

One representative case where it is clear that social alienation in the form of familial estrangement played a substantial role in shaping a patient's choice to opt for medical aid in dying is that of Nathan Verhelst, a Belgian 44-year-old who, in 2013 opted for medical euthanasia primarily on the basis of depression resulting from botched sex reassignment surgery (Nollet 2014; Hamilton 2013; Gordts 2013). It is important to note that, while the botched surgery was the proximate cause of Nathan opting for euthanasia, he was looking into seeking medical euthanasia even in advance of the surgery in question (Nollet 2014). An abusive and traumatic childhood coupled with continued estrangement from his emotionally unavailable mother contributed greatly to Nathan viewing his own life as not worth living. Ultimately, Nathan was approved for euthanasia on the basis of psychological and physical suffering resulting from his surgery, but it is clear that even in the absence of the physical suffering which resulted from the botched surgery, Nathan was deeply unhappy to the point of considering ending his life. Might Nathan have refrained from opting for medical euthanasia if he were able to reconcile with his mother (as he had with his father shortly before his father's death)? Might he have refrained if his brothers apologized for or even acknowledged the years of torment they inflicted on Nathan? It is impossible to know with certainty the answer to these questions. But it is nonetheless deeply troubling to think of the impact that psychological conditioning from abuse might play in determining the conception of the world and the worth of their own lives of patients like Nathan. It is also reasonable to think that social isolation may exacerbate preexisting mental illness.

Furthermore, even in standard EOL cases of PST, social isolation may be a factor that complicates both determinations of capacity and determinations of refractoriness of psycho-existential suffering. In a survey of palliative care physicians in Japan, Tatsuya Morita found that 22 percent of patients who received PST on the basis of psycho-existential suffering did so due to suffering which consisted in "isolation/lack of social support" (Morita 2004, 448). The cases under consideration took place in EOL contexts, so it is reasonable to think that there may simply not have been time for social integration of patients successfully to take place before they passed away from their underlying illnesses. But in cases of early PST, it seems that this is something that cannot be as easily determined. Here determinations of decision-making capacity and those of refractoriness of psychological suffering converge. Social alienation is only one of many considerations that may greatly affect a patient's conception of herself and the worth of her life, compound the effects of existing mental illness, and become more difficult to judge the refractoriness the further from anticipated death a patient is. In light of this, we should lean toward judgments of incapacity in cases such as that of Nathan and Elizabeth, for whom social alienation played a significant role in their decision to opt for medical aid in dying and cut short their considerable future lifespans. A blanket assumption of incapacity, like the one made for anorexic patients with regard to VPS specifically, may thus be warranted in such cases. However, to completely preclude mentally ill patients from having access to medical aid in dying in the absence of terminal illness and in advance of their anticipated deaths may be needlessly cruel in cases where suffering is extremely severe and genuinely refractory. It seems that any blanket presumption of incapacity should nonetheless allow for exceptions in cases of refractory and extremely severe (perhaps even debilitating) psychological suffering.

Should Decision-Making Capacity Always Matter?

But this prompts a further troubling question: if sufficiently severe suffering may override uncertainty regarding patient capacity, might severe enough suffering warrant taking drastic measures to relieve that suffering, *even in patients who are clearly incapacitated*? Sometimes the people who are suffering the most are also those who do not have capacity to make their own decisions. Consider Jukka Varelius's example of Mary:

> Mary is a psychiatric patient who has repeatedly tried to kill herself. Once again, her suicide attempt failed. . . . Though they are unable to have meaningful contact with her, the mental health-care providers are also convinced that, when she is not sedated to near unconsciousness, Mary is suffering unbearably. And they deem her condition incurable. Consequently, although this would be against the common psychiatric goal of suicide prevention to which they have adhered to so far, some of the mental health-care providers treating Mary have started to wonder whether they should assist her in ending her life rather than aim to prevent her from killing herself.
> (Varelius 2016, 228)

Mary is clearly suffering greatly, her condition has been deemed incurable, and although she does not possess the mental capacity to give genuine informed consent or to even make a request for physician-assisted suicide, Mary has clearly and persistently expressed a wish to die through her actions.

This presents the following problem: ending one's life early is an irrevocable decision of immense import, the sort of decision that seems to require that the person making it be able to do so rationally and in accordance with her own values and aims. Ending one's life early is also the sort of decision that requires weighty reasons in order to be justified. In medical contexts, extreme and intractable pain is often considered to constitute such a reason. However, in Mary's case, it seems that she has a very good reason to opt to end her life early in that she is suffering greatly, but the very thing causing her suffering also precludes her from being able to give informed consent to have her life ended.

It is unclear what we ought to do in a case like Mary's. On the one hand, she is clearly suffering greatly and wishes to die. This is apparent, even though she lacks capacity to consent to medical aid in dying. And, it seems that medical professionals do have a duty of beneficence to Mary, a duty that would be best fulfilled in such a case by aiding her in dying, either through PST or more direct means. On the other hand, providing medical aid in dying to suicidal but incapacitated psychiatric patients seems like an undesirable and even dangerous precedent to set. This is not to assume some nefarious motivations on the part of medical professionals. Rather, it is a hesitancy that is rooted in a concern for human fallibility. It would be unfortunate if patients whose suffering could have eventually been alleviated or who would in fact regain capacity at some point were aided in dying before this change had the opportunity to take place. Note that this does not mean that capacitated patients who are able to autonomously consent to PST due to psychological suffering ought to be kept alive in the hope of some treatment, however unlikely, being developed to alleviate their suffering. In such cases, the patient is consenting not only to receive medical aid in dying, but also to receive such aid in dying while knowing that *there is the possibility, however slight, that her pain may some day be alleviated*. Because there is no way for an incapacitated psychiatric patient to consent under such a caveat, considerations of eventual expansion of treatment options should take a greater role in deciding whether aid in dying is warranted.

One might be inclined to say here that the problem could be solved in many cases by simply allowing proxy consenters to choose a medically assisted death for patients like Mary. If such proxies are choosing out of a concern for Mary's interests and well-being, then they could make this choice on the assumption that it is best for those patients and in line with what those patients themselves would want, were they capacitated. (Although, if the patients were capacitated, they likely would not have the same weight of circumstances pushing them toward choosing death, so this may be seen as a bit of a puzzling standard under the circumstances.) However, I do not think that allowing a proxy consenter to make such a decision solves the underlying problem, at least not entirely. This is so for a couple of reasons. First, it may be unfair to saddle proxies with such a decision. While making life and death decisions on behalf of loved ones is always difficult, doing the same in a situation where not only is no terminal illness present, but additionally there is so much epistemic uncertainty regarding refractoriness of suffering and what the patient would want were she capacitated seems even more difficult. Second, the special relationships between most patients and their proxies (who are often parents, guardians, or other family members) may seriously and troublingly complicate decision making. For instance, the emotional and sometimes financial toll that severe mental illness can take on relationships and the lives of those who support mentally ill family members are the sort of things that might lead a proxy to rationalize aid in dying in situations that might be borderline, or in which medical aid in dying might be inappropriate, out of sheer exhaustion or frustration. This is especially so in places like the United States where mental health care is inadequately funded and so the financial burden of illness must be largely shouldered by families. Such circumstances compound the unfairness of saddling proxies with making this decision.

As uncomfortable as I am with such philosophical positions in general, I am inclined to say that in this sort of case providing medical aid in dying to incapacitated psychiatric patients whose suffering is refractory, severe, and continuous, and who have expressed a consistent, persistent, and unwavering wish to die through their actions and/or words might be the morally best choice on the part of *individual medical providers*. However, I am not sure I could accept the implications of legislating such aid and/or explicitly incorporating it into medical practice. Here I am endorsing something similar to what David Velleman proposed where medical euthanasia is permitted "by tacit failure to enforce the institutional rules that currently serve as barriers to justified euthanasia" rather than "an explicitly formulated permission" in the form of policy or law (Velleman 1992, 680). In Mary's case, her medical providers might be strictly speaking morally justified in assisting her suicide, but it might nonetheless set a dangerous precedent to incorporate such assistance into hospital or legal policy.

Conclusion

If VPS were the only available method of early palliative sedation, then it seems that the fundamental uncertainty regarding the motivations of any particular anorexic patient would justify a blanket judgment of incapacity in all such cases. Further, applied more broadly, it seems that similar uncertainty when coupled with further concerns such as the role social alienation may play in shaping a mentally ill patient's conception of the world and herself should give us pause when determining capacity for mentally ill patients to consent to medical aid in dying in the absence of terminal illness and far in advance of the patient's anticipated death. In the face of such troubling uncertainty, it seems that a blanket judgment of incapacity under such circumstances—with possible room for exceptions—may be justified as well.

Notes

1. As Paul Appelbaum notes, "Any diagnosis or treatment that compromises mentation may be associated with incompetence. However, since a range of severity is associated with most diagnoses, no diagnosis in which consciousness is retained is invariably predictive of incapacity" (Appelbaum 2007, 1835).
2. See Doernberg et al. (2016) for evidence of inconsistency in the way that capacity determinations are made for patients requesting euthanasia or physician-assisted suicide.
3. While in the United States "capacity" is characteristically used to refer to clinical judgments and "competence" to legal judgments, this usage is not standardized across the literature; some authors cited in this chapter use "competence" to refer to capacity.
4. One might make the case that withdrawing a patient's feeding tube while she undergoes PST demonstrates that the physicians intend the death of the patient (see, e.g., Jansen and Sulmasy 2002). However, it is commonly the case that the withdrawal of food and fluids would have taken place regardless of whether the patient was sedated or not (see, e.g., Morita et al. 2005).
5. The Belgian news article I rely upon here was originally published in Dutch, translated into English with the help of Google. While I acknowledge that some nuance may have been lost in translation, I have done my best to be careful in describing this case, and the bare facts of the case on their own are such that they provide a good illustration of the sort of patient this project centrally concerns.
6. I owe the terminology of "early" PST/Terminal Sedation to Victor Cellarius (2011).
7. Savulescu bases his claim that a competent person ought not be compelled to eat on a "moral principle of inviolability of the person" wherein it is "impermissible for one person, A, or several people B-D, to insert any part of their body, object or substance into the body of another competent person, X, without X's valid consent" (Savulescu 2014, 111). I think such a principle, as Savulescu formulates it, may be overstated. However, consideration of voluntary palliated starvation as a form of early PST is still warranted.
8. Ableism and misdiagnosis may play a part in this, as well as compounding factors stemming from intersectional identities. See the following chapters for more: Chapter 8: "Medical Over-testing and Racial Distrust" by Golemon, Chapter 9: "The Epistemology of Medical Error in an Intersectional World" by Shapiro, and Chapter 10: "Knowledge-based Medical Errors: The Case of Ableism" by Reynolds and Peña-Gúzman.

Works Cited

Adoue, Cyril, et al. 2015. "A Further Assessment of Decision-Making in Anorexia Nervosa." *European Psychiatry* 30 (1): 121–127.

Appelbaum, Paul. 2007. "Assessment of Patients' Competence to Consent to Treatment." *New England Journal of Medicine* 357: 1834–1840.

Beauchamp, Tom, and James Childress. 2009. *Principles of Biomedical Ethics, Sixth Edition*. New York: Oxford University Press.

Brock, Daniel. 1992. "Voluntary Active Euthanasia." *The Hastings Center Report* 22 (2): 10–22.

Bryden, Pier, et al. 2010. "The Ontario Experience of Involuntary Treatment of Pediatric Patients with Eating Disorders." *International Journal of Law and Psychiatry* 33 (3): 138–143.

Buchanan, Allen E., and Dan W. Brock. 1995. *Deciding for Others: The Ethics of Surrogate Decision Making*. New York: Cambridge University Press.

Cellarius, Victor. 2011. "'Early Terminal Sedation' Is a Distinct Entity." *Bioethics* 25 (1): 46–54.

Chater, Susan, et al. 1998. "Sedation for Intractable Distress in the Dying—A Survey of Experts." *Palliative Medicine* 12 (4): 255–269.

Chochinov, Harvey, et al. 2006. "Dignity in the Terminally Ill: Revisited." *Journal of Palliative Medicine* 9 (3): 666–672.

Doernberg, Sam, et al. 2016. "Capacity Evaluations of Psychiatric Patients Requesting Assisted Death in the Netherlands." *Psychosomatics* 57 (6): 556–565.

Dworkin, Ronald, et al. 1997. "Assisted Suicide: The Philosophers' Brief." *The New York Review of Books* 44 (5).

Dworkin, Ronald. 1994. *Life's Dominion: An Argument About Abortion, Euthanasia, and Individual Freedom*. New York: Vintage Books.

The Economist. 2015, November 10. "24 & Ready to Die." [Video File]. Retrieved from https://youtu.be/SWWkUzkfJ4M.

Gordts, Eline. 2013. "Nathan Verhelst Chooses Euthanasia After Failed Gender Reassignment Surgeries." *Huffington Post*. Retrieved from www.huffingtonpost.com/2013/10/05/nathan-verhelst-euthanasia-belgium_n_4046106.html

Hamilton, Graeme. 2013. "Terminally Transsexual: Concerns Raised Over Belgian Euthanized After Botched Sex Change." *National Post*. Retrieved from https://nationalpost.com/news/canada/terminally-transsexual-concerns-raised-over-belgian-euthanized-after-botched-sex-change

Jansen, Lynn, and Daniel Sulmasy. 2002 "Sedation, Alimentation, Hydration, and Equivocation: Careful Conversation About Care at the End of Life." *Annals of Internal Medicine* 136 (11): 845–849.

Mayo Clinic Foundation for Medical Education and Research. (2018). *Anorexia Nervosa*. Retrieved from www.mayoclinic.org/diseases-conditions/anorexia/symptoms-causes/syc-20353591

MacKenzie, Catriona, and Natalie Stoljar. 2000. *Relational Autonomy: Feminist Perspectives on Autonomy, Agency, and the Social Self*. New York: Oxford University Press.

McMahan, Jeff. 2002. *The Ethics of Killing: Problems at the Margins of Life*. New York: Oxford University Press.

Morita, Tatsuya. 2004. "Palliative Sedation to Relieve Psycho-Existential Suffering of Terminally Ill Cancer Patients." *Journal of Pain and Symptom Management* 28 (5): 445–450.

Morita, Tatsuya., et al. 2005. "Ethical Validity of Palliative Sedation Therapy: A Multicenter, Prospective, Observational Study Conducted on Specialized Palliative Care Units in Japan." *Journal of Pain and Symptom Management* 30 (4): 308–319.

Nollet, Roel. 2014. *Nathan—Free As A Bird* [Documentary Film]. Belgium: Trotwaar Production.

O'Gara, Eilish. 2015, June 29. "Physically Healthy 24-Year-Old Granted Right to Die in Belgium." *Newsweek*. Retrieved from www.newsweek.com/euthanasia-belgiumeuthanasiaassisted-dyingmental-illnessdr-marc-van-hoeyright-603019.

Oregon Health Authority, Public Health Division. 2018. "Oregon Death with Dignity Act: 2017 Data Summary." Retrieved from www.oregon.gov/oha/PH/

PROVIDERPARTNERRESOURCES/EVALUATIONRESEARCH/DEATH
WITHDIGNITYACT/Documents/year20.pdf
Oregon Health Authority. 2018. *Death with Dignity Act Requirements.* Retrieved
from www.oregon.gov/oha/PH/PROVIDERPARTNERRESOURCES/EVALUA-
TIONRESEARCH/DEATHWITHDIGNITYACT/Documents/requirements.pdf
Pasman, Roeline, M. Rurup, D. Willems, and B. Onwuteaka-Philipsen. 2009.
"Concept of Unbearable Suffering in Context of Ungranted Requests for
Euthanasia: Qualitative Interviews with Patients and Physicians." *The BMJ*
339: b4362.
Quill, Timothy, Rebecca Dresser, and Dan Brock. 1997. "The Rule of Double
Effect—A Critique of its Role in End-of-Life Decision Making." *New England
Journal of Medicine* 337 (24): 1768–1771.
Rietjens, Judith, Donald van Tol, Maartje Schermer, and A. van der Heide. 2009.
"Judgement of Suffering in the Case of a Euthanasia Request in the Nether-
lands." *Journal of Medical Ethics* 35 (8): 502–507.
Rousseau, Paul. 2000. "The Ethical Validity and Clinical Experience of Palliative
Sedation." *Mayo Clinic Proceedings* 75: 1064–1069.
Savulescu, Julian. 2014. "A Simple Solution to the Puzzles of End of Life? Volun-
tary Palliated Starvation." *Journal of Medical Ethics* 40 (2): 110–113.
Savulescu, Julian. 2015. "Autonomy, Interests, Justice and Active Medical Eutha-
nasia." In Michael Cholbi and Jukka Varelius (eds.), *New Directions in the
Ethics of Assisted Suicide and Euthanasia. International Library of Ethics,
Law, and the New Medicine 64.* Basel: Springer International Publishing Swit-
zerland: 41–58.
Sherwin, Susan. 2012. "A Relational Approach to Autonomy in Health Care."
In Elizabeth Gedge and Wilfred Waluchow (eds.), *Readings in Health Care
Ethics—Second Edition.* Buffalo: Broadview Press: 14–32.
Taylor, Robert, and Robert McCann. 2005. "Controlled Sedation for Physical
and Existential Suffering?" *Journal of Palliative Medicine* 8 (1): 144–147.
ten Have, Hank, and Jos Welie. 2013. "Palliative Sedation Versus Euthanasia: An
Ethical Assessment." *Journal of Pain and Symptom Management*: 1–14.
van de Perre, Kim, and Ward Daenen. 2016. "'Ik Wil Niet Meer Leven, Maar
Geef Me Tijd om te Sterven': De Tweestrijd van Elizabeth, Tussen Ondraaglijk
Leven en een Zachte Dood." *De Morgen.* Retrieved from www.demorgen.be/
lifestyle/-ik-wil-niet-meer-leven-maar-geef-me-tijd-om-te-sterven-be13a7e3/.
Varelius, Jukka. 2016. "On the Moral Acceptability of Physician-Assisted Dying
for Non-Autonomous Psychiatric Patients." *Bioethics* 30 (4): 227–233.
Velleman, J. David. 1992. "Against the Right to Die." *Journal of Medicine and
Philosophy* 17 (6): 665–681.
Verhagen, Eduard, and Pieter Sauer. 2005. "The Groningen Protocol—Euthan-
sia in Severely Ill Newborns." *New England Journal of Medicine* 352 (10):
959–962.
Williams, Sarah, and Marie Reid. 2010. "Understanding the Experience of
Ambivalence in Anorexia Nervosa: The Maintainer's Perspective." *Psychology
and Health* 25 (5): 551–567.
Williams, Sarah, and Marie Reid. 2012. "'It's Like There Are Two People in My
Head': A Phenomenological Exploration of Anorexia Nervosa and Its Rela-
tionship to the Self." *Psychology and Health* 27 (7): 798–815.

Part IV
Learning From Error

12 Medical Error as a Collaborative Learning Tool

Jordan Joseph Wadden

Why Should We Examine Medical Error?

The risk of medical error is positively correlated to the increasing work load placed on hospitals and medical teams (Elwahab and Doherty 2014). This makes medical error a prime candidate for research aimed at improving both medical encounters and patient well-being. Health-care professionals[1] and patients often have the same goal in health-care, but in some situations these groups deviate in their priorities. One such situation is when an error occurs. Both health-care professionals and patients want to be told when an error has occurred; however, only around one-third of medical errors are disclosed to patients and only about half are reported internally.[2] This is curious, as reporting an error seems to be a logical step in preventing the same error from occurring again. However, there are several reasons why a health-care professional might not report an error, ranging from: a fear of reprimand, a fear of what others might think of their error (residents might fear a loss of job, senior doctors might fear losing their credentials, etc.), or a belief that the error was not nearly as bad as it might seem, among others. In this sense, having a theory of error might be helpful to understand how we might use medical errors in a positive manner.

As of writing this chapter there are no philosophers who have done a comprehensive study on error in a sense relevant to this book.[3] This means there are several gaps that this chapter must traverse, alongside the work of others in this book. My contribution to filling these gaps is to develop how an understanding of medical errors might be an untapped resource for collaborative learning in medicine in both training and on-the-job experience.

Further motivating an analysis of medical error is the fact that health-care professionals' mental and emotional well-being often suffer when they recognize that they have caused an error.[4] These negative effects feed into the culture of blame and perfectionism in our health-care systems. The purpose of this chapter is to motivate the idea that we can create a better health-care system for all involved (patients, health-care professionals, policy makers, etc.) if we can mitigate this fear-laden culture and replace it with one in which we can collaboratively learn from errors.

My approach to this chapter is as follows. First, I will outline the problem of unknown evidence, as I believe this is crucial for understanding how to use medical errors in a positive sense. I then sketch a few different kinds of medical error that occur and then differentiate these medical errors from adverse events. The purpose of this is to delineate just how pervasive medical error is in our health-care systems and how many health-care professionals are affected by error. This is important for motivating the use of error as a collaborative learning tool. I then join this section to the first to develop an account of how medical error can, and I believe *should*, be used as a collaborative learning tool for medical students and professionals alike. Here I will show that, rather than ignoring or shaming those who commit errors, we ought to take these occurrences as opportunities to improve collective professionalism. This leads to my final section, where I conclude and discuss a recognition of how errors can help develop epistemic humility.

The Problem of Unknown Evidence

Epistemic Counterfactuals

To make any decision, the decider needs to rely on the relevant evidence. But just what *is* the relevant evidence? Deliberation on what counts as evidence can happen intentionally, by actively pouring over the various reasons one has for developing a belief, but this can also happen quickly and in an almost intuitive manner. However, the evidence we *do not* have for many topics comprises most of the relevant evidence for that topic. This realization alone should create doubt that we have all the relevant evidence. Once we have this doubt, we ought to adjust our credence in our initial belief (Nathan Ballantyne 2015). Otherwise, we risk obstinance.

This brings us to the concept of *epistemic counterfactuals*. Counterfactuals are statements that relate to or express something that has not happened or is not the case. Epistemic counterfactuals are a sub-type of these statements that are concerned with how our evidence and justification for events might change if some contrary-to-fact state had occurred.[5] We can use this alternate information to determine if our current evidence is enough to justify believing what we hold to be true, or if we need to adjust our credence in our beliefs. These can be simple statements, such as "if you had studied for your MCAT, then you might have gotten in to a better medical school." However, epistemic counterfactuals can be more complex statements, such as "if Henry the VIII had not created the Church of England, then there would be good reasons to believe that the English Reformation and subsequent separation from the Pope might never have happened."

These counterfactual statements present us with *defeaters* for beliefs we currently hold as true. A defeater is simply a new belief that is incompatible with some other belief we already hold. To illustrate these defeaters, suppose for a moment that we have a proposition *P*.[6] The first type of defeater presents a reason that attacks the connection between your belief in *P* and your justification for believing *P*. These are called undermining defeaters. Undermining defeaters are consistent with *P* being true, but by removing justification for believing *P* they leave your current belief in *P* unsupported (and therefore irrational). Suppose for a moment that *P* is the belief that your scrubs are red. If you suddenly learned that you were red–green color-blind, you now have reason to think your belief that your scrubs are red is defeated. They might very well be red, but you will need new evidence to justify believing this is true (such as the testimony of another nurse, for example). The second type of defeater acts as a reason against *P* itself. These are called rebutting defeaters and are inconsistent with *P* being true. Suppose now that *P* is the belief that your supervising physician is retiring on Tuesday. If your colleague then tells you that your supervisor is not retiring (perhaps they are just taking a much deserved vacation) you now have reason to think your belief *P* is incorrect. The main difference between a rebutting defeater and an undermining defeater is that a rebutting defeater suggests you ought to disbelieve *P*, whereas an undermining defeater suggests you should only suspend judgment in *P* and *not* that you should disbelieve *P*.

Epistemic counterfactuals present us with a significant problem: in most knowledge claims we have a reasonable counterfactual claim that challenges their truth. When we try to decide what to include in the relevant set of evidence for a medical decision, we need to ask whether we have overlooked anything and whether the evidence we do have comprises a fair sample of the total relevant evidence. Many of us will hold a belief while simultaneously realizing there is likely unpossessed evidence we may (or may not) have access to. Nathan Ballantyne calls this the Problem of Unpossessed Evidence and it is based in what he considers the reality of information overload (Nathan Ballantyne 2015, 317n1). For example, if a physician determines that a patient's results for a set of tests *must* be Disease X, another physician could present the counterfactual "If the lab had run an additional test, then you might have concluded that the patient has Disease Y instead." In fact, in many cases, there may be multiple alternatives *and* more health-care professionals might support an alternative the original physician did not conclude.

There are two ways I believe these defeaters could contribute to medical error. The first is if we overlook a defeater for some belief. This can happen if we realize (on our own or with the help of others) that we have likely missed reasons for *rejecting* a conclusion. For example, the physician above decided that their patient has Disease X because of the tests that they ordered. We can imagine that their resources might have been different if they were at an urban hospital, rather than a rural hospital. At an urban hospital they might have had access to additional tests. At a rural hospital these additional tests are overlooked not due to any physician negligence. Rather, they are overlooked due to a restriction to access that many rural hospitals face. Thus, the physician in this case very likely could have come to a different conclusion depending on where they are stationed, urban or rural.

The second way defeaters can contribute to medical error is if we come to doubt our evidence for some decision represents a fair sample of the possible evidence. The significance of this consideration is that it forces us to confront the fact that our evidence is always, at best, partial. Because of this, we can easily wonder whether our sample of evidence is fair. Recall the physician above once again. The decision to use the tests she ordered is an accident of her personal history. Had she been educated at a different university, she might have been taught to prefer a completely different method and set of tests to make her decision. This hypothetical shift has the potential to return a completely different result (say, diagnosing some disease instead of some other disease).

Using Counterfactuals in Medicine

Counterfactuals are not new to medical decision making. But what do counterfactuals have to do with medical error? Consider the following hypothetical situation: Yael is an emergency surgeon in an urban emergency ward. A patient arrives in a serious condition, and she realizes she needs to use either Treatment A or Treatment B to attempt to save this patient. She decides to use Treatment A, and unfortunately the patient dies. Yael now wonders whether she made a mistake in choosing Treatment A, and whether she should have gone with Treatment B.

In this hypothetical situation, Yael has presented herself with the counterfactual that, if she had chosen Treatment B, then the patient may have survived. Her worry about whether she has made an error presents her with an undermining defeater. This is because, while it is possible that Treatment A was indeed correct, and the patient was going to die due to some unrelated complication, Yael no longer has clear justification for the decision she made. John Petrocelli claims that the more likely a physician is to select their counterfactual alternative, "the more extreme the affective reaction he/she will experience in response to the unfortunate outcome" (Petrocelli 2013, 1). I will return to this affective element, as I believe it plays a role in why many do not report errors.

Petrocelli says that counterfactual thinking is most likely to emerge for health-care professionals when they experience unexpected outcomes, undesirable outcomes, repeatable situations, and when they come close (but do not reach) desirable outcomes (Petrocelli 2013, 5). What these situations share is that they all lend themselves to error. This makes sense because the act of considering whether some other course of action would have been better for a given situation implicitly suggests the presence of error. In the above thought experiment, for example, Yael is worried that she *incorrectly* chose Treatment A, and this deliberation comes following an undesirable outcome (the loss of her patient). This is not to say that Yael is incompetent; far from it, as a surgeon Yael has become an expert in the medical field. Instead, this uncertainty plays on the fact that there is undoubtedly evidence that she does not (or possibly *could not*) know at the time when she had to make her decision.

The Problem of Medical Error

Identifying Medical Errors

In an ideal world our health-care systems would operate smoothly and error free. However, any system involving human interaction will never be completely error free, so these systems need methods to identify and react to error. This is easier said than done. In this section I briefly outline that even the concept of "medical error" is difficult to pin down, making attempts at mitigating errors difficult. Understanding medical errors first involves drawing a distinction between medical errors and adverse events (sometimes called adverse outcomes). Medical errors can be defined as incorrect medical care that, either through inaction or improper action, have the potential to cause substantive harm. Adverse events, on the other hand, are any unintended substantive harm to a patient resulting from medical treatment and that is not attributable to their underlying condition (Proctor et al. 2003).[7] The occurrence of error is not itself an adverse event, as not all errors cause harm (they simply have the potential to cause harm).

The two most frequent classes of adverse events are postoperative infections and pressure ulcers (i.e., bedsores) (Schwendimann et al. 2018, 1). On the whole, these do not occur because of poorly performing physicians. Instead, these events appear to be a result of cost-cutting efforts that end up compromising patient safety. Adverse events can also appear because of an unknown complication, in addition to these cost-cutting efforts. These two causes of adverse events are different from those causes of medical errors. This is part of the difficulty involved in understanding, reporting, and mitigating medical errors and adverse events. Once an adverse event has been identified, it is not always easy to tell when it is due to a complication, some systematic problem, or an error on the part of a health-care professional.

Medical errors come in many different types. For the purpose of this chapter I will consider three: clinical errors, medication errors, and diagnostic errors. The first kind, clinical errors, can be defined as the failure to complete some planned action, or the use of the wrong action, in a plan to achieve some aim (Oyebode 2013, 323). Clinical errors occur predominately in intensive care units, operating rooms, and emergency departments. The following is a non-exhaustive list of some such errors: improper transfusions, adverse drug events, wrong-site-surgery, and mistaken patient identity. In current health-care systems, these are the least likely to be reported. This is because of the culture of blame and perfection that exists in health-care. This culture leaves health-care professionals unfortunately believing that reporting clinical errors will be perceived as a negative reflection on their skills or knowledge.

A second kind of error is medication errors. This category is sometimes considered a subset of clinical error, while other times it is considered its own proper set of errors. There are many reasons for medication error, such as faulty supply and labelling issues, but the most common medication errors involve poor prescribing and dosage errors. The actual rate of medication errors is difficult to determine, primarily because there are variations in how this kind of error is defined (Likic and Maxwell 2009, 656). In a systematic review, Sarah Ross and colleagues reported that error rates among junior doctors in hospitals were between 2 and 514 per 1000 items prescribed (Ross et al. 2009, 637).[8] This does not include more senior health-care professionals, but it does demonstrate that proper diagnosing is incredibly difficult. Proper prescribing involves diagnostic skills, knowledge of various medicines, communication skills, an appreciation of risk and uncertainty, and experience.

Diagnostic error is the last type of error I want to outline in this chapter. These are errors that result from misdiagnosis or the miscommunication of a diagnosis. Eta Berner and Mark Graber claim that through large-scale surveys of patients and health-care professionals we can conclude that diagnostic errors are quite common in daily hospital life (Berner and Graber 2008, S2). They claim that errors resulting in serious harm, such as death or prolonged treatment, have been reported by 35 percent of health-care professionals and 42 percent of patients in surveys examining experiences of error. What these statistics show is that diagnostic error is the most common worry, and most common error, experienced in health-care settings. While diagnostic errors have been found to be the leading cause of malpractice litigation (twice as many as medication error), the relationship between factors influencing medical decision making and diagnostic error are not as clear as the relationship between other types of error (Thammasitboon, Thammasitboon, and Singhal 2013, 227).

With these three types of errors outlined, it would be beneficial to consider the extent to which multiple people might achieve the same result from similar evidence pools. One way this can happen is when there is a problem with inter-rater reliability, or the likelihood that two (or more) agents will come to the same decision given identical sets of evidence. While there are several kinds of inter-rater reliability tests, I will be focusing on Cohen's kappa and Fleiss's kappa which consider the chance that the individuals will agree by chance.[9] Jacob Stegenga uses the following toy example to demonstrate how a kappa score shows inter-rater reliability. Two teaching assistants are grading the same class of 100 students where their only decision is to pass or fail the student. Beth passes half the class, while Sara passes 60 students. Independently, they managed to agree to pass 40 and fail 30. Through calculating the kappa with this information, there is only a 40 percent chance Sara and Beth will agree on whether any particular student should pass or fail (Stegenga 2018, 101).

In a hospital setting, however, judgment calls are not made on such a simple pass–fail criterion. There are many more considerations to account for, and many more health-care professionals involved, both of which will negatively impact the inter-rater reliability (and thus negatively affect the chance of coming to the same decision given the same information). So, even with the same set of evidence, two health-care professionals can easily come to drastically different conclusions.

Among these additional considerations is the fact that many conditions involve comorbid conditions. Comorbidities are additional diseases, illnesses, or conditions that occur in tandem with a primary disease or condition, and which have their own symptoms. These can sometimes occur subtly (or even invisibly), but they can also present with such a strong symptomology that the primary condition is masked. An example of a common comorbidity is the existence of a substance use disorder when a patient presents with an anxiety disorder. At times the substance use disorder may mask the anxiety disorder because of an appearance that they are solely "an addict." However, this patient's addiction may be masking their anxiety, which could be the real primary condition that needs to be addressed. This masking, as can be assumed, presents a significant possibility for error, since the health-care professionals may not have enough evidence to make an accurate diagnosis.

Issues Reporting Errors

In one set of surveys, health-care professionals in New Zealand claimed that their primary reasons for not reporting errors were the fear of public outcry and losing patient trust, while health-care professionals in the United States cited losing patient trust and the threat of litigation as their primary reasons (Huang and Soleimani 2010, 18–19). An additional article reports that "[t]here is a natural hesitancy to point out one's own mistakes for fear of being labeled incompetent and a reluctance to point out others' mistakes for fear of being labeled a whistleblower" (Leonard 2010, 154). Despite these stated fears, professionals in both New Zealand and the United States said that they believed reporting errors in the right way could *reduce* the chances of litigation and outcry. While this is admittedly a narrow set of data, it does indicate that reporting errors can be much more complicated than *simply* reporting when an error occurs. Health-care professionals often take into consideration factors outside of the error itself before deciding whether they should report the incident. These internal deliberations occur despite the confidentiality protocols in place within existing error reporting systems.

This said, it might help to examine these fears further before moving on. To start, consider the following claim reported by Rebecca Lawton and Dianne Parker:

> The culture of medicine—with its emphasis on professional auton-omy, collegiality, and self-regulation—is unlikely to foster the report-ing of mistakes. Moreover, the organisational culture of the NHS, with its emphasis on blame, and an increasingly litigious public may only serve to exacerbate the problem.
>
> (Lawton and Parker 2002, 15)

This statement highlights the social culture of the discipline. Health-care professionals work in a high-risk environment. This means they are more likely to experience social pressure driving them toward perfection; after all, they quite literally have the lives of their patients in their hands. But perfection is not possible, despite what this social pressure demands. This allows errors to cause dissonance between who the health-care profes-sional believes they must be and who the health-care professional is. This can then be exacerbated by fears of public outcry (in countries where there is a no-fault system in place) or litigation (in countries that do not have such protections).

Other high-risk industries have recognized several problems with exist-ing error management, including, but not limited to: focusing on active failures rather than latent conditions, focusing on the personal rather than the situational, and the employment of blame-laden terminology when discussing error (such as "carelessness," "irresponsibility," etc.) (Reason 1997, 126).[10] I believe medicine can learn from these recogni-tions in error reporting in other high-risk industries. One primary reason why I believe this is possible is because of the (often implicit or uninten-tional) connection between blame and error. James Reason claims that, because of our focus on individual free will and autonomy in the West, "errors are seen as being, at least in part, voluntary actions" (Reason 1997, 127). Blame relies on the attribution of responsibility to an indi-vidual. This means that, if errors are conceived as voluntary actions, and voluntary actions entail responsibility, then errors are blameworthy. The health-care professionals from New Zealand and the United States reported fears that are intimately connected to blame. So, to adequately learn from and collaboratively engage with errors, we will additionally need to address the current culture of blame that many health-care professionals have reported.

Beyond these issues of blame, reporting errors can also just be time consuming. Often, unless the health-care professional is incredibly lucky, writing and filing error reports is something that must wait to be completed until the end of shift. Typically, the most that can be done before the end of shift is for the individual to write some notes on a scrap piece of paper or a notebook (and this even depends on the confidentiality protocols at their place of work, as any notes that are not on official documentation could be considered an unnecessary risk to patient confidentiality). Time can be a factor in medical error because it presents a situational constraint on the health-care professional. Not only might an individual rush a report (because they want to go home), but they also might incorrectly report key information due to exhaustion at the end of their shift.[11]

Using Error for Collaborative Learning

Learning From Error

Learning in medicine happens both in school and in the professional world. However, there are some topics that are not covered as often as professionals might want, if at all. Daniel Rocke and Walter Lee note that most medical trainees do not receive any education on how to properly disclose medical errors, even though there is an overwhelming interest expressed in having such training (Rocke and Lee 2013, 551). Given that error rates can be uncomfortably high (see earlier sections), this seems like a problem area that ought to merit a more central focus in health-care education. If it is not possible in our schools, for whatever reason, then it ought to be considered as an avenue for continuing medical education credit. Rocke and Lee assert that current conferences tackling error tend *not* to even refer to errors *as errors*. They claim that this is because using the term "error" reinforces the idea that errors are something to be ashamed of. This brings Rocke and Lee to the conclusion that "this culture of perfectibility should be replaced by one in which mistakes can be openly admitted and discussed" (Rocke and Lee 2013, 551). Necessarily, this will involve a serious reconceptualization of error and the role it can play in health-care.

This said, learning beyond the classroom can be difficult. New residents do not always draw on the experiences of those health-care professionals they believe are "lesser-trained" (such as nurses or social workers). These non-physician health-care professionals have different sets of knowledge that physicians, both new residents and senior staff members, ought to engage with when treating a patient. Medical decisions are made in large part by the specific experiences a health-care professional has encountered throughout their training and work as professionals. Petrocelli states that a health-care professional's experiences shape their explanations of medical outcomes, which in turn "inevitably effects his/her decisions about diagnoses and treatments in future cases; each case can serve as an important learning experience" (2013, 5). Those who have not yet developed a set of experience in their field cannot rely on this part of typical medical decision making, and so ought to feel a responsibility to ask for help.[12]

One way to aid in learning on the job is through mentorship. In health-care settings, mentorship is one of the many available types of professional development one can draw on to continually improve in their practice. There are several kinds of mentorship, including formal (where a mentor is assigned to a health-care professional) and informal (such as peer-to-peer mentorship). Shelagh Keogh says that:

> If we ask ourselves a question, we may come up with an answer that meets our desires rather than our professional needs. Ask a respected friend or colleague a question and they are more likely to give you a different response, based on their knowledge of best practice; and thus your knowledge is expanded. One can therefore conceptualise a mentor as a respected friend.
>
> (Keogh 2015, 4)

If we recall the problem of unknown evidence (see § 2, above), then we ought to feel a duty to use both mentors and peer-mentors when trying to determine what to do in any given situation. This is because, no matter how much experience and knowledge an individual health-care professional possesses, there is always going to be relevant information they do not possess. Remember, this is the argumentative force behind both the ways defeaters can contribute to medical error (as outlined in the subsection "Epistemic Counterfactuals").

Relying on mentors and learning from (non-mentor) health-care professionals from different fields who have more experience (e.g., novice nurses looking to experienced social workers, or residents looking to senior administrators) seem to be good starting points for learning from medical error.

Rethinking Error

In one study, medical students who rethought a diagnosis after coming to their initial hypothesis were more likely to avoid diagnostic error and return a correct diagnosis (Coderre, Wright, and McLaughlin 2010). This study presented first-year medical students with two variations of four common clinical presentations (chest pain, jaundice, dyspnea, and anemia). Each common case had a set of primary data, such as a symptom or an abnormal test result, and two sets of secondary data (accounting for two variations on the presenting case). Primary data was presented first, and the students were asked to render a diagnosis. Following this judgment, the students were then presented with one of the two variations of secondary data and subsequently had to re-evaluate their diagnosis. This process determined that "querying does not harm a correct initial diagnosis; most often, [students] recognized their diagnosis as correct and retained it. But querying did seem to rescue students from an incorrect initial diagnosis" (Coderre, Wright, and McLaughlin 2010, 1128). What this demonstrates is that, at least for diagnostic error, embracing the possibility of error has net positive effects.

What this also demonstrates is that there is a place in health-care for collaborative learning. At its simplest, collaborative learning is a teaching strategy in which individuals work as a group to accomplish some educational goal. A more complex understanding of collaborative learning is detailed by Ming Ming Chiu. He assigns either the status of "knowing" or "unknowing" to all participants in a given group, depending on their relevant knowledge in a hypothetical situation (Chiu 2000, 40). If all participants are "unknowing," then the group will be in a joint construction interaction, wherein members present supportive and critical contributions, statements, questions, and many are rejected by the group. If at least one member is designated as "knowing." then the group is in a guided construction interaction. In this situation, the knowing person(s) provides responsive contribution questions and supportive statements with detailed explanation, while the unknowing person(s) provides supportive contributions, statements, and questions with few explanations. Finally, if all members are designated "knowing," they are in an automatic joint solution interaction, wherein everyone provides supportive additions to accepted ideas with few explanations.

Collaborative learning in some form has been used in public school and college-level education, including secondary-entry programs (such as in nursing schools).[13] Some benefits of collaborative learning include: aiding the development of critical reasoning, immediate feedback from peers, active participation in the learning environment, and it provides a responsibility toward one's own learning (Dambal et al. 2015).

Given the prevalence of medical error, coupled with the problem of unknown evidence, collaborative learning seems like a potential avenue for working with error to develop a greater and more effective health-care system. Health-care professionals understandably come from diverse backgrounds. Not only are there many professions that comprise this group, we also need to consider that each individual grew up under different circumstances, went to different schools, engages in different methods of continuing learning, etc. When an error occurs, rather than trying to cover it up, pretend it never happened, or dogmatically pushing on, these additional voices can collaborate with the initial health-care professional to determine what to do next, and how to grow as a team from the error that occurred.

To see how this could work, I want to bring back Yael from earlier, this time with the following modifications: Yael is an emergency doctor in an urban emergency ward. A patient arrives in a serious condition, and she realizes she needs to use either Treatment A or Treatment B to save this patient. She decides to use Treatment A, and unfortunately the patient dies. Following the patient's death, Yael notices that the nurse who connected the IV used a drug that is listed as a severe allergen on the patient's chart. Yael realizes that this death has resulted from a medication error caused by miscommunication somewhere between the pharmacist, the nurse, and the hospital's administration.

In this modified case, what is likely a simple miscommunication has caused a severe error, ultimately leading to the adverse event that was the patient's death. While the culture of blame and perfection might tempt Yael to cover up this mistake, or perhaps report this mistake without talking to the nurse, pharmacist, or administrator about the details, I believe that a different culture could promote a better option. While nothing can be done to fix this error and revive the patient, and while an explanation and reparation will need to be given to the family, this is also an opportunity to prevent future deaths from the same cause. Yael can bring the team together and collaboratively work through the complications of this unfortunate situation. Perhaps her instructions to the nurse were unclear; this is a potential background condition that paved the way for the error to occur. Or perhaps the patient's medical records were improperly managed by several preceding health-care professionals, none of whom were on staff during the incident. Regardless, by discussing as a team, health-care professionals could collaboratively determine what went wrong and what measures need to be put in place to mitigate future occurrences of the same error. Not only could this help everyone involved learn how to better perform their duties, but it also helps by slowly chipping away at the blame culture that exists in so many workplaces today.

There is one final, and potentially unexpected, collaboration I believe ought to be discussed before concluding, due to its unique opportunity for collaborative learning. This is the collaborative team formed between a patient and their health-care professional. Most patients do not have access to medical knowledge or vocabulary, which presents as a problem for health-care professionals who are trying to diagnose. In this type of collaboration, patients would understandably be labelled "unknowing." However, the patient does have information that a health-care professional needs to learn in order to properly treat this patient. This dissonance in knowledge can lead to error because the health-care professional might not ask the right questions, or the patient might not give all the relevant information. This, again, recalls the problem of unknown evidence and the two kinds of defeaters from earlier.

I believe that even these cases can function as collaborative learning opportunities, specifically through guided construction strategies. In these cases, health-care professionals, either alone or in a team, can build upon the statements and contributions of the patient to determine how an error occurred. The patient in turn can pose questions and offer contributions that help the health-care professionals determine what steps to take next. In so doing, the patient receives the additional benefit of feeling included in their own health-care decision-making process. This also presents a benefit for the health-care professional because their patient will be more willing to comply with their directions.

Embracing Error

Change is hard. This is especially true when trying to change something that exists in a high-stakes context. Changing health-care systems is particularly difficult due to the various combinations of factors (e.g., bedside charts) and agents (e.g., health-care professionals) involved in even the most mundane situations. Jeffrey Braithwaite asserts that this means "[w]hen advocates for improvement seek to implement change, health systems do not react predictably; they respond in different ways to the same inputs" (Braithwaite 2018, 1). As such, those reading a chapter in a book that advocates for the rethinking and embracing of medical error might be skeptical, at best, of the author's conclusions. Hopefully, though, my readers are a little more receptive to this.

I believe the problem of unknown evidence provides good reason for taking a humbler approach to error management in health-care systems. Currently, due to the culture of blame and perfection, "[h]ealth-care professionals must overcome the instinct to ignore, hide, or worst of all, deny when an adverse event occurs" (Leonard 2010, 154). Ignoring, hiding, or denying that errors have occurred prevents much of the potential for growth that arises after the event has occurred. If errors are embraced, and recognized as opportunities for collaborative learning, it might be possible to mitigate their prevalence *and* offer more patient-centered care at the same time. Necessarily, this means health-care professionals will need to be supported, rather than simply blamed, when errors have occurred. Blame presumes voluntary choice (see § 3.2), but this ignores situational factors and poor luck. So, if support is offered, and errors are embraced as collaborative learning tools, we can also offer health-care professionals a healthier work environment, alongside the patient benefits.

However, there are some who might resist the suggestion that blame and poor luck should be separated. Such an objector could ask "is it not possible for me to be unlucky (causing a medical error) *and yet I should still be blamed or punished*?"[14] Take the following possible case: Ghazal works in a busy cancer clinic and frequently runs behind schedule due to physician shortages. One day a patient arrives late to their appointment, but Ghazal decides to squeeze him in because she does not believe in letting a patient go unseen. In a hurry, she takes the medication from the tray prepared by her staff without comparing the label to the patient's chart. She learns a few days later that she administered the wrong drug, and the patient has died due to a severe adverse reaction.[15] Surely, despite Ghazal's error arising from poor luck (namely, that her staff prepared the medication tray incorrectly), we might still want to blame her for not being as careful as she should have been.

This is a case of what philosophers call moral luck. Such cases are defined as situations where an agent is blamed for things outside their control. In the above case, Ghazal did not have full control over her situation because: her clinic has physician shortages, her staff prepared the tray, and her patient was running late. An objection based on moral luck challenges the separation of voluntary action and blame because it shows that there are cases in which we intuitively feel like the agent's actions are more serious than if the agent had done the same thing in a different situation. For example, if Ghazal had acted identically, but her staff had properly prepared the tray resulting in the continued treatment of the patient, we might not even notice she made a protocol error. If we did notice, she would likely only have to attend safety training or have some mark placed in her employee file. Moral luck explains why we feel the original case is blameworthy, while the modified case is merely an accident.

I do not believe that moral luck objections should impact our overall decision to embrace medical errors. Instead, I believe these cases *highlight* the need for collaborative learning. This is because my earlier arguments about unknown evidence demonstrate that errors are inevitable in the health-care professions. In the case where Ghazal's patient dies, there is an imperative to figure out what happened and whether it was because of an error at the clinic. This can result in Ghazal being blamed for the death of her patient. But, if we only treat this as an investigation to blame or punish someone, then we have only addressed a symptom of the larger problem. This case can be developed into training and learning opportunities for those who work at this clinic, potentially reducing the likelihood that staff will stock trays incorrectly or physicians will fail to cross-check with their patient's chart. In this way, an event with a negative outcome can be utilized to create better future outcomes for other cases. By embracing the fact that an error will inevitably occur, we can be humbler in our assumptions and actions on the job.

Humility in Medicine

This leads to another take-away from this chapter: that we can begin to address errors more effectively if we start to include more humility in health-care. Specifically, health-care professionals can benefit from something called epistemic humility—namely, an attentiveness to one's own mental limitations and deficits, and the ability to work with the fact that there is relevant knowledge they lack. According to José Medina, epistemic humility is an important epistemic virtue that counters the vice of epistemic arrogance (Medina 2013, 43).[16] Given the problem of unpossessed evidence, which I suggest responsible health-care professionals ought to accept, epistemic humility seems like the most logical position to hold regarding one's own knowledge. Everyone has limitations, and many of these are due simply to situational factors (such as where one attended school, who one's teachers and mentors have been, etc.).

Epistemic humility is an important virtue to develop for health-care professionals, especially when phenomena such as the "July Effect" exist. Also called the "August killing season" in the United Kingdom, the July Effect occurs when hospitals undergo cohort turnover (this is when an organization loses many experienced workers and gains many inexperienced workers at roughly the same time).[17] This phenomenon is commonplace in many teaching hospitals, as well as other health-care settings. In these hospitals, July is typically the month that freshly minted MDs graduate from medical school and join the workforce. These new health-care professionals have the *knowledge* required for proper health-care, but they lack the *skill* that comes from experience and making mistakes. Skill and knowledge are vastly different. Knowledge is something that can be gained from studying books and attending lectures, but skill is something that only experience can grant. So, when new health-care professionals take over in these teaching hospitals, they know *what* to do, but they do not know *how* to do it. This naturally leads to a spike in medical errors.

The best health-care professionals will ask questions. Not everyone is willing to do this, and that can be because of the culture of blame and perfection in health-care today. But if health-care professionals can be more epistemically humble, maybe they can shift their perspective on medical errors. It is always unfortunate, and sometimes even tragic, when medical errors occur. No one doubts this. However, instead of hiding from or dismissing errors, I hope this chapter has convinced my readers that we can put errors to use as collaborative learning tools. Even the best health-care professionals are plagued by the problem of unknown evidence. By rethinking and embracing errors, I believe health-care professionals can strengthen the care patients receive and promote a healthier working environment for themselves and their colleagues.

Notes

1. When most people hear the term "health-care professional" they assume it refers to physicians, surgeons, specialists, and maybe nurses. However, I use the term to refer to a much wider range of professionals within the health-care system. This range includes, but is not limited to: physicians, surgeons,

specialists, nurses, pharmacists, dieticians, administrators, social workers, occupational therapists, physiotherapists, and so on. I use this wide category because I believe it is important to recognize the various stances and contributions of everyone involved in our health-care systems. This will make more sense as the chapter unfolds.

2. See: Hannawa, Shigemoto, and Little (2016), and Poorolajal, Rezaie, and Aghighi (2015), respectively. The statistic of one-third for patient disclosure may not surprise readers, but the idea that only half of the errors are reported internally is concerning. According to Poorolajal and colleagues, just over half of health-care professionals who *commit* an error *did not report* the error. This might be slightly offset by those who *do not commit* an error but *do report* them (which sits at roughly 68 percent); however, this still leaves a large gap in reporting and it does not make up for the fact that half of those who commit an error do not follow their obligation to report. This study outlines several reasons that health-care professionals believe are partially responsible for error underreporting, including: the lack of effective error reporting systems, a lack of support for a person who has commit an error, and a lack of personal attention to the importance of medical errors.

3. Or, at least, no study that is easily found by someone with decent institutional access. Doubtless, there is evidence I do not have or have access to. This ties into the problem of unknown evidence, which is a moderate real-world skepticism I take from Nathan Ballantyne (2015), and which I believe health-care professionals ought to accept. More information on this problem will be provided in the section "The Problem of Unknown Evidence."

    Additionally, part of the difficulty is that to philosophers "error theory" recalls a cognitivist problem in meta-ethics regarding whether morality exists or is just make-believe (Shafer-Landau 2005). Meta-ethics is the branch of ethics that seeks to understand the nature of ethical statements, attitudes, judgments, and so on. As this is not immediately relevant to a study of ethics and medical error, I will not be considering it further.

4. See: Hannawa et al. (2016).

5. The modifier "epistemic" connects these counterfactuals to the discipline of epistemology (as opposed to metaphysics or semantics). Epistemology is the name philosophers give to the theory of knowledge. As such, epistemologists are concerned with determining what distinguishes justified beliefs from mere opinions. So, when used to modify counterfactuals, "epistemic" means that we are interested in the justification or knowledge that would or might result had a different state of affairs occurred or had we made a different decision in a previous event.

6. What the proposition *P* stands for is not important, as this hypothetical case is just for demonstration purposes. I provide two example propositions in this paragraph to help clarify the types of defeaters, but these are also just meant to be stand-ins to help illustrate the concept.

7. Other researchers, such as Grober and Bohnen (2005), claim that it is only *preventable* adverse events that should be attributed to medical errors. On their understanding, preventable adverse events are those which occur when there is some failure to follow accepted practice at the individual or systems level. Such a distinction means that an allergic reaction due to improper medication choice (based on the patient's previous medical history) would be an adverse event, while an allergic reaction due to improper medication choice where *no chart was available* would *not* be an adverse event. Since this makes medical errors and adverse events much more nuanced, and my intentions in this chapter are not to trace a comprehensive taxonomy of what

is or is not an error or event, I will instead use the more broadly conceived definition of adverse event.

8. The vast range in error rates was due in large part to the different definitions of what counted as a medication error across the 24 studies included in this review. Ross and colleagues say that this leaves comparative analyses on medication error impossible because, even within those studies that had similar definitions, large differences were reported due to inconsistent methodology.

9. Cohen's kappa can be calculated by the following equation: κ = [p(a)—p(e)] / [1—p(e)], where p(a) is the observed frequency of some event and p(e) is the probability of a chance agreement between two (or more) agents. Fleiss's kappa is a modification of Cohen's kappa that instead uses the average p(a) and the average p(e) to calculate the kappa for multiple agents.

10. Industries that Reason includes as high-risk include: banks, insurance companies, nuclear power plants, oil exploration and production, chemical process installations, and transportation (e.g., air, sea, and rail). Because of how wide he has cast his net, I see no reason why health-care cannot take suggestions from his analysis.

11. To illustrate how time restrictions can create improper reporting, I want to elaborate on some personal experience with this matter. For two years I was a crew chief for the student branch of campus security. This branch was responsible for assisting the main branch of security on campus as well as filling the role of first responders for the campus (and sometimes even town) population. As a crew chief I had to make sure that if an incident occurred there was also proper documentation from every staff member involved, which I would then have to compile into a master report. This would frequently take until 5:00am (when shift normally ended around 3:30am). On particularly draining nights, many staff would try to quickly write their report so that they could leave faster. This often led to errors, *especially* in our medical incidents. Some crew chiefs were also known to pretend events were milder than they were in order to save time and to make their shift look more "in control." Creating this false sense of control, however, risked our collective credibility and the health of our patients because these reports were sent directly to the hospital (or campus clinic, for milder incidents) to inform the physicians and nurses who were responsible for the continued care of a patient.

12. Admittedly, asking for help is difficult for a variety of reasons that I will not be exploring in this chapter. However, as previously discussed, the culture of blame and perfection has a strong role to play in why many health-care professionals are reluctant to ask for help. The fear of looking incompetent can lead to artificially inflating one's own competence.

    However, there is another factor that might contribute to the reluctance some newer health-care professionals have with asking for help. This is due to the Dunning-Kruger effect, which is a cognitive bias wherein people with low experience present high self-confidence due to a failure to recognize their own lack of experience (Kruger and Dunning 1999). The more experience and individual gains, the less confident they become (due to a recognition that they can make mistakes). Eventually they reach a turning point in which they become more confident in their own judgments because they have a better grasp of the relevant experience. In this sense, an error in a novice's self-view can create a medical error due to a perceived competence that does not exist.

13. See: Sandahl (2010) and Levine et al. (2018).

14. I thank an anonymous referee for prompting me to think about this kind of objection.
15. This example is modified from the opening comparative cases in Hubbeling (2016). Hubbeling's cases, as well as the real-world case they are based on, are discussed in detail in his chapter with an emphasis on the connection between medical errors and moral luck. For more, see Chapter 2: "Medical Error and Moral Luck" by Allhoff.
16. Medina's analysis focuses on the epistemology of dominant (oppressive) groups and resistive (oppressed) groups. He believes that epistemic virtues occur more readily in the oppressed, and that epistemic vices occur more readily in oppressors. This does not, however, mean that members of an oppressed group cannot possess epistemic vice, or that members of a dominant group cannot possess epistemic virtue. While my analysis here does not explicitly engage with oppression or injustices of this type, I believe that the concepts of humility and arrogance have an appropriate application to health-care. I believe this is the case because of the culture of blame and perfection that causes health-care professionals to ignore, hide, deny, and fear medical errors. If a health-care professional does not embrace error, I believe they are acting with epistemic arrogance (in some manner), intentionally or unintentionally.
17. See: Phillips and Barker (2010) and Young et al. (2011).

Works Cited

Abd Elwahab, Sami, and Eva Doherty. 2014. "What about Doctors? The Impact of Medical Errors." *The Surgeon* 12 (6): 297–300.

Ballantyne, Nathan. 2015. "The Significance of Unpossessed Evidence." *The Philosophical Quarterly* 65 (260): 315–335.

Berner, Eta S., and Mark L. Graber. 2008. "Overconfidence as a Cause of Diagnostic Error in Medicine." *The American Journal of Medicine* 121 (5A): S2–S23.

Braithwaite, Jeffrey. 2018. "Changing How We Think About Healthcare Improvement." *BMJ* 361 (k2014): 1–5.

Chiu, Ming M. 2000. "Group Problem-Solving Processes: Social Interactions and Individual Actions." *Journal for the Theory of Social Behaviour* 30 (1): 27–50.

Coderre, Sylvain, Bruce Wright, and Kevin McLaughlin. 2010. "To Think Is Good: Querying an Initial Hypothesis Reduces Diagnostic Error in Medical Students." *Academic Medicine* 85 (7): 1125–1129.

Dambal, Archana, Naren Nimbal, Shanmukh T. Kalsad, R. K. Rajashekhar, Sunita Kalyanshetti, Gajanan Pise. 2015. "A Comparison of Collaborative Learning with Individual Learning in Retention of Knowledge Taught in Ethics and Professionalism Class of General Medicine." *Journal of Evolution of Medical and Dental Sciences* 4 (84): 14622–14628.

Grober, Ethan D., and John M. A. Bohnen. 2005. "Defining Medical Error." *Canadian Journal of Surgery* 48 (1): 39–44.

Hannawa, Annegret F., Yuki Shigemoto, and Todd D. Little. 2016. "Medical Errors: Disclosure Styles, Interpersonal Forgiveness, and Outcomes." *Social Science & Medicine* 156: 29–38.

Huang, Henry and Farzad Soleimani. 2010. "What Happened to No Fault? The Role of Error Reporting in Healthcare Reform." *Houston Journal of Health Law & Policy* 10 (1): 1–34.

Hubbeling, Dieneke. 2016. "Medical Error and Moral Luck." *HEC Forum* 28 (3): 229–243.

Keogh, Shelagh. 2015. "Mentorship and Professional Development." In Mary E. Shaw and John Fulton (eds.), *Mentorship in Healthcare, Second Edition*. Keswick, UK: M&K Publishing: 1–13.

Kruger, Justin, and David Dunning. 1999. "Unskilled and Unaware of It: How Difficulties in Recognizing One's Own Incompetence Lead to Inflated Self-Assessments." *Journal of Personality and Social Psychology* 77 (6): 1121–1134.

Lawton, Rebecca, and Dianne Parker. 2002. "Barriers to Incident Reporting in a Healthcare System." *BMJ Quality & Safety* 11 (1): 15–18.

Leonard, Michael S. 2010. "Patient Safety and Quality Improvement: Medical Errors and Adverse Events." *Pediatrics in Review* 31 (4): 151–158.

Levine, Ruth E., Nicole J. Borges, Brenda J. B. Roman, Lisa R. Carchedi, Mark H. Townsend, Jeffrey S. Cluver, Julia Frank, Oma Morey, Paul Haidet, Britta Thompson. "High-Stakes Collaborative Testing: Why Not?" 2018. *Teaching and Learning in Medicine* 30 (2): 133–140.

Likic, Robert and Simon R. J. Maxwell. 2009. "Prevention of Medication Errors: Teaching and Training." *British Journal of Clinical Pharmacology* 67 (6): 656–661.

Medina, José. 2013. *The Epistemology of Resistance: Gender and Racial Oppression, Epistemic Injustice, and the Social Imagination*. Toronto: Oxford University Press.

Oyebode, Femi. 2013. "Clinical Errors and Medical Negligence." *Medical Principles and Practice* 22 (4): 323–333.

Petrocelli, John V. 2013. "Pitfalls of Counterfactual Thinking in Medical Practice: Preventing Errors by Using More Functional Reference Points." *Journal of Public Health Research* 2 (e24): 136–143.

Phillips, David P., and Gwendolyn E. C. Barker. 2010. "A July Spike in Fatal Medication Errors: A Possible Effect of New Medical Residents." *Journal of General Internal Medicine* 25 (8): 774–779.

Poorolajal, Jalal, Shirin Rezaie, and Negar Aghighi. 2015. "Barriers to Medical Error Reporting." *International Journal of Preventative Medicine* 6 (1): 97.

Proctor, Monja L., Jennifer Pastore, Justin T. Gerstle, and Jacob C. Langer. 2003. "Incidence of Medical Error and Adverse Outcomes on a Pediatric General Surgery Service." *Journal of Pediatric Surgery* 38 (9): 1361–1365.

Reason, James. 1997. *Managing the Risks of Organizational Accidents*. London: Routledge.

Robertson, Jennifer J., and Brit Long. 2018. "Suffering in Silence: Medical Error and its Impact on Health Care Providers." *Journal of Emergency Medicine* 54 (4): 402–409.

Rocke, Daniel and Walter T. Lee. 2013. "Medical Errors: Teachable Moments in Doing the Right Thing." *Journal of Graduate Medical Education* 5 (4): 550–552.

Ross, Sarah, Christine Bond, Helen Rothnie, Sian Thomas, and Mary Joan Macleod. 2009. "What Is the Scale of Prescribing Errors Committed by Junior Doctors? A Systematic Review." *British Journal of Clinical Pharmacology* 67 (6): 629–640.

Sandahl, Sheryl S. 2010. "Collaborative Testing as a Learning Strategy in Nursing Education." *Nursing Education Perspectives* 31 (3): 142–147.

Schwendimann, René, Catherine Blatter, Suzanne Dhaini, Michael Simon, and Dietmar Ausserhofer. 2018. "The Occurrence, Types, Consequences and Preventability of In-Hospital Adverse Events – A Scoping Review." *BMC Health Services Research* 18 (521): 1–13.

Shafer-Landau, Russ. 2005. "Error Theory and the Possibility of Normative Ethics." *Philosophical Issues* 15 (1): 107–120.

Stegenga, Jacob. 2018. *Medical Nihilism.* Oxford: Oxford University Press.

Thammasitboon, Satid, Supat Thammasitboon, and Geeta Singhal. 2013. "Diagnosing Diagnostic Error." *Current Problems in Pediatric and Adolescent Health Care* 43 (9): 227–231.

Young, John Q., Sumant R. Ranji, Robert M. Wachter, Connie M. Lee, Brian Niehaus, and Andrew D. Auerbach. 2011. ""July Effect": Impact of the Academic Year-End Changeover on Patient Outcomes: A Systematic Review." *Annals of Internal Medicine* 155 (5): 309–315.

13 Inference to the Best Explanation and Avoiding Diagnostic Error

David Kyle Johnson

Introduction

Abduction is the form of reasoning where one considers, compares, and contrasts multiple hypotheses according to certain criteria to arrive at, and ultimately accept, the best one. For this reason, it is also known as "inference to the best explanation" (IBE). When it comes to medical diagnosis, as it is performed by family and hospital physicians, it is perhaps obvious that IBE most accurately describes the type of reasoning that they deploy. The possible causes of a patient's symptoms are the explanations that are considered, and the diagnosis upon which the physician arrives is the one the physician has concluded is best. Indeed, in his entry for the *Stanford Encyclopedia of Philosophy*'s entry on abduction, the only source Igor Douven cites for his claim that "Abduction is also said to be the predominant mode of reasoning in medical diagnosis," is a book about abductive inference that simply uses diagnosis to illustrate what abduction is in its first chapter.[1] In other works, such statements are asserted without argument or citation at all.[2]

This seemingly obvious truth, however, has escaped too many authors. In "Reasoning Foundations of Medical Diagnosis," for example, Ledley and Lusted restrict their description of diagnostic reasoning to deductive inferences, probabilistic calculus, and value judgments. They do acknowledge that, as a step in the process, physicians "list all the diseases which the specific case can reasonably resemble [and then] exclude one disease after another from the list," but do not fully appreciate all that goes into how such exclusion happens.[3] In "Diagnostic Reasoning," Jerome Kassirer categorizes diagnostic reasoning into three types—probabilistic reasoning, causal reasoning, and deterministic or categorical reasoning—and only briefly mentions that "it requires eliminating competing hypotheses in a process analogous to disproving competing scientific hypotheses (can any other diseases better explain the patient's findings)."[4] To be fair, Kassirer does mention, once, certain criteria—what he calls coherency, adequacy, and parsimony—that are (as we shall soon see) arguably similar to criteria that IBE employs. And both articles could be viewed as articulations of how the reasoning practices they describe help physicians arrive at the best explanation. But neither article appreciates the full extent of IBE's role in diagnostic reasoning, or the complex process that IBE is.

In "The Logic of Medical Diagnosis," Stanley and Campos rightly observe that articles in the medical literature have sorely neglected to address "improving diagnosis," and concentrated instead on "evaluating evidence" (Stanley and Campos 2013, 301). This, they argue, is a mistake because "diagnosis should trump evidence" (Stanley and Campos 2013, 301). To address this problem, they suggest that more attention should be paid, both in the literature and by physicians, to "abduction." But in using this word, they are not referring to IBE. They are using the more restrictive, less common, use of the term which refers simply to the production of hypotheses.[5] The literature, they argue, concentrates too much on how to test hypotheses, and not enough on how physicians figure out which hypotheses should be tested. With this I agree, but Stanley and Campos also neglect the role that IBE plays in the evaluation of hypotheses once they are selected for consideration.

Stanley and Campos are still correct, however, that "attention to . . . philosophy of science in general, can help medical doctors become better at diagnosis, for the conceptual clarification that results from the philosophical analysis will improve a doctor's reasoning" (Douven 2017). And this is much needed, given that "diagnostic error accounts for 40,000 to 80,000 deaths per year . . . the number of patients who are injured must be substantially higher, [and] 96% [of physicians feel] that diagnostic errors [are] preventable" (Douven 2017, 301). Indeed, as of 2015, it was still true that every person in America is likely to suffer from the consequences of at least one diagnostic error in their lifetime.[6] To make matters worse, Kohn's landmark *To Err is Human* and the Committee of Quality of Health Care in America's *Crossing the Quality Chasm*, that drew attention to the problem of diagnostic error, both commit the same error of *putting evidence evaluation before diagnosis* that Stanley and Campos identify, and both completely neglect the role of IBE in diagnostic reasoning.[7]

It is the purpose of this chapter, therefore, to argue that the role of IBE in diagnostic reasoning should be fully recognized by medical authors and practitioners. Because an appreciation and understanding of IBE could help reduce diagnostic error, further research should be dedicated to the role of IBE in medical diagnosis, and the method itself should be taught in medical textbooks. To accomplish this goal, I shall first describe IBE and briefly articulate how it is central to scientific reasoning in general. I will then articulate the direct similarities between the textbook descriptions of scientific reasoning and the textbook descriptions of diagnostic reasoning, and show that they do not fully represent what scientists or physicians are doing in the real world. This will set up a brief argument that indeed, in practice, diagnosis is IBE. Then, in an attempt to lay the groundwork for further research on this topic, I will demonstrate, both abstractly and with an example, how recognizing diagnosis as IBE can help avoid diagnostic error. Before a brief summarizing conclusion, I will also point out another benefit of recognizing diagnosis as IBE: it helps avoid so-called "Dr. House Syndrome" (Novella 2013).

What Is Inference to the Best Explanation (IBE)?

IBE is a method of reasoning by which one evaluates multiple hypotheses or explanations, compares them according to a set of criteria, and then accepts the one that best coheres with them. Because IBE is an inductive rather that deductive method of reasoning, IBE can never guarantee that the conclusion it suggests is true.[8] The best explanation might be wrong. Nevertheless, when the IBE clearly demonstrates that one hypothesis is the best explanation, rationally it is the explanation that should be accepted.

IBE's clearest formal articulation comes from Schick and Vaughn's textbook *How to Think about Weird Things* (2014). They give it a useful acronym: The SEARCH Method. State a hypothesis (i.e., possible explanation) as precisely as possible. Evaluate the evidence for the hypothesis. State and evaluate the evidence for at least one Alternative hypothesis. And then Rate according to the Criteria of adequacy each Hypothesis (Schick and Vaughn, 222–227).

That last step is key, and the five criteria of adequacy are best understood via the questions they pose. Does the hypothesis make novel predictions? If so, then it is *testable*. Does the hypothesis get those novel predictions correct? If so, then it is *fruitful*. How much does the hypothesis explain? Does it helpfully unify our knowledge, or unhelpfully invoke the inexplicable or raise unanswerable questions? The more it does the former and avoids the latter, the more *scope* the hypothesis has. How many new assumptions does the hypothesis require? Does it invoke the existence of entities or forces we do not already know exist? The less it does this, the *simpler* or more parsimonious it is. And how well does the hypothesis align with what we think we already know? The more it does, the more *conservative* it is (Schick and Vaughn, 171–181).

The production of hypotheses in this process can be rigid. As Thagard and Shelly point out, sometimes one will simply have a list of possible hypotheses, derivable from the relevant data, to choose from (Thagard and Shelley 1997, 416). And, as Stanley and Campos argue, considerations like scope can be used to eliminate especially bad hypotheses before evidence evaluation begins or further comparison is done. This is also true of considerations like whether it seems "simple, natural, and plausible to us," whether it is similar to existing explanations in other fields, and even "the question or economics of money, time, thought, and energy" (Stanley and Campos 2013, 307). But the process of hypothesis generation can also be non-scientific, requiring imagination or inspiration, and in this way is not unlike art (Schick and Vaughn 2014, 224). Indeed, creativity in hypothesis production is often what generates discovery, both in science at large and in medicine specifically.[9]

The evaluation of evidence will, obviously, involve many of the kinds of reasoning normally mentioned in the existing medical literature on diagnosis: probability calculus, deduction, etc. It is here that testing and experimentation is done. If the hypothesis fails to make accurate predictions, it will be deemed unfruitful in the next step of the process. But the evaluation of evidence for a hypothesis must also involve efforts to detect fallacious reasoning that might be thought to support it: logical fallacies, bad studies, misleading statistics, mere anecdotes, subjective observations, etc. Were any of the ways that our senses, memory, or intuitive reasoning can lead us astray involved?[10] Were authorities cited? Were they relevant? All these things must be considered.

The comparison of multiple hypotheses is essential. Because of confirmation bias, availability error, and evidence denial, simply considering one hypothesis can lead a person astray.[11] After all, it's easy to find evidence *for* a hypothesis. Absent any other alternatives, "Santa did it" would be the best explanation for the presents under your Christmas tree. It's only when you have honestly tried to prove something false and failed that you really have good reason to think that it is true. As Clendening and Hashinger put it, "the most brilliant diagnosticians . . . are the ones who do remember and consider the most possibilities."[12]

It is also essential to realize that a hypothesis can be the best among all relevant alternatives without adhering to all five criteria. The best explanation is simply the one that adheres to more or to a greater degree. For example, Einstein's Theory of Relativity was not conservative when it was first proposed because it conflicted with Newton's theories, but was eventually accepted because it was more fruitful, simple, and wide scoping.[13] Or take Newton's theories themselves. When his laws were unable to correctly predict the movement of the planet Uranus, astronomers did not abandon them. Because his theory was still simpler and more wide scoping than any alternative, they hypothesized the existence of another planet that was throwing Uranus's orbit off course—and that's how we discovered Neptune.[14] So a theory can even fail to make accurate predictions—it can fail tests and thus fail to be fruitful—yet still be the best explanation.[15]

Although we often do it unconsciously, most people employ IBE on a daily basis. Indeed, although philosophers still debate about *the definition* of "the scientific method," IBE undoubtedly lies at the heart of all scientific reasoning.[16] To be sure, in the history of science, there has been much disagreement about what constitutes the scientific method. Aristotle,[17] Galileo,[18] Francis Bacon,[19] John Stuart Mill,[20] William Whewell,[21] and C.S. Peirce[22] each had had their own unique method, which did not always cohere with the others. Bacon criticized Aristotle, Whewell criticized Bacon, Mill criticized Whewell.[23] But as McMullin points out, inference to the best explanation plays a core role in the reasoning of all of science's founders.[24]

Indeed, as Thomas Kuhn (1996) famously argued in *"The Structure of Scientific Revolutions,"* it is through IBE that scientific revolutions take place. Anomalies build up for which the "established" theory cannot account, new hypotheses are proposed and compared, and the best one wins out. This is, for example, how the germ theory of disease became accepted. It contradicted conventional wisdom and proposed the existence of new entities: germs. It was therefore not conservative or simple. But it proved itself over the competing hypotheses by being testable, monumentally fruitful, and wide scoping. Pasteur's tests of his anthrax "vaccine" on animals were widely successful, and his theory unified our understanding of disease.[25]

Given that IBE stands are the heart of scientific reasoning, it is all the more surprising that descriptions of diagnostic reasoning neglect it so profoundly. But in doing so, the authors of medical articles and textbooks are not alone. Those who write general science textbooks make a very similar mistake. And looking at the similarity of those mistakes will be very helpful in demonstrating that medical diagnosis is, indeed, IBE.

What's Wrong With the Science Textbooks?

The definition of diagnostic reasoning that seems to be endorsed in the journal research, such as Ledley and Lusted (1959) and Kassirer (1989), and that is most common in medical texts, such as Kohn (2000), Committee (2001), and Balogh (2015), is usually called "System 2 Reasoning" and mirrors the definition of the scientific method most commonly found in standard science textbooks:

The Standard Textbook Scientific Method	The Standard Model of Diagnostics
1. Observe	1. Cue Acquisition
2. Hypothesize	2. Working Diagnosis
3. Make predictions and test hypothesis	3. Cue Interpretation
4. Accept or reject/revise hypothesis[26]	4. Hypothesis Evaluation[27]

That the former is not an adequate description of the scientific method is perhaps most obviously revealed by the fact that anecdotal reasoning follows the same pattern.

I have a stomach ache. I think Tic Tacs cure stomach aches. If I'm right, my stomach ache will go away after I take a tic-tac. Let's test

that. (I swallow a tic-tac. Later my stomach ache subsides). Success!
My hypothesis is confirmed and I now accept that tic-tacs cure stom-
ach aches.

Clearly, even though this follows the textbook scientific method, it is not scientific reasoning. But to understand why The Standard Model of Diagnostics is not an accurate description of real-world diagnostic reasoning, it will first be helpful to understand exactly why The Standard Model of Diagnostics is inadequate as a description of real-world scientific reasoning.

First, it fails to recognize what Kuhn (1996) and Feyerabend (1959, 1969) taught us: observation is theory laden. Without a theory to inform what observations are important and relevant, observation has no direction and cannot produce anything useful. An entire lifetime could be spent observing facts in a room—the number of fibers in the carpet, and size and distance between objects—but no science would ever get done. One needs a theory to test, or a problem to solve, to even begin to know what observations are relevant. As Karl Popper put it, "the instruction 'Observe!' is absurd. . . . Observation is always selective. It needs a chosen object, a definite task, and interest, a point of view, a problem" (Popper 1965, 46). The prescription to begin the scientific process by simply "observing" will ensure that it never begins.

Second, the Standard Textbook Scientific Method neglects the process that lies behind hypothesis generation. As we've seen, sometimes the data might entail a certain limited number of possible explanations from which one can choose. Other times, creativity will be needed to generate hypotheses. But the Standard Textbook Scientific Method appreciates neither of these possibilities. It also says nothing about the comparison of competing hypotheses which, again as we have already seen, is essential to scientific reasoning.

Third, it says nothing about experimental design, replication, or guarding against fallacious reasoning, like confirmation bias or hasty generalizations. Experiments must be designed to guard against the many ways our experiences can lead us astray. This is why, for example, medical studies on medications must be double blinded and must be replicated before their conclusions can be accepted. This is why one must guard against logically fallacious thinking to make sure that one does not protect a favored falsified hypothesis, or unfairly criticize an unfavored proven one. None of this is mentioned in the textbook account.

The textbook account also suggests that one should accept a hypothesis if it passes the test, and revise or reject the hypothesis if it fails—but when it comes to scientific reasoning, things are far more complicated. For one, a hypothesis making an accurate prediction is not always a reason to accept it as true. For example, when the scientific community thought that Venus was cold, Veilkovsky successfully predicted that it was hot because he thought it had been ejected from Jupiter. But this was not a good reason to accept the latter as true.[28] Second, if a hypothesis fails to successfully predict the outcome of a test, there are many possible responses. One could reject it, revise it, or even suggest that the test was flawed. Consider when, contrary to the theory of relativity, the OPERA Particle detector measured neutrinos as going faster than the speed of light. Was that a reason to reject relativity? To revise it? Or should we conclude that the measuring apparatus was not functioning properly? In that case it turned out to be the latter, which was not surprising, given the massively unconservative nature of the notion that neutrinos travel faster than light.[29] But since the Standard Textbook Scientific Method says nothing about conservatism, it gives one no way to make this determination.

This last failure is primarily due to the textbook description's reliance on falsification. In his criticism of the theories of Karl Marx and Sigmund Freud, Karl Popper demonstrated that falsification is important in science. To be scientific, he argued, a theory needs to make observable, testable, predictions.[30] Later, however, Duhem and Quine famously revealed that no theory is completely falsifiable. Because every hypothesis' prediction is informed by other assumptions and theories, all predictive failures can be excused away by changing the background theory or assumptions.[31] For example, million-year-old fossils clear falsify the Biblical creationist hypothesis that the Earth is only 6000 years old. In an attempt to save their hypothesis, some creationists changed their background assumptions by suggesting that Satan planted the fossils and made them look older than they are. Clearly that is not scientific. But, as we've already seen, when irregularities in Uranus's orbit falsified Newton's laws of planetary motion, scientists saved his theory by suggesting that there was another planet pulling it off course—and that was scientific. But that's essentially the same move: changing the background theory to account for falsifying evidence. What makes the latter scientific but the former not? The textbook description of scientific reasoning is silent on the subject.[32]

Worse still, it is also silent about how we can and have decided scientifically between hypotheses that cannot be differentiated observationally. Geocentrism and heliocentrism, for example, can only be observationally distinguished via parallax yet we came to accept heliocentrism long before parallax could be observed.[33] Why? Because geocentrism is more parsimonious; it does not require epicycles.[34] Since parsimony is a key consideration in IBE, this example shows not only another shortcoming of the standard textbook description of the scientific method, but is yet another reason to think that IBE is central to scientific reasoning.

One might object, of course, that the textbook description's shortcomings are due simply to its oversimplified nature. "It leaves out the details but gets the basic idea right." But this objection falls short. According to the textbook description, many things that clearly are science would not be. Consider, for example, when astronomers infer the makeup of astronomical phenomena like stars, clouds, and planetary atmospheres by simply examining the spectrum of light they emit. This is clearly science but does not follow the textbook method at all. Indeed, one might argue that, on a strict interpretation of the textbook description of the scientific method, astronomy is not science because of its heavy reliance on observation and the fact that it does not test hypotheses by performing experiments like other sciences such as physics and chemistry. And yet, quite obviously, astronomy is science.[35]

What's Wrong With the Standard Model of Diagnostics?

The Standard Model of Diagnostics that describes "System 2 reasoning"—cue acquisition, working diagnosis, cue interpretation, and hypothesis evaluation—has the same shortcomings as the Standard Textbook Scientific Method.

For example, it fails to account for how observation is theory laden—how background assumptions dictate what observations or symptoms are deemed relevant or irrelevant. In medicine, the germ theory of disease and previous knowledge about how diseases present tells physicians what facts about a patient are relevant and which are not, and which symptoms need explaining and which do not. Without them, one could spend a year observing basic facts about a patient—skin color, number of hairs, exact length of finger nails—and never even notice that they are sick.

The Standard Model of Diagnostics also says nothing about how diagnoses/hypotheses are generated—a process which can require both experience and creativity. One might need to know what explanations the data entails are possible; in extremely difficult cases, where misdiagnosis is common, creativity might be needed. It also says nothing about how to guard against anecdotal reasoning or testing flaws, like false positives. Nor does it call for the direct comparison of hypotheses or give us guidelines for doing so. It says nothing about experimental design, replication, or when more than one test is needed.

Because it concentrates solely on falsification, it also completely neglects the role of things like simplicity, scope, and conservatism. Simplicity is why, all things being equal, physicians usually offer up a single condition as a diagnosis, instead of two or more. Per Ockham's razor, one should not multiply entities beyond necessity. Scope is why, all things being equal, the diagnosis of a new unknown disease for a single patent is not taken seriously. It can only explain one case and thus such a diagnosis's explanatory power is low. Conservatism is why, all things being equal, physicians do not entertain certain diagnoses, like chronic Lyme's disease. The existence of such diseases contradicts well-established knowledge. Indeed, physicians often correctly diagnose something because "it's going around" without even doing tests—and in doing so, they invoke all three of these criteria while completely ignoring falsification. And it is through the consideration of all the criteria that one can discover when all things are not equal and indeed the patient does have two conditions, a previously unknown disease, or that we were wrong about whether a disease exists. Clearly, the Standard Model of Diagnostics that describes "System 2 reasoning" is not an adequate description of diagnosis as it occurs in the real world.

To be fair, there are other descriptions of diagnostic reasoning in the medical literature, like System 1 reasoning and Bayesian probabilistic calculus, that pick up some of the slack.[36] Take System 1 reasoning, for example, which is common in veteran physicians and relies on experience and pattern recognition. Physicians observe certain symptoms, notice that they fit the pattern of a disease they are familiar with, and then offer that as a diagnosis. This clearly appreciates the role of background assumptions in diagnostic reasoning and somewhat accounts for diagnosis generation.

In addition, Bayesian reasoning—a formalized method for updating the likelihood of a hypotheses given new evidence—can be used to compare diagnoses and can guard against testing errors, like being misled by false positives.[37] For example, physicians commonly misdiagnosis cancer from a single positive test even though such a conclusion is unwarranted. Even if a test is 90 percent accurate, and false positives only happen 7 percent of the time, if the breast cancer rate in the general population is only 0.8 percent, a positive test only raises the probability that a patient has breast cancer to 9 percent.[38] Bayesian reasoning actually tells us why, and using Bayes's formula can help one avoid such errors.

But even when combined, these three "standard models" do not adequately describe real world diagnostics. For example, none involve a step which formally guards against logically fallacious reasoning, like anchoring, premature closure, affect bias, and confirmation bias. None lays out guidelines for how to decide between rejecting and revising a diagnosis if a test comes back negative, to decide whether the disease is absent, or is presenting a-typically. And none say anything about how one goes about deciding between two diagnoses that would give the same test results.

Why Diagnosis Is Inference to the Best Explanation

The reasons that IBE is a better description of diagnostic reasoning mirror the reasons that IBE is a better description of the scientific method.

Because IBE embraces the influence of our background assumptions, IBE appreciates the theory laden nature of observations in science and how creativity can be necessary for hypothesis generation, especially in difficult cases. In IBE, the comparison of hypotheses is essential, as is guarding against errors in reasoning. It explains why and when one should revise or reject a possible hypothesis in light of disconfirming evidence. And it is by comparing hypotheses to other criteria—like simplicity, scope, and conservatism—that one can scientifically confirm one hypothesis over another in the absence of distinguishing observational evidence. IBE even captures why astronomy is a science; astronomers are offering up explanations just like everyone else.

The same is true of IBE as a description of diagnostic reasoning. It articulates why and how physicians deem symptoms relevant and irrelevant, appreciates how diagnoses are generated, and why creativity can be necessary for diagnosis generation in difficult cases. It explicitly guards against fallacious and anecdotal reasoning and ensures reliable diagnosis testing procedures. Because it appreciates the role of non-observational criteria like simplicity, scope, and conservatism, it describes how and why physicians reject or revise a hypothesis in light of negative test results.[39] It also explains how physicians decide between diagnoses that produce the same test results and even why physicians universally reject demonic explanations for diseases.[40]

The main strength of IBE as a description of the scientific method is its inclusiveness and flexibility. In real world science, different kinds of reasoning are relevant and used in different situations—from inductive Bayesian reasoning to deductive hypothetical syllogisms. But because the evaluation of evidence and arguments for hypotheses is part of IBE, it can and does include all types of reasoning. Further, even though the relevance of different kinds of evidence varies, because none of the criteria of adequacy are essential—a hypothesis can fail on one or two counts, but still be the best explanation among the alternatives—IBE is flexible enough to describe why hypotheses come to be accepted in all circumstances.

The same is true of IBE as a description of diagnostic reasoning. Different factors are relevant in different situations. Notice that almost every source I have mentioned, that describes diagnosis, includes at least three different kinds of reasoning. Since IBE is flexible, it can include these methods of reasoning while also including all the other relevant elements of diagnostic reasoning that they exclude. IBE is therefore a description that fits in all circumstances.

Perhaps the most *convincing* reason why IBE better describes real world diagnostics is the fact that when one of the standard textbook models lead one astray, it is because it has neglected an essential element of the IBE process. For example, although specialists using System 1 can often diagnose what others cannot, when it goes wrong it's because one did not bother to properly test the proposed diagnosis, or because one got anchored to a particular hypothesis and did not compare it to a relevant rival. Similarly, Bayesian reasoning can also lead one astray if: (1) one mis-assigns the relevant prior probabilities, (2) one does not compare the relevant rival hypotheses or (3) the rival hypotheses are observationally equivalent. But, as we've seen, IBE has all these bases covered; the criteria of adequacy can even be used to accurately set the necessary prior probabilities.[41]

Using IBE to Avoid Diagnostic Error

A diagnosis that followed Schick's IBE "SEARCH" method formally would begin with (1) a patient presenting with symptoms that demand an explanation. The physician would then (2) generate a diagnosis that makes testable predictions, using creativity if obvious explanations were not suggested by the patient's symptoms. Next would come (3), the evaluation of the evidence for that hypothesis, which would include running tests, examining the results, and guarding against fallacious reasoning such as anchoring. The physician would then (4) consider alternative hypotheses, which are also consistent with the previous tests results, make additional predictions, perform additional tests that would delineate between the diagnoses in question, and consider the relevant evidence. Lastly would come (5) the comparison of the diagnoses using the criteria of adequacy to see, not only which one got the relevant predictions right, but to see which one is most consistent with what we know, explains the most, and is simplest.

Although steps (4) and (5) might seem like overkill if one is confident in the initial diagnosis, notice that the more one repeats steps (4) and (5), the more likely it would be that the initial diagnosis is correct. And this, it seems, would by itself reduce diagnostic error since it is overconfidence that often leads to misdiagnosis. Of course, one must determine when one is confident enough that the diagnosis is actionable. Such a determination will depend on many variables—the severity of the symptoms, the riskiness and costs of the treatments, etc.—but this is a separate issue that does not contradict my thesis that diagnosis is IBE.

If my thesis is correct, then the sharpening of one's "abductive skills"— the enhancement of one's ability to perform IBE—should greatly reduce one's chances of misdiagnosis. With that goal in mind, it's worth considering what Josephson and Josephson (1996) consider to be the five most common mistakes that people make when performing IBE.[42] The first is trying to explain something irrelevant or not trying try to explain something relevant. This can happen in diagnosis when a relevant symptom is ignored or a non-relevant one is not ignored. The second is not considering enough hypotheses. This happens when one's differential is not broad enough and thus the true diagnosis is not considered. The third is miscalculating how "adequate" a hypothesis is by either underrating the right hypothesis or overrating the wrong one. This might happen when one does not realize how rare a particular disease is or that there was a recent outbreak of another. The fourth is not evaluating the evidence for the hypotheses correctly. This can happen when one reads a test wrong or fails to recognize or guard against fallacious reasoning. And the fifth is miscalculating what the hypothesis could explain: thinking a hypothesis can explain what it cannot, or not realizing what it can. This can happen when one does not realize that a certain disease presents with a particular symptom.

Consequently, besides familiarizing oneself with IBE, to guard against misdiagnosis, one should be aware that observation is theory laden, think twice before dismissing a symptom as irrelevant, and realize that anchoring can make you overlook a symptom. One should also keep in mind that hypothesis generation is not always scientific. It's up to you to consider the right hypothesis, so stay up to date so you will have in mind all the relevant hypotheses. One should also know their "surroundings." Know, for example, how prevalent and likely diseases are in your area and keep current on advances. Judging a hypothesis as conservative is only worthwhile if one's medical knowledge is up to date. One should be careful while performing and reading tests and remind oneself often of common medical logical fallacies like availability error and confirmation bias. And one should know diseases and conditions, and how they present, both typically and atypically.

IBE Correcting a Diagnostic Error

As an example of how appreciating the central role of IBE in diagnosis can help avoid diagnostic error, consider how more formally using IBE could have avoided diagnostic error in the following real-world case (relayed to me by a colleague).

> An elderly patient returning from travel presented to a family physician with sudden symptoms of weakness, fever, cough, and shortness of breath. The patient was empirically diagnosed (via System 1 reasoning) with an infection (community acquired pneumonia) and an antibiotic was prescribed. No testing was done. After several days there was no response to the antibiotic and symptoms continued to worsen. The family physician referred the patient to the ED; a chest x-ray showed an infiltrate; a follow up CT scan (to rule out pulmonary embolus) was interpreted (by the radiologist) as consistent with lung cancer. Even though the patient was a non-smoker and two biopsies failed to confirm cancer, this became the accepted diagnosis. A bronchoscopy was recommended, but the patient refused and was discharged to hospice.
>
> When the patient reconsidered and was readmitted several days later, the admitting physician noted that a previous biopsy showed non-specific signs of possible infection. An infectious disease specialist was consulted and the differential diagnosis was expanded. More tests were ordered and another biopsy was performed. The

pathologist reviewing the biopsy also became suspicious of infection and requested an outside opinion. Special staining of the biopsy tissue resulted in the correct diagnosis of a specific pulmonary infection, which was consistent with the patient's recent travel history.

We can see how neglecting key elements of IBE specifically led to misdiagnosis in this case. Had the family physician been mindful of the theory laden nature of observation, he might have initially given more weight to the relevance of the travel history. Had he bothered to test his initial diagnosis of pneumonia, or compared it to a rival hypothesis, he would likely have avoided the initial misdiagnosis of CAP. Had he guarded against anchoring and premature closure, he might have recognized the relevance of the patient being a non-smoker and the fact that the symptoms had a sudden onset. This made the cancer diagnosis non-conservative, and thus not truly worth "protecting" in light of two negative biopsies.

But we can also see how IBE was crucial in arriving at a correct diagnosis. Not only did the (re)admitting physician generate a rival hypothesis for comparison before reaching a conclusion, but she tried to disprove that theory by consulting a specialist and performing more tests. The pathologist did something similar when she sought out a second opinion. Perhaps most importantly, both of these physicians recognized that the infection hypothesis deserved a "second chance" even though the initial round of antibiotics was ineffectual. Its explanatory power—the fact that it accounted for the symptoms, their sudden onset, and the negative test results—and its conservatism—the fact that it aligned with the patient's travel and the fact that he was a non-smoker—made the initial infection hypothesis deserving of revision instead of rejection.

IBE Also Helps Avoid "Dr. House Syndrome"

One weakness of all three of the "standard methods" is that they have a tendency to lead to what Yale neurologist Steve Novella calls "Dr. House Syndrome" (Novella 2013). According to Novella, Dr. House Syndrome is "largely learned from watching doctors on TV," like *House M.D.*, and can infect patients and physicians alike. Essentially, it's what one suffers from when one operates under the assumption that the goal of diagnostics is only to discover "the condition" you have such that, if that goal is not accomplished, the process is a failure. Novella points out that patients with this condition have actually been despondent about the fact that their test results for cancer came back negative. "I actually had one patient cry when I gave them the 'good news' that their test was negative [because they] were thinking diagnosis leads to treatment leads to cure—no diagnosis, no treatment" (Novella 2013).

But the goal of diagnostics should ultimately be good outcomes for patients, and that can be accomplished without always identifying specific conditions. Indeed, it is "sometimes better to have no diagnosis than to have a bad diagnosis" (Novella 2013). One wants to rule out especially bad conditions of course, but a non-specific diagnosis and the treatment of symptoms is often sufficient for a successful outcome. "Patients in whom all the tests come back negative (depending on the clinical situation) often do better than those with a specific diagnosis" (Novella 2013).

By their very nature, the three standard models can lead one to believe that the single goal of diagnostics is a specific diagnosis. But the IBE is perfectly compatible with multiple hypotheses being equally likely, because two hypotheses can be equally adequate. Perhaps they both measure up to the same criteria equally. Or perhaps they are equal in all other ways, but one is simpler and the other has wider scope. Consequently, in difficult cases, IBE can easily lead one to be satisfied with a non-specific non-serious diagnosis that simply leads to the treatment of symptoms. An emphasis on IBE in diagnosis reasoning can thus avoid Dr. House Syndrome.

Conclusion

I have argued that inference to the best explanation (IBE) is a better description of real-world diagnostic reasoning than the descriptions that are now most common in the medical literature. Often, when diagnostic reasoning goes wrong, it's because it has neglected some aspect essential to IBE. If my thesis is right, textbooks should describe diagnosis as such and emphasize the development of the relevant skills and methods. Research projects should also be opened that explore how an appreciation and understanding of IBE could help reduce diagnostic error.

Such steps would not eliminate diagnostic error of course, and would only be part of what should be a multifaceted solution. The identification and reporting of misdiagnosis will also have to be improved, for example, and better mechanisms will have to be put in place so physicians can learn from mistakes. To do so, hospitals will have to perform the delicate balancing act of holding physicians accountable while also making sure that physicians feel safe to report errors. But if physicians' diagnostic skills can be improved through the approach I have described, there will not be as many errors to learn from in the first place.

Notes

1. See Douven (2017). The book Douven cites is Josephson and Josephson (1996). He also mentions articles by Dragulinescu (2016, 2017), but these articles are about the use of IBE in medical research—particularly medical mechanisms in population studies—not diagnosis.
2. See, for example, Thagard and Shelley (1997, 413).
3. See Ledley and Lusted (1959, 9).

4. See Kassirer (1989, 894).
5. See Douven (2017), introduction.
6. See Balogh (2015).
7. See Committee (2001).
8. It should be noted that I have the modern conception of induction and deduction in mind here, not the ancient distinction identified by Aristotle that is often referenced in science textbooks. For Aristotle, an argument is inductive if it reasons from the specific to the general, and deductive if it reasons from the general to the specific. Today, philosophers consider an argument deductive if the person presenting it intends for its premises to guarantee its conclusion. It's inductive if the premises are merely intended to provide support. For more on this see Hawthorne (2018).
9. Consider, for example, the discovery of quarks, genes, and AIDS. See Thagard and Shelley (1997, 416–417).
10. See Schick and Vaughn (2014), Chapter 5.
11. See my articles "Availability Error," "Confirmation Bias," and "Suppressed Evidence" in Arp, Robert, Barbone, Steven, and Bruce, Michael. *Bad Arguments: 100 of the most importance fallacies in Western Philosophy.* 2019 Wiley-Blackwell, Hobken, NJ. pp. 128–132, 317–320, 399–402.
12. See Clendending and Hashinger (1947). I found this quote in Ledley and Lusted (1959), p. 9.
13. Relativity was more fruitful because it correctly predicted the appearance of a specific star during a solar eclipse on May 29, 1919. See O'Neil (2017). It was simpler because it did not require gravity to be an existing "force" in the universe. See Redd (2017). It has wider scope because it explained things like the perihelion of Mercury. See Conover (2018).
14. See Schick (2014, 169–171).
15. Of course, this is not true of all new theories. When proposing them, it is important to avoid the Galileo Gambit—a line of reasoning by which one believes that their hypothesis is true simply because it contradicts conventional wisdom. "You laugh at my theory, but they laughed at Galileo too, and he turned out to be right." For more, see my chapter on the Galileo Gambit in Arp (2018), pp. 152–156.
16. Elaboration on this point will follow, but for more on the debate regarding the definition of the scientific method see Andersen and Hepburn (2015).
17. See Aristotle (1883). See also Aristotle and Barnes (1976).
18. See Galilei et al. (1939).
19. See Bacon and Fowler (1889).
20. See Mill (1886).
21. See Whewell (1901).
22. See Peirce (1877).
23. The disagreement between these philosophers was often expressed in the primary sources footnoted earlier, but for a survey of such debates, and the issues surrounding the debate about what the scientific method is, see Nola (2000).
24. See McMullin (1992). For a complete defense of the idea that there indeed is a scientific method, see Nola and Sankey (2007).
25. For more on Pasteur's vaccination test on animals, see Giere (1997, 94). For a decent rundown of the history of germ theory, and the tests that helped prove it, see Garcia (2018).
26. For evidence that this is how science textbooks often articulate the scientific method, see Schick and Vaughn (2014, 161).
27. Ironically, these steps might have been inspired by the scientific method of the person who coined the term abduction, C.S. Pierce. For Pierce, scientific

reasoning begins with hypothesis generation (what he called abduction), moves to deriving testable consequences (what he called deduction), and then performing the tests (what he called induction). See Burch (2018), section 3. None of these terms are used in this way by modern logicians.

28. See Schick and Vaughn (2014, 176–177).
29. See Strassler (2012).
30. See Popper (1959), and Thornton (2018)
31. See Duhem (1954), Quine (1951), and Stanford (2017).
32. The answer in this case has to do with falsification. The "Satan did it" excuse itself cannot be tested; it is thus "ad hoc" and therefore unscientific. The "a new planet did it" excuse was testable—we could look to see if a planet was there—and thus was scientific. Ironically, this same excuse was proposed to explain irregularities in the orbit of Mercury, but even when a planet could not be found, scientists still did not reject Newton's laws. But their inadequacy was undeniable once Einstein's relativity explained the perihelion of Mercury without the need of any extra planets. See Schick and Vaughn (2014, 177–178).
33. Parallax is the apparent motion of distant stars. See *ibid.*, 179–180.
34. To account for the apparent retrograde of the planets in the night sky, geocentrism suggests that the planets orbit invisible points that orbit the earth.
35. A more controversial example would be string theory, which is not considered science by everyone, but because of its scope (its explanatory power), and the key role that scope plays in IBE, it probably should be. By the textbook definition it is not science simply because it makes no observable predictions.
36. See Balogh (2015, 53–66).
37. Bayes's theorem is expressed as such: $Pr(A \mid B) = [Pr(B \mid A) \times P(A)] / P(B)$. This is the kind of probabilistic reasoning mentioned by Ledley and Lusted (1959). See also Kassirer (1989).
38. See Balogh (2015, 65–66).
39. Think back to the example about the discovery of Neptune. If a diagnosis has already proven adequate, and the revision to it that accounts for the predictive failure is itself testable, then revision of a diagnosis in light of disconfirming evidence is warranted. Otherwise, one should reject the hypothesis.
40. "Demons did it" is, by its very nature, an untestable and un-parsimonious explanation.
41. See Lipton (2004).
42. See Josephson and Josephson's "Conceptual Analysis of Abduction" in Josephson & Josephson (1996, 1–26).

Works Cited

Andersen, Hanne, and Brian Hepburn. 2015. "Scientific Method." *Sandford Encyclopedia of Philosophy.* November 13, Accessed December 30, 2018. Retrieved from http://plato.stanford.edu/entries/scientific-method.

Aristotle, Octavius, Freire Owen, and Porphyry. 1883. *The Organon, or Logical treatises, of Aristotle.* London: G. Bell and Sons.

Aristotle. 1976. *Posterior Analytics,* Trans. Jonathan Barnes. Oxford: Clarendon Press.

Arp, Robert, Steven Barbone, and Michael Burce. 2018. *Bad Arguments: 100 of the Most Important Fallacies in Western Philosophy.* Hoboken, NJ: Wiley-Blackwell.

Bacon, Francis, and Thomas Fowler. 1889b. *Novum Organum*. Oxford: Clarendon Press.
Balogh, Erin, Bryan Miller, and John Ball. 2015. "Clinical Reasoning and Diag-
nosis." In Bryan Miller, John Ball, and Erin Balogh (eds.), *Improving Diagnosis
in Health Care*. Washington, DC: The National Academic Press: 53–66.
Burch, Robert. 2018. "Charles Sanders Peirce." In N. Edward and Zalta Win-
ter (ed.), *The Stanford Encyclopedia of Philosophy*. Accessed April 2, 2019.
Retrieved from https://plato.stanford.edu/archives/win2018/entries/peirce.
Clendening, Logan and Edward Hashinger. 1947. *Methods of Diagnosis*. St.
Louis: Mosby.
Committee on Quality of Health Care in America and Institute of Medicine.
2001. *Crossing the Quality Cchasm: A New Health System for the 21st Cen-
tury*. Washington, DC: National Academy Press.
Conover, Emily. 2018. "Einstein's General Relativity Reveals New Quirk of Mer-
cury's Orbit." *ScienceNews.org*. April 11, Accessed April 2, 2019. Retrieved
from www.sciencenews.org/article/einstein-general-relativity-mercury-orbit.
Douven, Igor. 2017. "Abduction." In N. Edward and Zalta Summer (ed.), *The
Stanford Encyclopedia of Philosophy*. Accessed April 2, 2019. Retrieved from
https://plato.stanford.edu/archives/sum2017/entries/abduction.
Dragulinescu, S. 2016. "Inference to the Best Explanation and Mechanisms in
Medicine." *Theoretical Medicine and Bioethics* 37 (3): 211–232.
Dragulinescu, Stefan. 2017. "Inference to the Best Explanation as a Theory for
the Quality of Mechanistic Evidence in Medicine." *European Journal for Phi-
losophy of Science* (7): 353–372.
Duhem, Pierre. 1954. *The Aim and Structure of Physical Theory*. Princeton, NJ:
Princeton University Press.
Feyerabend, Paul. 1959. "An Attempt at a Realistic Interpretation of Experi-
ence." In Paul Feyerabend (ed.), *Realism, Rationalism, and Scientific Method
(Philosophical Papers I)*. Cambridge: Cambridge University Press: 17–36.
Feyerabend, Paul. 1969. "Science Without Experience." In Paul Feyerabend (ed.),
Realism, Rationalism, and Scientific Method (Philosophical Papers I). Cam-
bridge: Cambridge University Press: 132–136.
Galilei, Galileo, Henry Crew, and and Alfonso de Salvio. 1939. *Dialogues Con-
cerning Two New Sciences*. Chicago: Northwestern University.
Garcia, Hector. 2018. "Louis Pasteur and the Germ Theory of Disease." *StMU
History Media*. May 10, Accessed December 30, 2018. Retrieved from www.
stmuhistorymedia.org/germ-theory-of-disease/.
Giere, Ronald. 1997. *Understanding Scientific Reasoning, Fourth Edition*.
Orlando, FL: Harcourt Brace College Publishers.
Hawthorne, James. 2018. "Inductive Logic." *Standord Enclyopedia of Philoso-
phy*. March 19, Accessed December 30, 2018. Retrieved from https://plato.
stanford.edu/entries/logic-inductive/.
Josephson, John, and Susan Josephson. 1996. *Abductive Inference: Computa-
tion, Philosophy, Technology*. Cambridge: Cambridge University Press.
Kassirer, Jerome. 1989. "Diagnostic Reasoning." *Annals of Internal Medicine*
110: 893–900.
Kohn, Linda, Janet Corrigan, and Molla Donaldson. 2000. *To Err Is Human:
Building a Safer Health System*. Washington, DC: National Academy Press.

Kuhn, Thomas. 1996. *The Structure of Scientific Revolutions*. Chicago, IL: University of Chicago Press.

Ledley, Robert, and Lee Lusted. 1959. "Reasoning Foundations of Medical Diagnosis." *Science, New Series* 130 (3366): 9–21.

Lipton, Peter. 2004. *Inference to the Best Explanation, Second Edition*. London: Routledge, Taylor and Francis Group.

McMullin, Ernan. 1992. *The Inference That Makes Science*. Milwaukee, WI: Marquette University Press.

Mill, John. 1886. *A System of Logic Ratiocinative and Inductive: Being a Connected View of the Principles of Evidence and the Methods of Scientific Investigation*. London: Longmans, Green.

Nola, Robert, and Howard Sankey (ed.). 2000. *After Popper, Kuhn and Feyerabend: Recent Issues in Theories of Scientific Method*. London: Springer.

Nola, Robert and Howard Sankey. 2007. *Theories of Scientific Method: An Introduction*. Stocksfield: Acumen.

Novella, Steven. 2013. "Clinical Decision Making: Part I." *Science-Based Medicine*. March 6, Accessed December 30, 2018. Retrieved from https://sciencebasedmedicine.org/clinical-decision-making-part-i/.

O'Neill, Ian. 2017. "How a Total Solar Eclipse Helped Prove Einstein Right About Relativity." *Space.com*. May 29, Accessed April 2, 2019. Retrieved from www.space.com/37018-solar-eclipse-proved-einstein-relativity-right.html.

Peirce, Charles. 1877. "The Fixation of Belief." *Popular Science Monthly* 12 (1): 1–15.

Popper, Karl. 1959. *The Logic of Scientific Discovery*. London: Hutchinson.

Popper, Karl. 1965. *Conjectures and Refutations: The Growth of Scientific Knowledge*. New York: Basic Books.

Quine, Willard. 1951. *Two Dogmas of Empiricism*. Cambridge, MA: Harvard University Press.

Redd, Nola. 2017. "Einstein's Theory of General Relativity." *Space.com*. November 7, Accessed April 2, 2019. Retrieved from www.space.com/17661-theory-general-relativity.html.

Schick, Theodore, and Lewis Vaughn. 2014. *How to Think About Weird Things: Critical Thinking for a New Age*. New York, NY: McGraw-Hill.

Stanford, Kyle. 2017. "Underdetermination of Scientific Theory." *Stanford Encyclopedia of Philosophy*. October 12, Accessed December 30, 2018. Retrieved from https://plato.stanford.edu/entries/scientific-underdetermination/.

Stanley, Donald, and Daniel Campos. 2013. "The Logic of Medical Diagnosis." *Perspectives in Biology and Medicine* 56 (2): 300–315.

Strassler, Matt. 2012. "Of Particular Significance: Conversations about Science with Theoretical Physicist Matt Strassler." *Profmattstrassler.com*. April 2, Accessed December 30, 2018. Retrieved from http://profmattstrassler.com/articles-and-posts/particle-physics-basics/neutrinos/neutrinos-faster-than-light/opera-what-went-wrong.

Thagard, Paul, and Cameron Shelley. 1997. "Abductive Reasoning: Logic, Visual Thinking, and Coherence." In Dalla Chiara, M. Doets, D. Mundici and J. van Benthem (eds.), *Logic and Scientific Methods*. Amsterdam, The Netherlands: Kluwer Academic Publishers: 413–427.

Thornton, Stephen. 2018. "Karl Popper." *Stanford Encyclopedia of Philosophy.* August 7, Accessed December 30, 2018. Retrieved from http://plato.stanford.edu/entries/popper/.

Whewell, William. 1901. *History of the Inductive Sciences from the Earliest to the Present Time.* New York: D. Appleton and Company.

14 Psychopathy Treatment and the Stigma of Yesterday's Research[1]

Rasmus Rosenberg Larsen[2]

Introduction

Psychopathy is one of the most studied and recognized psychiatric diagnoses in mental health research (Hare, Neumann, and Widiger 2012). The clinical prototype of a psychopathic patient includes traits of grave antisocial conduct, pathological lying, and a callous lack of empathy (e.g. Cooke, Hart, Logan, and Michie 2012). Relatedly, psychopaths are believed to be overrepresented in the criminal populace. Whereas psychopaths are estimated to make up about 1 percent of the general population, it is projected that some 30 percent of all incarcerated individuals might be psychopaths (Hare and Neumann 2008). As a result of these estimates, the psychopathy diagnosis has predominantly been researched and applied in forensic settings, yielding actuarial non-trivial information about behavior prediction, risk evaluation, treatment amenability, institutional placement, parole decision, etc. (e.g. Gacono 2016; Hare, Black, and Walsh 2013).

While many of the traits associated with psychopathy also overlap with other personality and conduct disorders (e.g. Crego and Widiger 2015), psychopaths are nevertheless considered importantly unique on a number of parameters. One such central difference is the prevailing belief that—different from most psychiatric conditions—psychopathy is an essentially chronic, untreatable disorder (e.g. Hare et al. 2013). For example, in a survey of Swedish forensic practitioners (n = 90), Sörman et al. (2014) found that participants generally endorsed the view that (a) psychopaths cannot change, (b) that there is no treatment that can cure a psychopath, and (c) that criminal psychopaths cannot be rehabilitated (2014, 411). These findings were consistent with a 1993 survey of UK forensic practitioners (n = 515) that found that only 1 percent thought that psychopathic personality was always remediable; most answered that only in some cases could patients benefit from treatment (Tennent, Tennent, Prins, and Bedford 1993).

The view that psychopaths are immune to various forms of psychiatric intervention and rehabilitation is not a new development, but echoes a long-standing truism in the research history (e.g. Cleckley 1988; Hare 1998; Harris and Rice 2006; Maibom 2014; McCord and McCord 1964; Suedfeld and Landon 1978). Presumably as an effect of these beliefs, researchers have reported on widespread evidence that the psychiatric diagnosis is generally applied, not as an indicator of psychiatric treatment, but moreover as a discriminator for treatment and rehabilitation programs (e.g. Polaschek and Skeem 2018). As was recently argued by a team of leading researchers, forensic practitioners are better off considering *management* a more appropriate goal than *treatment* when dealing with psychopathic patients, given that there is "no evidence that treatment programs results in a change in the personality structure of psychopathic individuals" (Hare et al. 2013, 244–245).

Mirroring a growing sentiment among researchers, this contribution argues that the *untreatability view* about psychopaths is medically erroneous due to insufficient support of scientific data. Moreover, the aggregate of recent research appears to paint a comparatively more optimistic picture of psychopaths' response to psychiatric intervention. Such a perspective, if reasonable, raises novel ethical concerns expedient to the field of forensic psychiatry; for example, whether the clinical narrative and forensic practice concerning psychopathy meets the ethical standards for proper psychiatric professionalism. Speaking to this suspicion, new cautionary directions for future practices and research are discussed.

The Psychopathy Diagnosis and Its Forensic Application

The psychopathy diagnosis is arguably among the historically and currently most researched psychiatric conditions (Hare, Neumann, and Widiger 2012), and as a result, its research paradigm has become an increasingly large and challenging affair to navigate. These complexities are further amplified by pop-cultural and unscientific anecdotes that surround the field, colorfully portraying psychopaths as vile intraspecies predators, sometimes deviating wildly from the basic tenets of the empirical research (e.g. Berg et al. 2013). Thus, one strategy for a sober and informative discussion of psychopathy research is to start with some basic perspectives in terms of what exactly psychopathy *is* and *is not*.

It should be noticed that psychopathy is not an "official" psychiatric diagnosis in the sense that its details are recognized by the broader psychiatric community. For instance, the diagnosis is not explicitly included in the latest (fifth) edition of the *Diagnostic and Statistical Manual of Mental Disorders* (DSM-5). Instead, the DSM-5 includes canonical psychopathic personality traits as *specifier* criteria under the diagnosis of *Antisocial Personality Disorder* (ASPD), ostensibly cataloging psychopathy as a subcategory to ASPD (for a discussion of the differences, see Crego and Widiger 2014). This should not necessarily be seen as a problematic aspect, though. Some researchers have argued that our understanding of psychopathy has greatly surpassed our understanding of ASPD, since the majority of research efforts (and funding) has migrated away from ASPD to the psychopathy diagnosis (e.g. Gacono 2016; Hare and Neumann 2008).

More fundamentally, though, classificatory descriptions of psychopathy in the psychiatric nomenclature can vary depending on the researchers we consult. For instance, some describe psychopathy as a *personality disorder*, others as a *clinical construct*, and some have argued that psychopathy is merely an *adaptive lifestyle* (e.g. Glenn, Kurzban, and Raine 2011; Hart and Cook 2012). In addition to these perspectives, the many different scientific theoretical accounts of the diagnosis are multifaceted. For instance, some posit psychopathy to be a cognitive disability, and others think it is an impairment of emotion dispositions (for a discussion of the contemporary accounts, see Brazil and Cima 2016). While these disagreements in the field are substantial, a more generous interpretation might be that they reflect a growing suspicion among researchers that psychopathy is a much more heterogenous disorder than previously assumed; that the diagnosis might consist of, or be divided into several sub-types (e.g. Hicks and Drislane 2018) with varying underlying etiologies (e.g. Jurjako and Malatesti 2018; Stratton, Kiehl, and Hanlon 2015).

However, aside from these divergences, the more fundamental motivation for applying the diagnosis is that the diagnosis itself aims at signifying a common patient stereotype encountered in the psychiatric clinic. That is, over the decades of psychiatric professional practices, clinicians have come to a sort of consensus that there exists a specific class of patients who demonstrate a peculiar constellation of personality and behavior; namely, a markedly callous personality disposition (e.g. lack of empathy, glibness, grandiosity) and strong antisocial tendencies (e.g. violence, pathological lying, impulsivity). These are the concrete individuals that clinicians aim to demarcate when they apply the term *psychopathy* (i.e. regardless of whether they see it as a *disorder*, *construct*, or something else).

More decisively, though, the majority of researchers generally agree that the syndromic constellation of so-called *psychopathic traits* is a sign of abnormality, positing that the homogeneity of observed traits across this particular "patient class" is caused by a discrete and shared underlying etiology (or a suite of different, yet discrete etiologies). Importantly, psychopaths are not seen as merely ill-behaved people with a socially appalling character. Certainly, there is not necessarily something psychologically abnormal about being deceitful and violent; we might even say this is what eventually differentiated *Homo sapiens* from other mammals (e.g. Wolin 1963). Rather, when psychologists refer to psychopathy as a psychiatric diagnosis, what is conveyed is a claim about a discrete *condition* or *symptom*, hypothesized to be caused by one or more likewise discrete etiological mechanisms (e.g. genes, neurobiological structures, cognitive functions, emotion deprivations, etc.) (e.g. Hare and Neumann 2008). Thus, when average people are deceitful and violent, this would be different from when psychopaths are so, since their behavior is caused/premediated by their psychological abnormality. Furthermore, this hypothesis also substantiates the larger forensic and criminological interest in psychopathy insofar that if psychopathy has discrete etiological mechanisms, we might be able to intervene medically with the violent antisocial behavior allegedly associated with psychopathy (e.g. Reidy et al. 2015).

When we speak of the field of psychopathy research, then, what we are really referring to is a largely coordinated scientific effort to corroborate this main hypothesis: that the observed patient stereotype makes up a homogenous class of individuals, undergirded by one or more discrete etiologies.[3] Although this research effort is multifaceted, it can be roughly divided into three interrelated, yet independent, research efforts: (1) *theoretically accounting* for what exactly makes psychopaths' psychology abnormal compared to normal individuals (e.g. Blair, Mitchell, and Blair 2005; Fowles and Dindo 2006; Hamilton and Newman 2018); (2) *empirically measuring* the etiological mechanisms of psychopathy (e.g. Ferguson 2010; Stratton, Kiehl, and Hanlon 2015; Werner, Few, and Bucholz 2015); (3) and an applied effort to build reliable and valid *assessment tools* capable of distinguishing psychopaths from non-psychopaths in the populace (e.g. Hare 2003; Lilienfeld and Widows 2005; Patrick, Fowles, and Krueger 2009).

In light of these different efforts, one common ground of confusion when speaking about psychopathy is when the various branches of research are conflated or mistaken with one another; for example, when (1) theoretical accounts of psychopathy are conflated with (3) the work of building valid assessment tools. Indeed, the former is concerned with accounting for the *mechanics behind* observed traits, while the latter regards the methods to reliably and validly demarcate psychopaths from non-psychopaths *based on* observable traits. Analogously, this example equals comparing theoretical studies of diabetes (e.g. accounting for the mechanics of cellular abnormalities in the pancreatic islets) with the diagnostic testing for diabetes (e.g. measuring blood sugar levels). Although the two are importantly related, they are obviously two very different things. The former regards what diabetes *is*, while the latter is a proxy measure *of* diabetes. Conflating the former into the other in psychopathy research and practices will result in the mistaken belief that a psychopathy measure *is* psychopathy (indeed, a common misconception, e.g. Skeem and Cooke [2010]).

Why is this nuance important? Because most of the times when the psychopathy diagnosis is introduced in forensic settings, what is really being discussed is (3) the *measure* of psychopathy. And as it is with all forms of psychiatric diagnostic assessments, there exists the very real possibility that the individuals we *measure* to have psychopathy are, in fact, not psychopaths (i.e. that they do not carry the hypothesized etiology). In such cases, we would be dealing with false positives, and many of our scientific inferences that we make about the psychiatric condition would not apply to the patient. It equals falsely asserting that a person has diabetes based on irregularities in blood sugar levels, which likewise would make him/her respond very differently to insulin injections (for a discussion of such *false positives* in psychopathy research, see: Larsen 2018; Skeem and Cooke 2010).

This point should not be taken easily, since there are good reasons to believe that our psychiatric assessments in general yield a high number of such inaccurate diagnoses. Compared to biomedical diagnostic assessment tools, say, a test for diabetes, psychiatric assessment tools are much less accurate for a number of reasons. First, researchers broadly disagree on how exactly to account for an alleged disorder (i.e. theoretical disagreement). Second, research in psychiatric etiology is scarce and ambiguous (i.e. disagreement and unfamiliarity about causality). Third, because of theoretical disagreement and lack of etiological insight, the assessment tools being developed will naturally have fundamental inbuilt uncertainties. For instance, when we do not have a clear theoretical understanding of a disorder, let alone know its cause(s), it trivially follows that we cannot know with certainty that our assessments measure what they purport to measure. While it is obvious that many medical disorders seem straightforward to measure even in the absence of theoretical and etiological insight (e.g. scientists were relatively accurate when demarcating diabetic patients before they knew what diabetes was), psychiatric conditions are presumably theoretically and etiologically more complex, and its signs and symptoms relatively more elusive than "somatic" disorders. So, where a traditional biomedical diagnostic method (e.g. measuring diabetes) yields a surprisingly high number of false diagnoses notwithstanding its comparatively high accuracy rates,[4] we can soundly assume that psychiatric tools are comparatively much more erroneous due to both the *basic nature* and our *epistemic limitations* about what we are measuring.

With this cautionary note on psychiatric diagnostics in mind, the term "diagnosed psychopath" shall in the following refer to a person who meets the, so to speak, *clinical standard* or *threshold* of psychopathy, namely, a person who has been assessed to be psychopathic with official field-specific assessment tools.

The most widely used psychopathy assessment method is the *Hare Psychopathy Checklist-Revised* (PCL-R) (R. D. Hare 2003) (see *Figure 14.1*). The PCL-R consists of 20 trait items, of which 18 load on two factors (and four facets). The assessment is carried out by analyzing patient records and conducting a semi-structured interview with the patient,

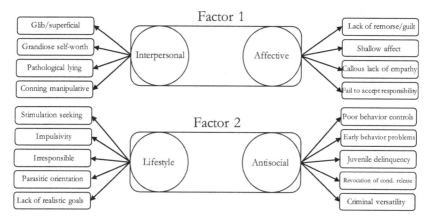

Factor 1

Glib/superficial

Grandiose self-worth

Pathological lying

Conning manipulative

Interpersonal

Affective

Lack of remorse/guilt

Shallow affect

Callous lack of empathy

Fail to accept responsibility

Stimulation seeking

Impulsivity

Irresponsible

Parasitic orientation

Lack of realistic goals

Factor 2

Lifestyle

Antisocial

Poor behavior controls

Early behavior problems

Juvenile delinquency

Revocation of cond. release

Criminal versatility

Figure 14.1 The Hare Psychopathy Checklist-Revised, two-factor and four-facet model (adapted from: Hare and Neumann 2008). In addition to these 18 factor-correlated traits, the PCL-R also includes: Many short-term marital relationships and promiscuous sexual behavior; although these two traits do not load on any factor, they are nevertheless believed to depict a shared characteristic of the patient class.

scoring each of the 20 items from 0–2 points. The score *zero* is given if the trait is not present in the patient; score *1* if the trait is partially present; or score *2* if the trait is a stable mark of the patient. Thus, the PCL-R score ranges from 0–40, where a conventionally decided cut-off score of a proper diagnosis is understood to be somewhere between 25–30 points. The diagnostic cut-off, however, is not implied as a hard line between *psychopathic* and *non-psychopathic*. Instead, the psychopathy diagnosis is broadly considered to be dimensional, where a score is better representative of the level of psychopathy in a patient (i.e. score 40 is considered "full blown" psychopathy) (for a peer-reviewed discussion of the PCL-R as a valid diagnostic tool, see: Hare and Neumann 2008).

One of the advantages of the PCL-R is its *clinical reliability*, i.e. the extent to which two or more clinicians independently give the same patient a similar score (e.g. Blais, Forth, and Hare 2017). This makes the PCL-R particularly apt at discerning the patient class (i.e. so-called psychopaths) based on the aforementioned observable traits. Notice, again, that this does not mean that the PCL-R selects *actual* psychopaths (i.e. those who carry the hypothesized etiologies). It merely means that, if we take a random group of people, the PCL-R can reliably pinpoint which individuals *belong*, so to speak, to the patient class.

Because of this reliability, the PCL-R has been considerably effective in actuarial scientific research, measuring specific behavioral tendencies correlated with the patient class across various demographics. For example, one forensically useful type of information that can be derived from applying the PCL-R is its correlation with violent recidivism in the criminal populace (e.g. Serin, Brown, and Wolf 2016; Yang, Wong, and Coid 2010). Thus, when we point to such correlations, what is really communicated is a data-driven statistical probability about future behavior (e.g. violence) insofar that one belongs to a reliably demarcated patient class. This process is methodologically identical to how, say, an insurance company calculates the risk of driver accident probability; namely, associating the assessed person with generalized data on specific traits, e.g. age, gender, address, occupation, etc. (e.g. Serin et al. 2016).

It is primarily because of such actuarial data-driven efforts that the psychopathy diagnosis has gained its reputation as a legitimate tool for forensic application, not only for violence prediction, but also on a suite of other related issues, such as (though not limited to): child custody hearings, parole hearings, capital sentencing hearings, preventative detention, culpability, institutional placement, and treatment amenability (DeMatteo et al. 2014a, 2014b; Edens and Cox 2012; Hare et al. 2013; Walsh and Walsh 2006).

Treating the "Untreatable"

One particularly widespread usage of the psychopathy diagnosis (e.g., a PCL-R assessment) is to introduce it when making decisions regarding psychiatric treatment and rehabilitation program placements. In this context, a high psychopathy score (e.g., 25 or higher on the PCL-R) will thus be interpreted as indicating unamiable qualities in terms of successful treatment outcomes, which may then bar such a person from entering said programs (e.g., Polaschek and Skeem 2018). This practice expresses a deep *clinical pessimism* about diagnosed psychopaths insofar as the diagnosis is not invoked for treatment purposes, but, instead, for justifying clinical passivity (i.e., mere clinical management). In this section, the validity of the so-called clinical pessimism surmounting diagnosed psychopaths will be reviewed, demonstrating that the belief is scarcely supported by the scientific research. Such a finding raises pressing ethical concerns for forensic psychiatrists, which will be discussed in the final section.

The clinical pessimism concerning psychopathy is not only alive and well today, but has arguably been the prevailing view for the better part of the research history. One of the *founders* of contemporary psychopathy theories, Hervey Cleckley, famously characterized the paradoxical nature of treating psychopaths. In his five-edition opus, *The Mask of Sanity* (first published in 1941), Cleckley spent several pages musing about the difficulties of treating psychopathic patients. According to Cleckley, one peculiarity about psychopaths was that, contrary to his other psychiatric patients, psychopaths did not appear to find their attitudes and behaviors problematic, let alone psychologically vexing—to Cleckley (2015) a strong indicator of futility in treatment efforts (26–32). Although Cleckley actually concluded his work with a hair of optimism on future treatment options, his overall assumption about the current state of clinical efforts was short and dire: there is not really much that can be done (p. 439).[5]

The clinical pessimism also made it into the single most read and cited book about psychopathy, Robert Hare's 1993 *Without Conscience*, which concludes with a snub:

> Many writers on the subject have commented that the shortest chapter in any book on psychopathy should be the one on treatment. A one-sentence conclusion such as, "no effective treatment has been found," or, "nothing works," is the common wrap-up to scholarly reviews of the literature.
>
> (Hare 1993, 194)[6]

Along these lines, the PCL-R *manual*—which makes up the foundation of the professional training of clinicians administering the PCL-R diagnoses—includes a similarly unenthusiastic section on treatment efforts (Hare 2003, 158–162). Here, the leading narrative is that, in general, "clinicians and researchers are rightly pessimistic about the treatability of psychopaths with traditional methods" (p. 158). But, on top of this, the PCL-R manual also emphasizes a discomforting phenomenon in treatment research; namely, that diagnosed psychopaths have shown *iatrogenic*, or adverse reactions, to treatment efforts. Treatment actually makes them more antisocial, prompting institutional violence and post-release recidivism.

The particular study mentioned in the PCL-R manual showing adverse effects is a retrospective follow-up study by Rice, Harris, and Cormier (1992). This research examined the recidivism rates of 176 treated offenders and 146 untreated offenders from a maximum-security institution over the course of 10.5 years. Among these patients were 92 diagnosed psychopaths, of which 46 received treatment (i.e. an intensive therapeutic community treatment program [e.g. Barker 1980]). Expectedly, the study found a significant difference in the *general* recidivism rates between psychopaths and non-psychopaths. However, the more interesting (and surprising) finding was that *violent* recidivism rates were substantially larger for treated psychopaths (77 percent), compared to non-treated psychopaths (55 percent). As such, violent recidivism was positively (i.e., adversely) associated with treatment efforts in diagnosed psychopaths. The study concluded on a speculative note: that community treatment programs that generally seek to cultivate pro-social empathic and caring qualities might inadvertently make psychopaths better equipped to "facilitate the manipulation and exploitation of others" and such treatment efforts could, therefore, be "associated with novel ways to commit violent crime" (Rice et al. 1992, 409).

The study by Rice, Harris and Cormier (1992) was based on a relatively small number of patients with a specifically non-diverse demographic, yielding unique and surprising results. Therefore, its generalizability should have been interpreted with caution. Nevertheless, the impact of the study has turned out to be nothing short of profound. As was noted in a review of the treatment literature on psychopathy, the study by Rice and colleagues effectively "slammed the lid shut for many on the advisability of even attempting treatment" (Polaschek and Daly 2013, 195).

Despite their own, and a community-wide, inability to replicate these adverse effect findings, the authors accentuated their conclusion in a 2006 review article of the psychopathy treatment literature (Harris and Rice 2006). In conclusion, they highlighted their 1992 findings, emphasizing that there was no compelling evidence for positive treatment outcomes of psychopaths, and that there were potential adverse outcomes of treating psychopaths: "We believe that the reason for these findings is that psychopaths are fundamentally different from other offenders and that there is nothing 'wrong' with them in the manner of a deficit or impairment that therapy can 'fix'. Instead, they exhibit an evolutionarily viable life strategy that involves lying, cheating, and manipulating others" (Harris and Rice 2006, 568). The larger point is that actual *treatment* might be too optimistic; instead, practitioners should focus on *managing* the antisocial patterns of diagnosed psychopaths. Hence, practitioners should use the psychopathy diagnosis as a discriminator for clinical treatment.

If we pause for a moment and consider these adverse effect perspectives, they should, as a minimum, give ground to critical suspicion. One initial problem is that, while we might be satisfied with the claim that the patient class selected by using the PCL-R potentially could be associated with adverse treatment effects, the way researchers here seem to qualify this view is, not with a reference to a patient class, but, rather, with reference to an underlying belief about the *nature* of psychopathy. But if it is the etiological aspect—i.e., psychopathy proper—that is correlated with adverse effects, we are left wondering how exactly this effect can be strongly correlated with a patient class that, all things considered, must include a great number of false positives. It is important to emphasize that, when we make actuarial projections based on a patient class (e.g. PCL-R score >25), these projections are entirely mute to any theory about underlying etiology (i.e., the actuarial claim is in and by itself a mere statistical observation). It therefore amounts to a logical leap of faith when these claims are translated into a narrative about adverse effects due to etiology that recommends management over treatment for the *entire* patient class (e.g. Hare et al. 2013). It is not that such claims are unintelligible from a hypothetical standpoint, though; it is, rather, that they seem insufficiently paired with critical scrutiny.

However, another problem with this narrative about untreatability and adverse treatment effects is that it is simply not supported by the overall research data, or, at least, the evidence in support of the widespread clinical pessimism is greatly disproportionate to the extent of the claim. For one, the study by Rice, Harris, and Cormier (1992)—which arguably serves as the most compelling, fundamental evidence in favor of clinical pessimism—was based on patients undergoing an infamously problematic treatment program at the *Oak Ridge Social Therapy Unit* in Ontario, Canada. The treatment program was so harrowing that a class lawsuit was raised against the institution and its practitioners in 2000. In May 2017, a Canadian judge ruled in favor of the plaintiffs, comparing the alleged treatment to *torture* (*Barker v. Barker* 2017; Fine 2017).[7] The details of the lawsuit confirmed widespread denigrating treatment procedures, such as chaining nude patients together for up to two weeks, keeping patients locked up in windowless rooms, feeding patients liquid food through tubes in the wall, experimenting with hallucinogens and delirium-producing drugs, and a complete disrespect and rejection of patient rights (Berg et al. 2013; D'Silva, Duggan, and McCarthy 2004; Ronson 2011).

In a 2016 interview, a former (recidivating) psychopathic patient from *Oak Ridge*, Jim Motherall, said that, when he was released from the institution in 1976, he was literally broken down and dysfunctional: "I wasn't ready to be on the street, I couldn't function on the street [. . .] I was angry. I hated them [the practitioners]. I hated what they did, I hated what they stood for. And I couldn't control the anger. I had lost any ability to get hold of that anger" (Sherren 2016). To Motherall, and presumably many of his fellow patients forced through the torturous "treatment" program, that anger led to multiple violent offences after his release, and decades of additional confinement.

The remaining question is, of course, whether (psychopathic) patients such as Motherall had their hypothesized condition exacerbated and, therefore, recidivated faster and more violently, or whether the violent frequencies were a result of some other factors related to their treatment. To answer this question in an accurate scientific manner, we would have to look closer at the psychological profiles of each recidivating patient and also know the details of the exact treatment program they underwent. For example, perhaps we would find that only certain personality traits (and not PCL-R psychopathy as such) were correlated strongly with elevated aggression. Unfortunately, such details are not present in the research data of Rice, Harris and Cormier (1992), nor have we seen any serious efforts in re-evaluating the research conclusion in light of the malpractice disclosure; for example, either retracting the study or further qualifying the data collection, methods, research results, etc. (which, of course, is common practice when the integrity of a study is compromised).

But perhaps asking these questions about adverse effects, let alone trying to answer them, is also rather futile. For instance, Polaschek and

Tadgh (2013) have argued that there is ample evidence that, in generalized and trivial ways, some treatment methods can potentially generate adverse outcomes in any patient class regardless of psychological disorder (e.g. Lilienfeld 2007; Skeem, Polaschek, and Manchak 2009). However, this is qualitatively different from claiming that specific treatment efforts (e.g. concrete maltreatment), or more profoundly, conventional treatment, *generally* makes diagnosed psychopaths at higher risk of recidivating—a grand view that needs more evidence than what can be drawn from a single compromised study (Polaschek and Daly 2013, 595). So far, Rice et al. (1992) remains the only cited evidence for the belief about adverse-effects,[8] raising the question why it continues to play a significant role in the treatment literature.

Notwithstanding the discussion of potential adverse effects, there is actually evidence suggesting that the overall clinical pessimistic conclusions about psychopaths are too precarious. The first study to suggest this was by Robert Salekin (2002), who reviewed 42 treatment studies, positing the unambiguous conclusion that the clinical pessimism associated with psychopathy has little scientific basis. Salekin highlighted a number of aggravating factors; mentioning a few should suffice. First, the study found a clear lack of valid generalizable data. For instance, out of the 42 studies, only four studies (9 percent) were based on the PCL-R, raising the question whether the different studies were actually studying individuals with the same traits/condition (i.e. unknown diagnostic compatibility). Second, although treatment outcomes varied greatly across studies, only one study reported adverse effects; namely, the study by Rice and colleagues (1992). This suggested to Salekin—presumably unaware that this treatment method would later be described as *torture* by a Canadian court—that the specific program of therapeutic community treatment administered by that particular institution was only *possibly* worsening the psychopathy condition (p. 105).

Curiously, although Salekin (2002) was arguably the most comprehensive large-scale review of the treatment literature of its time,[9] the publication of the second edition of the PCL-R in 2003 barely mentions these findings, merely declaring that: "Although some reviewers (e.g., Salekin 2002) have suggested that clinical pessimism might be replaced with clinical optimism, most clinicians and researchers are rightly pessimistic about the treatability of psychopaths with traditional methods" (Hare 2003, 158). Thus, even though there was poor scientific basis for making such a claim—as demonstrated by Salekin (2002)—the creators of the PCL-R manual continued to insist on the speculative perspective that:

> Some clinicians and administrators hold the uncritical view that psychopaths who have participated in prison treatment programs must have derived some benefit. This may help to lull the criminal justice system and the public into the false belief that the psychopaths with

whom they must deal have derived tangible benefits from treatment, simply because they and their therapist say so. Many psychopaths take part in all sorts of prison treatment programs, put on a good show, make "remarkable progress," convince the therapists and parole board of their reformed character, are released, and pick up where they left before they entered prison [Hare 1998].[10]

(Hare 2003, 158)

It is difficult to see such a narrative as anything else than incongruent with scientific standards, and thus, at best, anecdotal. Not only does the PCL-R cite the Salekin (2002) study, but it fails to acknowledge it as compelling, which, of course, is odd given that the study is a substantial peer-reviewed survey of the research literature. If extensive reviews and meta-analyses are not compelling scientific evidence, what is? Further, the literature raised in support of this alternative perspective in the PCL-R manual includes an extensive discussion of the study by Rice, Harris and Cormier (1992). We must assume, then, that the creators of the PCL-R, at the time of writing, were unaware of the fact that two to three years earlier to publication, a class action had been raised against the institution where Rice, Harris and Cormier (1992) collected their data, making public a mountain of evidence about disturbing psychiatric malpractices at *Oak Ridge Social Therapy Unit*.

For the past five to 10 years, however, a comparatively clearer, nuanced, and more optimistic picture about psychopathy and treatment has started to take shape. First, a few years after Salekin (2002), a review was published by D'Silva et al. (2004) that specifically sought to investigate the hypothesized adverse effects of treatment associated with the PCL-R diagnosis. The team systematically evaluated 24 studies and found that, above all, the aggregate of research was in such a condition that it was poorly equipped to answer their basic question about adverse effect (e.g., lack of control groups, lack of methodological rigor, poor data quality). They argued that, when researchers actually do draw the conclusion that psychopathy is related to adverse treatment outcomes (i.e. untreatability), such an interpretation amounts to a "logical error" (D'Silva et al. 2004, 175). Therefore, they expressed regret about the common practice that diagnosed psychopaths "are now being denied treatment on the basis that they are either untreatable or that treatment might make them worse" (D'Silva et al. 2004, 175).

Less than a decade after the publication of Salekin (2002) and D'Silva et al. (2004), a review study by Salekin, Worley and Grimes (2010) stressed a number of salient points. First, although they saw emerging developments in the field toward addressing the unique challenges related to treatment of diagnosed psychopaths, the collective research effort did not make a "strong case for the notion that psychopathy is untreatable" (Salekin et al. 2010, 255). Second, there was ample evidence that (adult) diagnosed psychopaths could indeed benefit significantly from *standard* treatment programs (Salekin et al. 2010, 255). Although researchers and practitioners still battle with overcoming the seeming unwarranted clinical pessimism, the two points stressed by Salekin and colleagues (2010) can now be traced broadly in the *research* field, though it is allegedly still far from a prevailing viewpoint among *practitioners* (e.g. Sörman et al. 2014).

Indeed, in the most recent and detailed evaluation of the treatment literature, Polaschek and Skeem (2018) notice that perhaps the strongest barrier for scientifically answering the question about treatability is, ironically, the notable "dearth of research," perhaps propelled in part by the prevailing belief among both researchers and practitioners that the question about treatability has long been answered; namely, that psychopaths *cannot* be treated (Polaschek and Skeem 2018, 710). What makes all of this ironic is that, instead of being a ground for neglecting treatment, diagnosed psychopaths should—according to canonical treatment guidelines—be viewed as prime targets for treatment efforts due to their common status as high-risk patients. Generally, treatment efforts are directed where it is likely to make an actual robust impact (i.e. the *Risk-Need-Responsivity* model); namely, treatment should be aimed at individuals who, for example, are likely to recidivate. Naturally, high-risk patients, such as diagnosed psychopaths, would fall within this group (Polaschek and Skeem 2018, 712).

With regard to effective treatment, Polaschek and Skeem (2018) underline that knowledge about concrete treatment methods is so far scarce, but notice that there is evidence of positive treatment outcomes across the literature (e.g. Polaschek 2011; Skeem, Monahan, and Mulvey 2002; Wong et al. 2012). So, while research is certainly lacking, and, therefore, increased efforts should be expected to shed further light on the issue, Polaschek and Skeem (2018) also stress the importance of simply beginning to encourage and facilitate treatment efforts. Such attempts may "restore faith among members of the public that psychopathic individuals are not intractable threats who must be indefinitely detained," promoting the view that our justice system ought to "provide access to rehabilitation for all adjudicated individuals in need of it" (Polaschek and Skeem 2018, 726).

In addition to the studies highlighted by Polaschek and Skeem (2018), novel approaches to treatment programs have in recent years shown that optimism is generally warranted. For example, Wong et al. (2012, 2015) developed a model using the PCL-R *factor scores* to guide treatment efforts insofar that some cognitive-behavioral treatment strategies[11] tend to be more efficient in psychopathic patients scoring high in Factor 2 items (i.e. typical criminogenic behavioral features), suggesting "that psychopaths and violent offenders in general have qualitatively similar treatment targets" (Wong and Olver 2015, 305). Utilizing this model,

Sewall and Olver (2019) examined the correlation between psychopathy, treatment, and sexually violent recidivism in a group of men (n=302) and found that diagnosed psychopaths benefitted equally from treatment compared to non-psychopaths (consistent with other results, e.g. Polaschek and Ross 2010). The authors concluded that their study "fuels optimism about the potential for psychopathic men to make meaningful risk-related changes akin to their nonpsychopathic counterparts" (Sewall and Olver 2019, 68). Similarly, Baskin-Sommers and Curtin and Newman (2015) tested a training program that purported to improve robust deficits found in psychopaths (e.g. attention deficits), and results strongly indicated that psychopaths "are capable of overcoming their subtype-specific deficits with practice and that receiving deficit-matched training results in generalizable change in these subtype-specific deficits" (Baskin-Sommers, Curtin, and Newman 2015, 51). Echoing this optimism, Brazil et al. (2018) highlighted the somewhat commonsensical point that as cognitive and behavioral research progresses, and new etiological insights about psychopathy are disclosed, such information is expected to yield comparatively much more precise intervention strategies.

As has been demonstrated, the research literature is rather clear with respect to two main points. First, there is virtually no concrete evidence that the psychopathy diagnosis should be adversely correlated with treatment efforts. Second, while there is significant evidence (though limited in scope) of successful treatment efforts, there is next to no scientifically based evidence in support of the thesis that psychopaths are generally immune to psychiatric intervention. In other words, the widespread *untreatability view* pertaining to diagnosed psychopaths is medically erroneous. Now, if the *untreatability view* is rejected by the research record, but forensic practitioners still maintain a widespread adherence to the precarious conclusions of outdated research narratives, it should raise a suspicion about the professional and ethical standards in the field.

Psychopathy and the Stigma of Yesterday's Research

In the remainder of this contribution, ethical perspectives and issues related to administering the psychopathy diagnosis will be discussed with a special focus on the matters concerning its use as a treatment amenability assessment. The aim of this final section, however, is not only to draw conclusions from the foregoing analysis, but also to add some general remarks to a growing sentiment in psychopathy research of encouraging contributions in ethics (e.g. Edens et al. 2018; Lyon, Ogloff, and Shepherd 2016; Pickersgill 2009). It should be underlined, though, that ethical discussions in forensic psychiatry are somewhat meager due to its status as a relatively young field (e.g. Appelbaum 2008). More so (and perhaps due to its even younger status), thoughtful discussions about the ethics of psychopathy research and practices is not only meager but next to non-existing, and a serious discourse has yet to manifest broadly across the paradigm (although, some admirable efforts have been made analyzing the role of psychopathy with respect to specific *legal* issues [e.g. Edens et al. 2018]).

Before examining the specific ethical challenges that emerge in the practice of utilizing the psychopathy diagnosis, a short comment is needed in order to establish what exact *ethical principles* we shall hold the following discussion up against. While the *American Psychiatric Association* provides a general set of guidelines for the psychiatric profession (i.e. the so-called *The Principles of Medical Ethics*), some researchers have sought to amend these guidelines with crucial nuances specifically applicable to forensic psychiatry (for an overview, see Austin, Goble, and Kelecevic 2009; Niveau and Welle 2018).[12] For example, Paul Appelbaum (1997, 2008) has with his so-called *standard position* argued that two basic principles in particular define the ethical obligations of forensic psychiatric practitioners:

The first principle is that of *truth-telling*; namely, that practitioners' testimony must always reflect their truthful, honest opinion. But not just any true opinion. If that were the case, ignorant psychiatrists would then be able to serve any side and any objective, as long as their statement were genuinely believed. Rather, Appelbaum (2008) stressed that there is an ethical obligation for forensic psychiatrists to accurately base their testimony on concrete "scientific data on the subject at hand and the consensus of the field," regardless of which side in the adversarial court system their comments may favor or disadvantage (Appelbaum 2008, 196). At first glance, this principle sets an increasingly high standard for an ethical guideline, since the scientific data of psychiatric research can be unreliable, and its theories often non-validated and disputed, raising the question whether there really are scientifically truthful psychiatric claims. However, Applebaum holds that when psychiatric research has established something akin to a consensus, practitioners may report on such information regardless of it being robustly validated. For example, where different forms of psychotherapy might lack peer-reviewed validity, some practitioners and clients may still benefit from such procedures, making them perfectly justified in terms of ethical standards. Indeed, one can still *do good* with unestablished science.

The second principle is that of *respect for persons*; namely, that in the quest of giving truthful, scientifically accurate testimonies, forensic psychiatrists must qualify their expertise so they always "respect the humanity of the evaluee," refraining from engaging in "deception, exploitation, or needless invasion of the privacy" of the people being examined, reported, or testified about (Appelbaum 2008, p. 197. This principle has several moderating applications. For one, if this principle is not applied, it would then follow that practitioners could engage in any practice as long as it were connected to seeking or conveying the truth; for instance, deceitfully exploiting an unprepared witness to get to the truth. Another qualification of the second principle is that of setting limits for what and how specific information is introduced to various stakeholders (e.g. in the adversarial court system). Where scientific truths might be conveyed with a genuine incentive, the forensic practitioner ought also to exert some standard awareness of, say, what potentially negative effects such information may have on the individual.[13]

With these ethical principles in mind, let us briefly consider the common practice with regards to applying the psychopathy diagnosis in *treatment amenability* processes. As mentioned, the psychopathy diagnosis is introduced in court or a correctional setting primarily as a way to provide data-driven actuarial testimonies about a patient; namely, by correlating and inferencing the specific patient to a reliably established patient class (i.e. PCL-R diagnosed psychopaths). That is, by assessing a patient with psychopathy (i.e. a particular PCL-R score), we can thereby, due to established empirical research, make an inference to the specific behaviors that are tested for in the research. This practice, of course, deviates markedly from drawing inferences based on mere "professional opinion." As such, the practice of making said data-driven (i.e. actuarial) inferences are seemingly on par with the first principle in the standard position (i.e. *truth-telling*) since it is based on widely accepted scientific procedures (e.g. Serin et al. 2016).[14]

Notice, though, that according to the *standard position* the scope of what exactly can be inferred from a psychopathy diagnosis will be fully contingent on the actual peer-reviewed research. That is, the psychopathy diagnosis—for example, the PCL-R assessment—can only be used as an inference about issues that have been tested for and validated by the research community. For example, it has been shown that there is a weak to moderate correlation between a high PCL-R score and violent recidivism (e.g. Yang et al. 2010). With this knowledge in hand, a forensic psychiatrist can therefore *truthfully* inform the court or correctional system of such specific probabilities and the extent to which they translate to the concrete case. Again, what makes such an inference truthful is simply that it is a scientific peer-reviewed qualified statement.

Regretfully, though, there is growing evidence that the psychopathy diagnosis has been used to make inferences to actuarial issues that have never been tested for. In a review study of how the psychopathy diagnosis has been introduced in court cases, Lyon, Ogloff, and Shepherd (2016) found a number of problematic applications; for example, one case in which the psychopathy diagnosis was introduced in court to argue that the patient (due to his high PCL-R score) was incapable of reading and comprehending intricate information (194). As the authors stressed, since there are no particular studies that test for such a hypothesis in the patient class, that inference is invalid. In accordance with the first principle in the *standard position*, then, introducing such invalid references (e.g. reading and comprehension capabilities) will thus amount to an instance of unethical practice due to it being scientifically *untruthful*.

Similarly, then, it appears clear that the use of the psychopathy diagnosis as a treatment amenability discriminator, specifically as an instrument to explicitly prohibit diagnosed psychopaths from entering rehabilitation and treatment programs, fails to meet the ethical demands of the first principle in the standard position. As it was shown, not only is the evidence for the untreatability hypothesis scarcely supported, but evidence of the stronger narrative about adverse effects is also insufficient. Instead, it was shown that the research literature has yielded increasing positive evidence for treatment and intervention effects on diagnosed psychopaths (e.g. Polaschek 2011; Polaschek and Skeem 2018; Sewall and Olver 2019; Skeem, Monahan, and Mulvey 2002; Wong et al. 2012). As a minimum, it is safe to say that there is no established consensus that psychopaths are untreatable.

Moreover, the case for unethical practices might be stronger than a mere misinformation to the court and correctional institutions. Not only does the practice of treatment discrimination fail on the first principle (i.e. truth-telling), but it also appears to fail on the second principle (i.e. respect for persons). Indeed, the patients in question are not offered the treatment they rightfully need. This omission effectively eclipses the broader standing guidelines of administering psychiatric intervention; namely, that high-risk patients are fundamentally high-priority individuals (i.e., the *Risk-Need-Responsivity* model). Arguably, such practices are not only problematic from the patient's perspective (i.e. his/her well-being is neglected), but, from the perspective of the greater good of society, such practices effectively increase social risks, as high-profile dangerous individuals are eventually released back into society without a proper attempt at rehabilitating treatment.

In addition to this deeper ethical suspicion, it is perhaps worth noticing that the *psychiatric pessimism* that appears to frame practitioners' dealings with psychopaths does not only boil down to a question of actual treatment, but may amount to a kind of harmful stigma. Its effects may transport deeply into the judicial system, well beyond the psychiatrist–patient relationship. Indeed, the belief that psychopaths are unlikely to rehabilitate, or, so to speak, are untreatable, seems to also have stabilized among lay people. For example, in a survey of people attending jury duty (n=400), Smith, Edens, Clark, and Rulseh (2014) found that respondents were generally doubtful about whether criminal psychopaths could successfully rehabilitate back into society, and remained largely undecided about the scenario of curing or treating psychopaths (Smith, Edens, Clark, and Rulseh 2014, 496). Although one might argue that lay people are outside of the proper forensic psychiatric concern, there are reasons to treat such findings seriously. Indeed, non-experts are importantly involved in everything from jury duty to parole decisions to the forming of public policies, which makes them central stakeholders for forensic psychiatrists.

Speaking to this suspicion of a broader stigmatizing effect of the untreatability narrative, Edens et al. (2018) noted that many key decisions in the legal system (e.g. parole decisions, capital sentencing, institutional placement, permanent detention) rest pointedly on evaluating whether the patient will be dangerous in the *future*. When a high-risk patient is assessed with psychopathy and, therefore, considered psychiatrically untreatable (as opposed to treatable), it is not far-fetched to suggest that this is taken to imply the aggravating notion that such a person is highly unlikely to change, let alone be responsive to correctional restraint and deterrence, and thus represents as a *chronic* future institutional and social risk (for similar perspectives, see DeMatteo et al. 2014a, 2014b; Edens, Davis, Smith, and Guy 2013).

In sum, there are good reasons why we should be ethically worried about the practice of introducing the psychopathy diagnosis for treatment amenability purposes. One, it is insufficiently based in scientific research. Second, it seems to violate the respect psychiatrists ought to have for their patients, unjustifiably stripping patients of serious rehabilitation efforts (with potential harm to them and the broader society). In addition, we may speculate that the untreatability perspective transports unto judges and jurors an aggravating, stigmatizing perspective of chronic antisocial behaviors, unloading extrajudicial, unfair hurdles unto the patient's process in the judicial and correctional system (i.e. the probative value of a PCL-R assessment is outweighed by the prejudicial effects).

In light of such a conclusion, we might ask what ought to be done in forensic psychiatry to alleviate this seemingly unethical procedure. Although one obvious recommendation is to stop using the psychopathy diagnosis in treatment amenability assessments, there might be reasons to suggest more critical and wider ranging recommendations. In their recent article, which surveyed a handful of important legal and ethical issues related to psychopathy and violence risk assessment, Edens et al. (2018) concluded with a critical question; namely, whether forensic psychiatrists should "abandon the use of psychopathy assessments, particularly PCL-R scores, to influence decision making" in court and correctional settings, given a growing evidence of forensic misuse and limited scientific validity. Their question seems to signal a growing skepticism in the field about the broader motivations and incentives behind the use of the psychopathy diagnosis, as well as a scientifically critical attitude toward the alleged *truths* communicated by the diagnosis. Perhaps it is time for the field to stop and more profoundly take status of the research and practices regarding the psychopathy diagnosis. Indeed, it is becoming increasingly clear that, although researchers might find it unproblematic to study this alleged pathology through their lenses in the *ivory tower*, the nuances and complexities that immerse this diagnostic category are precariously lost in the adversarial process of court and correctional settings.

Notes

1. Larsen, Rasmus. "Psychopathy Treatment and the Stigma of Yesterday's Research." *Kennedy Institute of Ethics Journal* 29 (3). pp. 247–272. © 2019 Johns Hopkins University Press. Reprinted with permission of Johns Hopkins University Press.
2. I would like to acknowledge the reviewers for their constructive feedback, which led to substantial improvements of the initial manuscript. All potential mistakes are entirely my own.
3. Notice that when researchers pursue the view that psychopathy is *not* homogenous, but instead a heterogenous construct that covers over several subtypes, these subtypes are then hypothesized to make up a homogenous (sub)class, with one or more discrete etiologies.
4. For an example of how to estimate the extent of false positive in diagnosis, see van Stralen et al. (2009).
5. Ironically, the first person to suggest the existence of the psychopathy diagnosis, the American polymath Benjamin Rush, was rather optimistic about the role of the psychiatrist, professing that medical insight into this disorder eventually would contribute to eradicating social evils at large (Rush, 1972, 37 [first published in 1786]).
6. Hare is here paraphrasing a well-known quote from Suedfeld and Landon (1978).
7. In an official statement, Judge Perell said: "I appreciate that apart from professional renown and advancement, there was no self-serving gratification for the Defendant physicians at the expense of the Plaintiffs [but] it is a breach of a physician's ethical duty to physically and mentally torture his patients even if the physician's decisions are based on what the medical profession at the time counts for treatment for the mentally ill" (Fine, 2017).
8. One study has reported adverse effects associated with specific PCL-R traits (i.e. Factor 1), although adverse effects were not correlated with the total PCL-R score (Hare, Clark, Grann, and Thornton 2000). This finding, however, has not been replicated. For the opposite findings; namely, that the same PCL-R traits can be associated with *positive* treatment outcomes, see Burt, Olver, and Wong (2016). Another study found *indications* of adverse effects (Seto and Barbaree 1999). This study, however, was later retracted after a follow-up study (Barbaree 2005).
9. However, there were some attempts at reviewing the treatment literature before Salekin (2002). For instance, a study by Garrido, Esteban and Molero (1995) reported on two separate meta-analyses, though without providing the needed detail on references and methods. A book by Dolan and Coid (1993) offered a comprehensive review of the treatment literature and concluded that the collective research suffered from lack of stable diagnostic criteria, had problematic sampling procedures, ill-described treatment processes, and an unsystematic measure of treatment outcomes, making it difficult to draw any scientifically meaningful conclusions. For a similar portrayal of the research efforts before Salekin (2002), see Harris and Rice (2006).
10. For what it is worth, the reference included at the end of this quote from the PCL-R manual is to Hare (1998), a book chapter that includes a

three-paragraph section titled "Recidivism Following Treatment." In this section, Hare includes an extensive discussion of the study by Rice and colleagues (1992).

11. For an anthology on cognitive-behavioral treatment, see Kazantzis, Reinecke, and Freeman (2010).

12. Notice that forensic psychiatry is a *subspecialty* in psychiatry insofar as the profession deals with mental functioning and behavior in legal and correctional settings (Bloom and Schneider 2016). Although the concrete role of a forensic psychiatrist can vary, it typically involves providing non-trivial information to the court and correctional settings, assisting the evaluation of fitness to stand trial, responsibility, sentencing, institutional placement, parole decisions, treatment, rehabilitation, etc. (e.g. Bloom & Schneider 2016, 693–718).

13. While the *standard position* has been broadly endorsed by practitioners and theorists, it is not without its strong critics. Alan Stone (2008) has argued that the *standard position* can never claim any neutral ethical worth. For instance, as Stone argued, due to the adversarial system in a court setting, forensic psychiatrists are bound to deliver statements that can potentially be both good and bad for the patient in question. As Stone puts it: "Psychiatrists are immediately over the [ethical] boundary when they go into court" (Stone 2008, 168).

14. This is not necessarily an unproblematic claim. Although the forensic psychiatric profession is ethically challenging (in both practical and theoretical affairs), we might here stress that it is not obvious that *actuarial data* meet the standard of "truth telling." Indeed, actuarial science is inherently uncertain due to its probabilistic nature. As one reviewer of this contribution pointed out, maybe the overall actuarial data on diagnosed psychopaths is simply too weak to make any *truthful* assertions about the patient class (this concern is also raised in Serin et al. 2016). Such a reservation would be even stronger if we weigh in the possibility of large-scale false positives within the PCL-R patient class (e.g. Larsen 2018).

Works Cited

Austin, Wendy, Erika Goble, and Julija Kelecevic. 2009. "The Ethics of Forensic Psychiatry: Moving Beyond Principles to a Relational Ethics Approach." *The Journal of Forensic Psychiatry & Psychology* 20 (6): 835–850. doi:10.1080/14789940903174147

Appelbaum, Paul. 1997. "A Theory of Ethics for Forensic Psychiatry." *Journal of the American Academy of Psychiatry and the Law Online* 25 (3): 233–247.

Appelbaum, Paul. 2008. "Ethics and Forensic Psychiatry: Translating Principles Into Practice." *Journal of the American Academy of Psychiatry and the Law Online* 36 (2): 195–200.

Barbaree, Howard. 2005. "Psychopathy, Treatment Behavior, and Recidivism: An Extended Follow-Up of Seto and Barbaree." *Journal of Interpersonal Violence* 20 (9): 1115–1131. doi:10.1177/0886260505278262

Barker, Elliott. 1980. "The Penetanguishene Program: A Personal Review." In Hans Toch (ed.), *Therapeutic Communities in Corrections* (pp. 73–81). New York: Praeger.

Baskin-Sommers, Arielle, John Curtin, and Joseph Newman. 2015. "Altering the Cognitive-Affective Dysfunctions of Psychopathic and Externalizing Offender

Subtypes with Cognitive Remediation." *Clinical Psychology Science* 3 (1): 45–57. doi:10.1177/2167702614560744

Barker v. Barker, ONSC 3397 C.F.R. 2017.

Berg, Joana, Sarah Smith, Ashley Watts, Rachel Ammirati, Sophie Green, and Scott Lilienfeld. 2013. "Misconceptions Regarding Psychopathic Personality: Implications for Clinical Practice and Research." *Neuropsychiatry* 3 (1): 63–74. doi:10.2217/npy.12.69

Blair, Rachel, Derek Mitchell, and Karina Blair. 2005. *The Psychopath: Emotion and the Brain*. Malden: Blackwell Publishing.

Blais, Julie, Adelle Forth, and Rober Hare. 2017. "Examining the Interrater Reliability of the Hare Psychopathy Checklist-Revised Across a Large Sample of Trained Raters." *Psychological Assessment* 29 (6): 762–775. doi:10.1037/pas0000455

Bloom, Hy, and Richard Schneider. 2016. "Forensic Psychiatry." In Caitlin Pakosh (ed.), *The Lawyer's Guide to the Forensic Sciences* (pp. 669–718). Toronto: Irwin Law Inc.

Brazil, Inti, and Maaike Cima. 2016. "Contemporary Approaches to Psychopathy." In Maaike Cima (ed.), *The Handbook of Forensic Psychopathology and Treatment* (pp. 206–226). New York: Routledge.

Brazil, Inti, Josanne van Dongen, Joseph Maes, Rogier Mars, and Arielle Baskin-Sommers. 2018. "Classification and Treatment of Antisocial Individuals: From Behavior to Biocognition." *Neuroscience and Biobehavioral Reviews* 91: 259–277.

Burt, Grant, Mark Olver, and Stephen Wong. 2016. "Investigating Characteristics of the Nonrecidivating Psychopathic Offender." *Criminal Justice and Behavior* 43 (12): 1741–1760. doi:10.1177/0093854816661215

Cleckley, Hervey. 1988. *The Mask of Sanity: An Attempt to Clarify Some Issues about the So-Called Psychopathic Personality, Fifth Edition*. St. Louis: Mosby.

Cleckley, Hervey. 2015. *The Mask of Sanity: An Attempt To Clarify Some Issues About the So-called Psychopathic Personality, Second Edition*. Mansfield Centre, CT: Martino Publishing.

Cooke, David, Stephen Hart, Caroline Logan, and Christine Michie. 2012. "Explicating the Construct of Psychopathy: Development and Validation of a Conceptual Model, the Comprehensive Assessment of Psychopathic Personality (CAPP)." *International Journal of Forensic Mental Health* 11 (4): 242–252. doi:10.1080/14999013.2012.746759

Crego, Cristina, and Thomas Widiger. 2014. "Psychopathy, DSM-5, and a Caution." *Personality Disorders-Theory Research and Treatment* 5 (4): 335–347. doi:10.1037/per0000078

Crego, Cristina, and Thomas Widiger. 2015. "Psychopathy and the DSM." *Journal of Personality* 83 (6): 665–677. doi:10.1111/jopy.12115

DeMatteo, David, John Edens, Meghann Galloway, Jennifer Cox, Shannon Smith, and Dana Formon. 2014a. "The Role and Reliability of the Psychopathy Checklist-Revised in US Sexually Violent Predator Evaluations: A Case Law Survey." *Law and Human Behavior* 38 (3): 248–255. doi:10.1037/lhb0000059

DeMatteo, David, John Edens, Meghann Galloway, Jennifer Cox, Shannon Smith, Julie Koller, and Benjamin Bersoff. 2014b. "Investigating the Role of the Psychopathy Checklist-Revised in United States Case Law." *Psychology Public Policy and Law* 20 (1): 96–107. doi:10.1037/a0035452

Dolan, Bridget, and Jeremy Coid. 1993. *Psychopathic and Antisocial Personality Disorders: Treatment and Research Issues.* London: Gaskell.

D'Silva, Karen, Connor Duggan, and Lucy McCarthy. 2004. "Does Treatment Really Make Psychopaths Worse? A Review of the Evidence." *Journal of Personality Disorders* 18 (2): 163–177. doi:10.1521/pedi.18.2.163.32775

Edens, John, John Petrila, and S.E. Kelley. 2018. "Legal and Ethical Issues in the Assessment and Treatment of Psychopathy." In Christopher Patrick (ed.), *Handbook of Psychopathy, Second Edition.* New York: The Guilford Press: 732–751.

Edens, John, and Jennifer Cox. 2012. "Examining the Prevalence, Role and Impact of Evidence Regarding Antisocial Personality, Sociopathy and Psychopathy in Capital Cases: A Survey of Defense Team Members." *Behavioral Sciences & the Law* 30 (3): 239–255. doi:10.1002/bsl.2009

Edens, John, Karen Davis, Krissie Smith, and Laura Guy. 2013. "No Sympathy for the Devil: Attributing Psychopathic Traits to Capital Murderers Also Predicts Support for Executing Them." *Personality Disorders: Theory, Research, and Treatment* 4 (2): 175–181. doi:10.1037/a0026442

Ferguson, Christopher. 2010. "Genetic Contributions to Antisocial Personality and Behavior: A Meta-Analytic Review From an Evolutionary Perspective." *The Journal of Social Psychology* 150 (2): 160–180. doi:10.1080/00224540903366503

Fine, Sean. 2017, June 7. "Doctors Tortured Patients at Ontario Mental-Health Centre, Judge Rules." *The Globe and Mail.* Retrieved from www.theglobeandmail.com/news/national/doctors-at-ontario-mental-health-facility-tortured-patients-court-finds/article35246519/

Fowles, Don, and Lilian Dindo. 2006. "A Dual-Deficit Model of Psychopathy." In Christopher Patrick (ed.), *Handbook of Psychopathy, First Edition.* New York: The Guildford Press: 14–34.

Gacono, Carl. (ed.) 2016. *The Clinical and Forensic Assessment of Psychopathy: A Practitioner's Guide, Second Edition.* New York: Routledge.

Garrido, Vicente, Cristina Esteban, and C. Molero. 1995. "The Effectiveness in the Treatment of Psychopathy: A Meta-Analysis." *Issues in Criminological and Legal Psychology* 12: 57–59.

Glenn, Andrea, Robert Kurzban, and Adrian Raine. 2011. "Evolutionary Theory and Psychopathy." *Aggression and Violent Behavior* 16 (5): 371–380. doi:10.1016/j.avb.2011.03.009

Hamilton, Rachel, and Joseph Newman. 2018. "The Response Modulation Hypothesis: Formulation, Development, and Implications for Psychopathy." In Christopher Patrick (ed.), *Handbook of Psychopathy, Second Edition.* New York: The Guilford Press.

Hare, Robert. 1993. *Without Conscience: The Disturbing World of the Psychopaths Among Us.* New York: The Guilford Press.

Hare, Robert. 1998. "Psychopaths and Their Nature: Implications for the Mental Health and Criminal Justice System." In Theodore Millon, Erik Simonsen, Morten Birket-Smith and Roger Davis (eds.), *Psychopathy: Antisocial, Criminal, and Violent Behavior.* New York: Guilford Press: 188–212.

Hare, Robert. 2003. *Hare Psychopathy Checklist—Revised, Second Edition.* Toronto: Multi Health System.

Hare, Robert, Pamela Black, and Zach Walsh. 2013. "The Psychopathy Checklist-Revised: Forensic Applications and Limitations." In Robert Archer and

Elizabeth Wheeler (eds.), *Forensic Uses of Clinical Assessment Instruments, Second Edition*. New York: Routledge: 230–265.

Hare, Robert, Danny Clark, Martin Grann, and David Thornton. 2000. "Psychopathy and the Predictive Validity of the PCL-R: An International Perspective." *Behavioral Sciences & the Law* 18 (5): 623–645. doi:10.1002/1099–0798(200010)18:5 < 623::Aid-Bsl409 > 3.0.Co;2-W

Hare, Robert, and Craig Neumann. 2008. "Psychopathy as a Clinical and Empirical Construct." *Annual Review of Clinical Psychology* 4: 217–246. doi:10.1146/annurev.clinpsy.3.022806.091452

Hare, Robert, Craig Neumann, and Thomas Widiger. 2012. "Psychopathy." In Thomas Widiger (ed.), *The Oxford Handbook of Personality Disorder* (pp. 478–504). New York: Oxford University Press.

Harris, Grant, and Marnie Rice. 2006. "Treatment of Psychopathy: A Review of Empirical Findings." In Christopher Patrick (ed.), *Handbook of Psychopathy, First Edition*. New York: The Guilford Press: 555–572.

Hart, Stephen, and Alana Cook. 2012. "Current Issues in the Assessment and Diagnosis of Psychopathy (Psychopathic Personality Disorder)." *Neuropsychiatry* 2 (6): 497–508. doi:10.2217/Npy.12.61

Hicks, Brian and Laura Drislane. 2018. "Variants ('subtypes') of psychopathy." In Christopher Patrick (ed.), *Handbook of Psychopathy, Second Edition* (Vol. 555–572). New York: The Guilford Press: 297–332.

Jurjako, Marko, and Luca Malatesti. 2018. "Neuropsychology and the Criminal Responsibility of Psychopaths: Reconsidering the Evidence." *Erkenntnis* 83: 1003–1025.

Kazantzis, Nikolaos, Mark Reinecke, and Arthur Freeman. 2010. *Cognitive and Behavioral Theories in Clinical Practice*. New York: Guilford Press.

Larsen, Rasmus. 2018. "False Positives in Psychopathy Assessment: Proposing Theory-Driven Exclusion Criteria in Research Sampling." *European Journal of Analytic Philosophy* 14 (1): 33–52.

Lilienfeld, Scott. 2007. "Psychological Treatments That Cause Harm." *Perspectives on Psychological Science* 2 (1): 53–70. doi:10.1111/j.1745–6916.2007.00029.x

Lilienfeld, Scott, and Michell Widows. 2005. *Psychopathic Personality Inventory—Revised: Professional Manual*. Lutz: Psychological Assessment Resources.

Lyon, David, James Ogloff, and Stephanie Shepherd. 2016. "Legal and Ethical Issues in the Assessment of Psychopathy." In Carl Gacono (ed.), *The Clinical and Forensic Assessment of Psychopathy: A Practitioner's Guide, Second Edition*. New York: Routledge: 193–216.

Maibom, Heidi. 2014. "To Treat a Psychopath." *Theoretical Medicine and Bioethics* 35 (1): 31–42.

Mathieu, Cynthia, and Paul Babiak. 2016. "Corporate Psychopathy and Abusive Supervision: Their Influence on Employees' Job Satisfaction and Turnover Intentions." *Personality and Individual Differences* 91: 102–106.

McCord, William, and Joan McCord. 1964. *The Psychopath: An Essay on the Criminal Mind*. Princeton, NJ: Van Nordstrand.

Niveau, Gerard, and Ida Welle. 2018. "Forensic Psychiatry, One Subspecialty with Two Ethics? A Systematic Review." *BMC Medical Ethics* 19 (1): 1–10. doi:10.1186/s12910-018-0266-5

Otto, Randy, and Kirk Heilbrun. 2002. "The Practice of Forensic Psychology: A Look Toward the Future in Light of the Past." *American Psychologist* 57 (1): 5–18. doi:10.1037/0003–066X.57.1.5

Patrick, Christopher, Don Fowles, and Robert Krueger. 2009. "Triarchic Conceptualization of Psychopathy: Developmental Origins of Disinhibition, Boldness, and Meanness." *Development and Psychopathology* 21 (3): 913–938. doi:10.1017/S0954579409000492

Pickersgill, Martyn. 2009. "NICE Guidelines, Clinical Practice and Antisocial Personality Disorder: The Ethical Implications of Ontological Uncertainty." *Journal of Medical Ethics* 35 (11): 668–671. doi:10.1136/jme.2009.030171

Polaschek, Devon. 2011. "High-Intensity Rehabilitation for Violent Offenders in New Zealand: Reconviction Outcomes for High- and Medium-Risk Prisoners." *Journal of Interpersonal Violence* 26 (4): 664–682. doi: 10.1177/0886260510365854

Polaschek, Devon, and Tadgh Daly. 2013. "Treatment and Psychopathy in Forensic Settings." *Aggression and Violent Behavior* 18 (5): 592–603. doi:10.1016/j.avb.2013.06.003

Polaschek, Devon, and Elizabeth Ross. 2010. "Do Early Therapeutic Alliance, Motivation, and Stages of Change Predict Therapy Change for High-Risk, Psychopathic Violent Prisoners?" *Criminal Behaviour Mental Health* 20 (2): 100–111. doi:10.1002/cbm.759

Polaschek, Devon, and Jeniffer Skeem. 2018. "Treatment of Adults and Juveniles with Psychopathy." In Christopher Patrick (ed.), *Handbook of Psychopathy, Second Edition*. New York: The Guilford Press: 710–731.

Reidy, Dennis, Megan Kearns, Sarah Degue, Scott Lilienfeld, Greta Massetti, and Kent Kiehl. 2015. "Why Psychopathy Matters: Implications for Public Health and Violence Prevention." *Aggression and Violent Behavior* 24: 214–225. doi:10.1016/j.avb.2015.05.018

Rice, Marnie, Grant Harris, and Catherine Cormier. 1992. "An Evaluation of a Maximum Security Therapeutic Community for Psychopaths and Other Mentally Disordered Offenders." *Law and Human Behavior* 16 (4): 399–412. doi:10.1007/bf02352266

Ronson, Jon. 2011. *The Psychopath Test: A Journey Through the Madness Industry*. New York: Riverhead Books.

Rush, Benjamin. 1972. *Two Essays on the Mind: An Enquiry into the Influence of Physical Causes upon the Moral Faculty, and on the Influence of Physical Causes in Promoting an Increase of the Strength and Activity of the Intellectual Faculties of Man*. New York: Brunner, Mazel Publishers.

Salekin, Randall T. (2002). "Psychopathy and therapeutic pessimism: Clinical lore or clinical reality?" *Clinical Psychology Review* 22 (1): 79–112. doi:10.1016/S0272-7358(01)00083-6

Salekin, Randall, Courtney Worley, and Ross Grimes. 2010. "Treatment of Psychopathy: A Review and Brief Introduction to the Mental Model Approach for Psychopathy." *Behavioral Sciences & the Law* 28 (2): 235–266. doi:10.1002/bsl.928

Serin, Ralph, Shelley Brown, and Angela Wolf. 2016. "The Clinical Use of the Hare Psychopathy Checklist—Revised (PCL-R) in Contemporary Risk Assessment." In Carl Gacono (ed.), *The Clinical and Forensic Assessment of*

Psychopathy: A Practitioner's Guide, Second Edition. New York: Routledge: 293–310.

Seto, Michael, and Howard Barbaree. (1999). "Psychopathy, treatment behavior, and sex offender recidivism." *Journal of Interpersonal Violence* 14 (12): 1235–1248. doi:10.1177/088626099014012001

Sewall, Lindsay, and Mark Olver. 2019. "Psychopathy and Treatment Outcome: Results From a Sexual Violence Reduction Program." *Personality Disorders-Theory Research and Treatment* 10 (1): 59–69. doi:10.1037/per0000297

Sherren, Reg. (Writer). 2016. *The Secrets of Oak Ridge.* In C. B. Corporation (ed.), Canada: Canadian Bradcast Corporation.

Skeem, Jennifer, and David Cooke. 2010. "Is Criminal Behavior a Central Component of Psychopathy? Conceptual Directions for Resolving the Debate." *Psychological Assessment* 22 (2): 433–445. doi:10.1037/a0008512

Skeem, Jennifer, Devon Polaschek, and Sarah Manchak. 2009. "Appropriate Treatment Works, But How? Rehabilitating General, Psychopathic, and High-Risk Offenders." In Jeniffer Skeem, Kevin Douglas, and Scott Lilienfeld (eds.), *Psychological Sciene in the Courtroom: Consensus and Controversy* (pp. 358–384). New York: Guilford Press.

Skeem, Jennifer, John Monahan, and Edward Mulvey. 2002. "Psychopathy, Treatment Involvement, and Subsequent Violence Among Civil Psychiatric Patients." *Law and Human Behavior* 26 (6): 577–603. doi:10.1023/A:1020993916404

Smith, Shannon, John Edens, John Clark, and Allison Rulseh. 2014. "So, What Is a Psychopath?" Venireperson Perceptions, Beliefs, and Attitudes About Psychopathic Personality. *Law and Human Behavior* 38 (5): 490–500. doi:10.1037/lhb0000091

Sörman, Karolina, John Edens, Shannon Smith, Olof Svensson, Katarina Howner, Marianne Kristiansson, and Hakan Fischer. 2014." Forensic Mental Health Professionals' Perceptions of Psychopathy: A Prototypicality Analysis of the Comprehensive Assessment of Psychopathic Personality in Sweden." *Law and Human Behavior* 38 (5): 405–417. doi:10.1037/lhb0000072

Stone, Alan. 2008. "The Ethical Boundaries of Forensic Psychiatry: A View from the Ivory Tower." *Journal of the American Academy of Psychiatry and the Law Online* 36 (2): 167.

Stratton, John, Kent Kiehl, and Robert Hanlon. 2015. "The Neurobiology of Psychopathy." *Psychiatric Annals* 45 (4): 186–194.

Suedfeld, Peter, and P. Bruce Landon. 1978. "Approaches to Treatment." In Robert Hare and Daisy Schalling (eds.), *Psychopathic Behavior: Approaches to Research.* Chichester, UK: Wiley: 347–376.

Tennent, Gavin, Duncan Tennent, Herbert Prins, and Anthony Bedford. 1993. "Is Psychopathic Disorder a Treatable Condition?" *Medicine Science and the Law* 33 (1): 63–66. doi:10.1177/002580249303300111

van Stralen, Karlijn, Vianda Stel, Johannes Reitsma, Friedo Dekker, Carmine Zoccali, and Kitty Jager. 2009. "Diagnostic Methods I: Sensitivity, Specificity, and Other Measures of Accuracy." *Kidney International* 75 (12): 1257–1263. doi:https://doi.org/10.1038/ki.2009.92

Walsh, Tiffany, and Zach Walsh. 2006. "The Evidentiary Introduction of Psychopathy Checklist-Revised Assessed Psychopathy in US Courts: Extent and Appropriateness." *Law and Human Behavior* 30 (4): 493–507. doi:10.1007/s10979-006-9042-z

Werner, Kimberly, Lauren Few, and Kathleen Bucholz. 2015. "Epidemiology, Comorbidity, and Behavioral Genetics of Antisocial Personality Disorder and Psychopathy." *Psychiatric Annals* 45 (4): 195–199. doi:10.3928/00485713-20150401-08

Wolin, Sheldon. 1963. "Violence and the Western Political Tradition." *American Journal of Orthopsychiatry* 33 (1): 15–28. doi:10.1111/j.1939-0025.1963.tb00355.x

Wong, Stephen, Audrey Gordon, Deqiang Gu, Kathy Lewis, and Mark Olver. 2012. "The Effectiveness of Violence Reduction Treatment for Psychopathic Offenders: Empirical Evidence and a Treatment Model." *International Journal of Forensic Mental Health* 11 (4): 336–349. doi:10.1080/14999013.2012.746760

Wong, Stephen, and Mark Olver. 2015. "Risk Reduction Treatment of Psychopathy and Applications to Mentally Disordered Offenders." *CNS Spectrums* 20 (3): 323–331.

Yang, Min, Stephen Wong, and Jeremy Coid. 2010. "The Efficacy of Violence Prediction: A Meta-Analytic Comparison of Nine Risk Assessment Tools." *Psychological Bulletin* 136 (5): 740–767. doi:10.1037/a0020473

15 Reducing Medical Errors Through Simulation

An Ethical Alternative for Training Medical Practitioners

T.J. Broy, Maureen Hirthler, Robin Rockhold and Ralph Didlake

Ethics of Medical Education

The ethical issues surrounding training new physicians are not new. Traditional teaching is based upon didactics, observation, and graduated practice. It has always been a challenge to balance the rights of patients to competent care with the need for trainees to gain experience. Supervising physicians alone have borne the responsibility for determining when a student or resident was prepared for independent decision-making or action. No standardization across medical schools and residencies existed; the style and amount of training varied widely (Beck 2004, 2139). The accepted dictum of "See one, do one, teach one" often prevailed, with residents teaching skills to medical students and other residents (Cooke et al., 2006, 1342). No policies and procedure manuals or examples of best practices existed. From history taking and physical examination through procedures, there was little direct supervision or feedback. Practice was on real patients. Patients were often unaware of the level of training or the experience level of their providers.

As the field of bioethics has expanded, medical schools and residencies are redesigning their curricula to provide optimal treatment and to ensure patient safety and well-being while still allowing for adequate training experience (Miles et al. 1989). The increased demand for patient safety has also pushed educational institutions to rethink the medical education system (Swanwick 2013, 4). Recent attention to preventable medical errors has also led to increased scrutiny of training practices and a discussion of the acceptable risk of human error. In many cases, this results in less actual experience for trainees. The competing values of the need for appropriately training new physicians and ensuring patient safety are often in conflict.

It is essential, then, to understand the principles of ethics which should guide our actions. There are several frameworks by which to analyze the subject of medical ethics. The four principles of Beauchamp and Childress—autonomy, non-maleficence, beneficence, and justice—form the basis of the field (Page 2012).

Autonomy, described as deliberate self-rule, requires us to consult people and obtain their agreement before we embark on a course of action (Gillon 1994, 185). The days of paternalistic treatment decisions should be over. Autonomy mandates true informed consent and a respect for the patient's decision, even when it conflicts with our own value system. It also requires us to not deceive patients, and to keep confidential the information shared with us. All of this is facilitated by good communication skills and the provision of adequate information. This respect for autonomy is called "shared decision making" (Charles, Gafni, and Whelan 1997).

In medical education, autonomy provides the patient with the right to know the training and skill level of their providers and to decide the degree, if any, in which they participate in the education of medical students and residents. It is essential to recognize that patients, especially those who are disadvantaged, are not training subjects. It also requires us to respect patients' education, economic and social status, and life-style choices, and provide optimum care within that framework.

Beneficence and non-maleficence are closely related. These are often summarized as "Do what is best for the patient" or "Do no harm," but multiple complex obligations are involved (Gillon 1994, 185). We must be certain that we can provide, to the best of our ability, the benefits we are stating. We need to be clear about the risks of a certain course of treatment, as well as the probabilities of success or failure. This information has to be based on effective and current medical research and implies life-long continuing education. We must be open-minded to innovations in patient care and treatment, even if they are not consistent with our training or experience, without blindly accepting new medications or procedures without due diligence in reviewing and understanding the studies that support their efficacy.

Research protocols must be rigorously analyzed by multidisciplinary boards such as an Institutional Review Board (IRB), which should be composed of ethicists, non-medical representatives, and clergy if so indicated, along with the scientists and health-care providers. Informed consent should be written and in detail. Risks and benefits (or the lack of personal benefit) must be explained in clear and unambiguous language.

All physicians and trainees are human; errors will be made. The ethical obligations associated with beneficence and non-maleficence require that we aggressively pursue methods to decrease the chance of harm to a patient through inadequate skill or knowledge. And yet, we must train new physicians, and some of this training must be done on human beings. The principle of informed consent again plays a key role.

Justice is perhaps the most difficult principle and can be summarized as the moral obligation to act on the basis of fair adjudication between competing claims (Gillon 1994, 185). Most often, we think of this in terms of distributive justice; that is, the fair distribution of scarce resources.

But medical education presents its own dilemma. We must balance an individual's right to choose not to participate in the training of doctors, our imperative to reduce the risk of harm to our patients, and our moral obligation to train medical students and residents to be the best physicians they can in order to provide care for future patients.

Simulation-Based Medical Education

Simulation-based medical education (SBME) can be a valuable tool in mitigating these ethical tensions and practical dilemmas (Ziv et al. 2003, 783). SBME can be defined as any educational activity that utilizes simulative aids to replicate clinical scenarios (Ziv, Ben-David, and Ziv 2005, 193). Recently a new formulation of an ethical framework for simulation-based medical education has been proposed: best standards of care and training, error management and patient safety, patient autonomy, and social justice and resource allocation (Ziv, Ben-David, and Ziv 2005, 195).

The challenge of SBME is to simulate an authentic health-care environment. This includes the physical set-up, the human set-up and the medical tasks to be performed (Ziv, Ben-David, and Ziv 2005, 195). The degree of fidelity depends upon the type of training needed. Simple task trainers may be used for routine procedural skills such as phlebotomy, urinary catheter placement, and endotracheal intubation. High-fidelity simulators are more suited to team training (Reese et al. 2010). These simulations may have operating rooms, an ICU, an ER, labor and delivery suites, post-anesthesia care units, and regular patient rooms, all providing verisimilitude. Manikins are computerized and interactive. Sham medications are placed in actual vials and boxes (clearly labeled "Not for patient use"). Working defibrillators are employed. Occasionally, simulations such as mass casualty drills occur "in-situ," that is, in the actual patient care areas (Sørensen et al. 2017).

The traditional focus on cognitive skills has slighted the skills of communication, management, cooperation, and interviewing. Deficiencies in these skills are causal factors in adverse outcomes (Ziv et al. 2003, 785). Simulation is an excellent technique for team training, also called crisis resource management (CRM). Team composition should mirror the actual care process; that is, nurses, pharmacists, respiratory technicians, and support staff. External stressors such as gunfire, sirens, distracting bystanders, or unnecessary or belligerent health-care professionals can also be added. Multiple complex tasks can be required simultaneously, adding to the potential for error and extending the value of the simulation.

Harm to patients as a byproduct of training or lack of experience is justified only after maximizing approaches that do not put patients at risk (Ziv et al. 2003, 785). SBME promotes standardization of both teaching practice and student experience; education is independent of preceptor variation and patient availability. Students are exposed to best practices for all common procedures and scenarios and are allowed unlimited time to become proficient. In addition, simulation provides exposure to a variety of clinical presentations and procedural contexts, including atypical patterns, rare diseases, critical incidents, near misses, and crises, many of which students and residents may not encounter during training (Ziv et al. 2003, 786). Students then interact with actual patients at a point further along in their education after significant practice of processes and procedures.

Error Management and Patient Safety

Students and residents often handle medical mistakes by denial, discounting personal responsibility, or distancing themselves from the consequences (Ziv et al. 2003, 787). Realistically simulating the anxiety, confusion, and lack of confidence that are characteristic of extreme and hard-to-handle cases is an important means to improve the ability to cope with similar instances in real life (Ziv, Ben-David, and Ziv 2005, 197). SBME provides a safe environment in which students can commit medical errors without causing harm to patients. Mishaps can be reviewed openly without concern of liability, blame or guilt. Trained facilitators are essential, though, to respond to the responses the scenario may cause in learners. Facilitators' recognition of extreme distress or triggers related to the scenario may lead to a change in the exercise or even to its termination. Skilled debriefing, using a validated tool such as DASH (Debriefing Assessment for Simulation in Health care), is imperative for placing these experiences into an educational and supportive context (Simon 2010).

SBME also provides a unique opportunity for multidisciplinary team training. In the past, training has been provided within each discipline, for example, medicine, nursing, respiratory. Current medical care is much more complex and occurs more often in team settings. It is essential for team members to understand their roles and the roles of others. Knowing in advance what is available and where it is located reduces anxiety and adds efficiency to the team. Practicing the cooperative and complimentary division of labor can lead to smoother, safer, and more efficacious patient care.

SBME can provide same or next-day critical incident debriefing. The interaction between providers, information systems, and technology can be assessed and system errors identified. A repeat scenario can be presented to make corrections and experience better understanding of the event. SBME is also valuable for continuing medical education and recertification in American Heart Association courses such as ACLS and PALS. Specialty boards such as Anesthesiology and Surgery are increasingly utilizing simulation in their certification process.

Nishisaki et al. reviewed the available literature on the question of whether simulation improves patient safety. They used a conceptual framework consisting of four elements: self-efficacy, competence, operational performance, and patient outcome (Nishisaki, Keren, and Nadkarni 2007, 228). Self-efficacy involves a trainee's self-assessment of their confidence in performing a particular procedure or providing care. Although simulation clearly improves self-efficacy, there is poor correlation of the self-assessment with competence or communication skills (Nishisaki, Keren, and Nadkarni 2007, 229). Competence, the capability to perform a particular task, can be measured during simulation by either a detailed checklist or by independent observation and global scoring of real-time or video recorded scenarios. Multiple studies suggest that simulation-based assessment can measure competence with good reliability and validity, and can improve trainee procedural and team-based competence (Nishisaki, Keren, and Nadkarni 2007, 230).

Operational performance measures should be able to quantify the degree to which competent care in simulation training sessions translates into competence in real clinical care settings (Nishisaki, Keren, and Nadkarni 2007, 231). There have been few studies in this area. However, there is some good evidence that procedural simulation improves actual operational performance in clinical settings (Nishisaki, Keren, and Nadkarni 2007, 232). The difficulty of controlling clinical variables is obvious. Recently, SBME has been shown to improve team operational performance and clinical outcomes in a meta-analysis by Boet (2014).

Patient Autonomy

Medical science has violated the ethical principle of autonomy throughout its history. Incidents such as the *Tuskegee Study of Untreated Syphilis in the Negro Male* and the case of Henrietta Lacks are just two examples of medical hubris. Medical education has both instilled and perpetuated this disregard of the patient's right to self-determination. In clinical settings, patients were often unaware of being cared for by medical students or residents. Unconscious, heavily sedated, or dead patients have been vulnerable subjects for medical training (Ziv et al. 2003, 787). True informed consent has been lacking, especially in regard to procedures. SBME provides an effective mode of training that leads to enhanced patient autonomy by significantly reducing the need to "practice" on real patients. In addition, skill trainers provide a variety of pathological conditions that may not be seen with frequency in live patients, reducing the number of patients that need to be examined in order to encounter pathology. The use of simulated patients can improve the quality of informed consent, especially in ethically challenging situations (Ziv et al. 2003, 787).

Social Justice and Resource Allocation

The basic bioethical principle of distributive justice requires that citizens equally share risks of medical innovation, research, and practitioner training (Ziv et al. 2003, 787). SBME can significantly reduce the overall need for human subjects in medical education, and improve awareness of ethical considerations in patient care. Historically, via the county hospital system, the disadvantaged have borne the burden of medical training. Academic health centers still see a disproportional number of the underprivileged population. SBME can reduce the proportion of indigent patients used as objects of medical training (Ziv et al. 2003, 788). Simulation training with standardized patients provides trainees with the opportunity to practice the allocation of finite resources (hospital capacity), scarce resources (organs for transplant), and physician time (critical care areas). Patient-care priorities can also be explored through simulated triage and mass-casualty drills.

Weighing the Costs and Benefits of SBME

The benefits to patient safety and reduction in number and significance of medical errors make for compelling points in favor of SBME. While it might be tempting to draw the conclusion that all medical training ought to incorporate at least some aspects of SBME, further reflection allows for a more nuanced give and take. How great a share of medical resources ought to be devoted to wide spread implementation of SBME? How much of a medical student's training should be replaced or augmented with simulations? What effects might SBME have in addition to reducing the risk of medical errors? Are there any downsides? While confronting these questions will muddy the waters surrounding SBME, the resulting analysis will allow for a more comprehensive and holistic understanding of the ethical impacts of SBME.

As with the implementation of any medical protocol, SBME carries along with it both costs and benefits. The benefits, as has been discussed, include reducing the risk of medical errors resulting from medical students training on live patients. Getting clear on the costs is more difficult. While incorporating SBME into medical training programs is becoming more common, rigorous investigation of the economic costs and benefits of these programs is much more rare (Lin et al. 2018, 151). With the considerable costs associated with constructing and operating health-care simulation centers, any justification of that cost must be made in terms of benefits relative to alternatives. Further research is necessary to establish, in economic terms, how much benefit is gained by implementing SBME over other alternatives. Any investment into SBME involves the allocation of resources which might be utilized elsewhere in the health-care system.

Insistence on considering only economic costs and benefits, however, might paint an incomplete picture. For example, SBME may have an effect on a medical student's ability to learn how to better communicate with patients and colleagues. Reducing the complexity of the training environment (when repeatedly using simulation to train one task-specific skill, for example) may have unintended consequences on how those skills can be applied in new contexts, how those skills are passed on to others, or in many other unpredictable effects on a medical student's training (Nestel et al. 2018, 140).

Because SBME relies on developing simulation technologies like robotics and virtual reality, many of its effects are difficult to predict. This further complicates the ethical analysis of whether or not we ought to implement SBME universally. This is not a problem unique to SBME, however. All ethical analysis involving emerging technologies operates under this sort of opacity. Because medicine as a whole relies on emerging technologies, medical ethics will always involve some amount of uncertainty regarding future developments or the effects of technological applications. Because of promised or possible benefits, this is less a reason to avoid these developments than it is a reason to urge care in developing the policies which surround them.

Simulation-based medical education separates a significant portion of teaching and learning from patient care. It has distinct ethical benefits by reducing the exposure of real people to health-care practitioners in the early stages of training or when learning new clinical skills. Encounters with real patients will always remain essential in exposing health providers to the full complexity of practice (Ziv et al. 2003, 788). Although SBME can never replace actual experience with patients, it can allow trainees to approach patients after obtaining exposure to various skills and practicing those skills to a degree of comfort.

Research in the ethics of robotics has pointed out the importance of human interaction in medical care (Sharkey and Sharkey 2011, 273–277). The motivations driving the development of robot care givers is much like the motivation driving the adoption of SBME, greater efficiency and risk reduction. If these concerns are given consideration to the exclusion of all others, however, there are possible negative effects for the patient. For example, feeling empathy from health-care providers is an important factor in patients reporting satisfaction with their health care (Naidu 2009, 367–368). Empathetic behavior may also lead to benefits such as increased diagnostic accuracy, increased patient compliance, and increased quality of life (Neumann et al. 2011, 996). With such benefits, training empathy seems like an important goal for any medical training. There are serious questions surrounding the study of empathy in medicine. For example, is it really empathy we need to train in order to see these results or merely empathetic physician behavior (Smajdor et al. 2011)? The concerns raised here do not depend on answers to these questions, but will apply equally to these different conceptions of empathy in medical practice.

Intuitively, reducing a medical student's exposure to patients might inhibit the development of empathy. If substantial parts of medical training are replaced by simulation, we might worry about medical students' ability to develop empathy. As we learn in the ethics of robotics literature, technological developments do not merely concern our interactions with technology, but also our interactions with other people (Borenstein and Pearson 2011, 252). Research on empathy in medical students actually shows decreases in empathy after beginning clinical interactions with patients (Neumann et al. 2011, 998). Hypotheses explaining why this is involve medical students deploying defense mechanisms to avoid distressing interactions. Because medical students are not prepared to encounter their patients' suffering, they retract away from it. At first glance, it seems that this problem will not be solved by implementation of SBME. Whether or not decreasing patient interactions by replacing training procedures with simulations will exacerbate this problem requires further research.

A first attempt at a solution is to add simulations on top of the existing amount of patient interaction medical students have during their training. This has both the benefit of preserving the value of medical students gaining experience interacting with patients and the benefit of delaying that interaction until the students have gained the skills provided by SBME. The problem with this solution is similar to many problems in medicine, the distribution of resources. This involves both financial and institutional resources, for example, having a fully functional simulation center in addition to traditional training infrastructure, and the investment of medical students' time. Modern medical school curricula are already under pressure to include all of a medical student's necessary training so that either extending the time required or replacing another part of the curriculum in order to train both with patients and on simulations is unlikely a feasible solution.

A more feasible solution might be found upon reflecting on the possibility of using simulations themselves to train empathy and thus both dispel the possible negative effects of SBME on empathy development and help to solve the broader problem of training empathy in medical students. As Neumann et. al hypothesize, medical students report a decrease in empathy after beginning clinical interactions with patients because they are unprepared for those interactions (Neumann et al. 2011, 998). SBME may have a role to play in preparing medical students for these interactions and so widespread implementation of SBME may well increase rather than decrease empathy. Research has been conducted using both standardized patients and virtual patients finding increases in trainers' assessments of empathetic patient interactions (Teherani, Hauer, and O'Sullivan 2008; Kleinsmith et al. 2015; Foster et al. 2016). Using simulations in this way allows for medical students to take their time assessing the situation and formulating their responses without the pressure of patients waiting for an answer. By learning first how to interact empathetically in this low stakes environment, students may then be better prepared to interact empathetically in their interactions with actual patients.

This proposal draws skepticism from some regarding whether training empathy is possible at all without interacting with actual patients outside of a context of assessment (Perrella 2016). Empathy, it might be thought, is a trait independent of the particular details of a physician's interactions with her patients. Not all of the benefits of empathy are had by acting empathetically. Inauthentic empathy might carry its own costs in terms of losing trust or developing resentment in the doctor–patient relationship. Thus, training empathetic interactions can only truly be had by training empathy in addition to particular actions. It is not enough for a physician to behave as if they empathize with their patient, rather they ought to actually empathize with their patients and then behave accordingly.

This objection to implementing SBME in training empathy only holds insofar as the end goal of using simulated patients is an empathetic physician. The benefits of SBME in training empathy, however, need not be so direct. Even if it is true that simulations could never train true empathy, that they help give more medical students the tools necessary to develop empathy over the course of their clinical experience is reason enough to support it. While empathetic behavior is not the whole of genuine empathy, it is certainly a part. If SBME can contribute to this part of developing empathy, then many of the goods of widespread implementation of SBME relating to empathy will be had. If empathy is impossible to train, then this is not a special problem for SBME. By these lights, all medical training protocols will struggle to promote the development of genuine empathy. SBME may help to gain ground where there is ground to be gained.

Training evaluations of SBME are based upon Kirkpatricks' four levels of training evaluation (Kirkpatrick and Kirkpatrick 2016). Level 1 is reaction. This is an assessment of how trainees felt about the evaluation. Level 2, learning, assesses trainees' knowledge, skills, and confidence before and after the simulation. Valid studies of the benefits of SBME are currently limited to trainee self-assessment and competence in the actual training scenario, that is, Levels 1 and 2. Level 3 studies behavioral change, and Level 4 analyzes outcomes. These are very difficult to do in the area of SBME. Studies of improvement in clinical outcomes, error reduction, and patient safety have been limited at single institutions both in homogeneity of students, facilitators, and the institution, and heterogeneity of patient populations and institutional protocols. Multi-center trials, with set practices, procedures, and assessment tools are needed. Meta- analysis of studies with clinical outcome data will be essential in order to make conclusions that justify the expense in money and time for a fully operational simulation center.

SBME has the potential to decrease the number and effects of patient errors, to facilitate open exchange in training situations, to enhance patient safety, and to decrease the reliance on vulnerable patients for training (Ziv et al. 2003, 787). In those ways it can enhance adherence to the basic principles of medical ethics—autonomy, non-maleficence, beneficence, and justice.

Future Directions for SBME

Simulations provide a valuable resource for medical education. Medical students can learn important technical, personal, and cooperative skills without endangering patients. The widespread employment of simulations in medical training is not without costs. Whether or not the advantages of simulation-based medical education are worth those costs is an important question. While an attempt at a preliminary answer has been made here, a conclusive answer will require more research into the effects of SBME as well as a full accounting of the associated costs.

The future development of SBME will also require more attention. Technical advances in fields like VR and robotics are sure to have an impact on medical simulations. What is less clear is how that development should be guided. At first pass, it seems plausible to promote increasing fidelity in medical simulations. But as the history of SBME shows, the pursuit of fidelity is not so clear cut as a long term goal (Rosen 2008; Bradley 2006). For example, standardized patients offer a high degree of fidelity insofar as interactions with standardized patients closely resemble real clinical interactions. They do not, however, provide the sort of skill training that a low-fidelity task trainer would. Concerns like this motivate some to reject fidelity as a desirable feature of medical simulations in favor of features like functional correspondence (Hamstra et al. 2014). The future of SBME will rely on research aimed at answering questions like these. So too, therefore, will any ethical benefits of SBME rely on answers to questions like these.

Works Cited

Beck, Andrew H. 2004. "The Flexner Report and the Standardization of American Medical Education." *Journal of the American Medical Association* 291 (17): 2139–2140.

Boet, Sylvain, Dylan Bould, Lilia Fung, Haytham Qosa, Laure Perrier, Walter Tavares, Scott Reeves, and Andrea Tricco. 2014. "Transfer of Learning and Patient Outcome in Simulated Crisis Resource Management: A Systematic Review." [In eng]. *Canadian Journal of Anesthesia* 61 (6): 571–582.

Borenstein, Jason and Yvette Pearson. 2011. "Robot Caregivers: Ethical Issues across the Human Lifespan." In Patrick Lin, Keith Abney and George Bekey (eds.), *Robot Ethics: The Ethical and Social Implications of Robotics*. Cambridge: MIT Press: 251–266.

Bradley, Paul. 2006. "The History of Simulation in Medical Education and Possible Future Directions." *Medical Education* 40: 254–262.

Charles, Cathy, Amiram Gafni, and Tim Whelan. 1997. "Shared Decision-Making in the Medical Encounter: What Does it Mean? (or It Takes at Least Two to Tango)." *Social Science & Medicine* 44 (5): 681–692.

Cooke, Molly, David M. Irby, William Sullivan, and Kenneth M. Ludmerer. 2006. "American Medical Education 100 Years After the Flexner Report." *The New England Journal of Medicine* 355: 1339–1344.

Foster, Adriana, Neelam Chaudhary, Thomas Kim, Jennifer Waller, Joyce Wong, Michael Borish, Andrew Cordar, Benjamin Lok, and Peter Buckley. 2016. "Using Virtual Patients to Teach Empathy: A Randomized Controlled Study to Enhance Medical Students' Empathetic Communication." *Simulation in Healthcare* 11 (3):181–189.

Gillon, Ranaan. 1994. "Medical Ethics: Four Principles Plus Attention to Scope." [In eng]. *BMJ* 309 (6948): 184–188.

Hamstra, Stanley J., Ryan Brydges, Rose Hatala, Benjamin Zenderjas, and David A. Cook. 2014. "Reconsidering Fidelity in Simulation-Based Training." *Academic Medicine* 89 (3): 387–392.

Kirkpatrick, James, and Wendy Kirkpatrick. 2016. *Kirkpatrick's Four Levels of Training Evaluation*. Alexandria, VA: ATD Press.

Kleinsmith, Andrea, Diego Rivera-Gutierrez, Glen Finney, Juan Cendan, and Benjamin Lok. 2015. "Understanding Empathy Training with Virtual Patients." *Computers in Human Behavior* 52: 151–158.

Lin, Yiqun, Adam Cheng, Kent Hecker, Vincent Grant, and Gillian Currie. 2018. "Implementing Economic Evaluation in Simulation-based Medical Education: Challenges and Opportunities." *Medical Education* 52: 150–160.

Miles, Steven H., Laura Weiss Lane, Janet Bickel, Robert M. Walker, and Christine K. Cassel. 1989. "Medical Ethics Education: Coming of Age." *Academic Medicine* 64 (12): 705–714.

Naidu, Aditi. 2009. "Factors Affecting Patient Satisfaction and Healthcare Quality." *International Journal of Health Care Quality Assurance* 22 (4): 366–381.

Nestel, Debra, Victoria Brazil, and Margaret Hay. 2018. "You Can't Put a Value on That . . . Or Can You? Economic Evaluation in Simulation-based Medical Education." *Medical Education* 52: 139–141.

Neumann, Melanie, Friedrich Edelhäuser, Diethard Tauschel, Martin Fischer, Markus Wirtz, Christiane Woopen, Aviad Haramati, and Christian Scheffer. 2011. "Empathy Decline and Its Reasons: A Systematic Review of Studies with Medical Students and Residents." *Academic Medicine* 86 (8): 996–1009.

Nishisaki, Akira, Ron Keren, and Vinay Nadkarni. 2007. "Does Simulation Improve Patient Safety? Self-Efficacy, Competence, Operational Performance, and Patient Safety." *Anesthesiology Clinics* 25 (2): 225–236.

Page, Katie. 2012. "The Four Principles: Can They Be Measured and Do They Predict Ethical Decision Making?" *BMC Med Ethics* 13: 10.

Perrella, Andrew. 2016. "Fool Me Once: The Illusion of Empathy in Interactions with Standardized Patients." *Medical Teacher* 38 (12): 1285–1287.

Reese, Cynthia E., Pamela R. Jeffries, and Scott A. Engum. 2010. "Learning Together: Using Simulations to Develop Nursing and Medical Student Collaboration." *Nursing Education Perspectives* 31 (1): 33–37.

Rosen, Kathleen R. 2008. "The History of Medical Simulation." *Journal of Critical Care* 23: 157–166.

Sharkey, Noel and Amanda Sharkey. 2011. "The Rights and Wrongs of Robot Care." In Patrick Lin, Keith Abney and George Bekey (eds.), *Robot Ethics: The Ethical and Social Implications of Robotics.* Cambridge: MIT Press: 267–282.

Simon, R. 2010. "Debriefing Assessment for Simulation in Healthcare (Dash) © Rater's Handbook." Center for Medical Simulation, Boston, MA. Retrieved from https://harvardmedsim.org/wpcontent/uploads/2017/01/DASH.handbook.2010.Final.Rev.2.pdf.2010.

Smajdor, Anna, Andrea Stöckl, and Charlotte Salter. 2011. "The Limits of Empathy: Problems in Medical Education and Practice." *Journal of Medical Ethics* (37): 380–383.

Sørensen, Jette Led, Doris Østergaard, Vicki LeBlanc, Bent Ottesen, Lars Konge, Peter Dieckmann, and Cees Van der Vleuten. 2017. "Design of Simulation-Based Medical Education and Advantages and Disadvantages of In Situ Simulation Versus Off-Site Simulation." *BMC Medical Education* 17 (20).

Swanwick, Tim. 2013. "Understanding Medical Education." In Tim Swanwick (ed.), *Understanding Medical Education: Evidence, Theory and Practice, Second Edition.* London: Wiley Blackwell.

Teherani, Arianne, Karen E. Hauer, and Patricia O'Sullivan. 2008. "Can Simulations Measure Empathy? Considerations on How to Assess Behavioral Empathy via Simulations." *Patient Education and Counseling* (71): 148–152.

Ziv, Amitai, Shaul Ben-David, and Margalit Ziv. 2005. "Simulation Based Medical Education: An Opportunity to Learn from Errors." *Medical Teacher* 27 (3): 193–199.

Ziv, Amitai, Paul Wolpe, Stephen Small, and Shimon Glick. 2003. "Simulation-Based Medical Education: An Ethical Imperative." *Academic Medicine* 78 (8): 783–788.

Contributors

Editors

Fritz Allhoff, J.D., Ph.D., is Professor in the Department of Philosophy at Western Michigan University and Community Professor in the Program in Medical Ethics, Humanities, and Law at Western Michigan University Homer Stryker M.D. School of Medicine. He received his Ph.D. in Philosophy from the University of California, Santa Barbara and his J.D., *magna cum laude*, from the University of Michigan Law School. Following law school, he clerked for the Honorable Chief Justice Craig F. Stowers of the Alaska Supreme Court and was a Fellow in the Center for Law and the Biosciences at Stanford Law School. His bioethics work has been published in the *American Journal of Bioethics*, *Cambridge Quarterly of Healthcare Ethics*, and *Kennedy Institute of Ethics Journal*. His monographs have been published by Oxford University Press, University of Chicago Press, and Routledge.

Sandra L. Borden, Ph.D., is Professor in the School of Communication and Director of the Center for the Study of Ethics in Society at Western Michigan University. Her work has been published in several scholarly books and journals, including *The Handbook of Mass Media Ethics*, the *Journal of Media Ethics*, *Journalism: Theory, Practice & Criticism*, *Communication Monographs*, and *Communication Theory*. Her book, *Journalism as Practice: MacIntyre, Virtue Ethics and the Press*, won the 2008 Clifford G. Christians Ethics Research Award and the National Communication Association's 2008 top book award in applied ethics. She has served as a member of the executive board of the Association for Practical and Professional Ethics and as Associate Editor of the journal *Teaching Ethics*. Borden, who teaches ethics and media criticism, earned her Ph.D. in Mass Communications from Indiana University.

Contributors

T.J. Broy, M.A., is a philosophy instructor at Western Michigan University, teaching classes including biomedical ethics, aesthetics, philosophy of art, and ethics of war. He is interested in ethics in many applied fields, including medicine, law, and business, as well as more abstract questions, such as how to attain virtue and various meta-ethical debates. Broy has presented his research at several regional and national conferences on topics, such as the relation between music, emotion differentiation and virtue, and the political implications for the Electoral College in light of its current state and our conceptions of democracy.

Ralph Didlake, M.A., M.D., F.A.C.S., is Vice Chancellor for Academic Affairs at the University of Mississippi Medical Center, Jackson, Mississippi. In 2008, he was appointed director of the UMMC's newly established Center for Bioethics and Medical Humanities, a position he continues to hold. He is also professor of surgery. He is a fellow of the American College of Surgeons and is a member of the American Society for Bioethics and Medical Humanities, among many other organizations. He is the author of numerous peer-reviewed articles, book chapters, and abstracts and has been principal investigator or co-investigator on a number of National Institutes of Health and foundation grants.

Jeremy R. Garrett, Ph.D., is Research Associate in Bioethics at Children's Mercy Bioethics Center, Children's Mercy Kansas City with appointments in the Departments of Pediatrics and Philosophy at the University of Missouri-Kansas City. Garrett has edited or co-edited three books, published more than three dozen articles in peer-reviewed journals and books, presented research more than 75 times at conferences and other professional venues around the world, and been PI of research on the ethics of returning individual results in genomic research (NHGRI R21HG006613). He has served on both an Institutional Review Committee and a Hospital Ethics Committee and began serving on the Data Safety Monitoring Board for the Prevention of Pediatric Asthma for the National Heart, Blood, and Lung Institute (NHLBI) in May 2018.

Kelsey Gipe, Ph.D., is Lecturer in Philosophy at the University of Maryland, College Park. Her primary areas of research are biomedical ethics and ethical theory, with a particular emphasis on ethical problems that arise in the context of clinical care. Her current research projects focus on distribution of scarce health resources, medical aid in dying, and issues of informed consent pertaining to vulnerable patient populations, such as children, the elderly, and the mentally ill.

Luke Golemon, M.A., is a Ph.D. student in the Department of Philosophy at the University of Arizona. His interests are in metaethics, philosophy of science, and metanormativity, as well as biomedical ethics, including their intersection with law and religion. He has a keen interest in clinical ethics and the problems of inequity in medicine. He has participated in several sessions of Methodist Medical School's Roundtable program and has presented his research at several regional and national conferences. Golemon was also the lead developer of a biomedical ethics course at Western Michigan University, which will be deployed to approximately 1,000 students per year, across various colleges and professional backgrounds.

Maureen Hirthler, M.D., M.F.A., has just retired from being an Assistant Professor of Physical Diagnosis at the Lake Erie College of Osteopathic Medicine in Florida and the Director of Accreditation, Office of Interprofessional Simulation, Training, Assessment, Research, and Safety, University of Mississippi Medical Center, Jackson, Mississippi. She received her medical degree from Perelman School of Medicine at the University of Pennsylvania and has been in practice for more than 20 years. Her work has appeared in several journals, most recently in the *Yale Journal of Medical Humanities* and the University of Oklahoma School of Medicine's *Blood and Thunder*.

Alexander Hyun, Ph.D., is Assistant Professor at Minerva Schools at the Keck Graduate Institute. He received his B.A. in Philosophy at the University of California Berkeley, and his M.A. and Ph.D. in Philosophy at the University of Wisconsin-Madison. Hyun has published in *Journal of Philosophy*, *Journal of Ethics and Social Philosophy*, and *Religious Studies*. His research primarily focuses on issues related to moral error theory, moral realism, and practical normativity.

Megan Hyun, Ph.D., is Assistant Professor in the University of Nebraska Medical Center's Radiation Oncology department. She received her B.S. in Physics at Taylor University and her M.S. and Ph.D. in Medical Physics at the University of Wisconsin-Madison. Hyun has published in *Medical Physics*, *Journal of Applied Clinical Medical Physics*, and *Radiation Oncology*. Her research has focused on improving the safety and accuracy of radiation-based cancer treatments.

David Kyle Johnson, Ph.D., is Professor of Philosophy at King's College and also produces philosophy courses for *The Teaching Company*'s "The Great Courses." He specializes in logic and reasoning (both formal and scientific), metaphysics, and philosophy of religion. He has published in journals such as *Sophia*, *Religious Studies*, *Think*,

Philo, and *Science, Religion and Culture.* His latest publication was 11 entries for *Bad Arguments: 100 of The Most Important Logical Fallacies in Western Philosophy* (Wiley-Blackwell, 2018). His courses for "The Great Courses" include *Sci-Phi: Science Fiction as Philosophy* (2018), *The Big Questions of Philosophy* (2016), and *Exploring Metaphysics* (2014).

Rashmi Kudesia, M.D., M.Sc., is a practicing reproductive endocrinologist and infertility (REI) specialist at CCRM Fertility Houston in Houston, Texas, where she is also Director of Patient Education and Sugar Land Site Director, as well as Assistant Clinical Professor of Obstetrics & Gynecology at Houston Methodist Hospital. Kudesia completed her M.D. with honors from the Duke University School of Medicine, trained at Weill Cornell and Montefiore Medical Centers, and was previously on the faculty at the Icahn School of Medicine at Mount Sinai. Kudesia has held many national leadership roles in organized medicine, presented scientific research nationally and internationally, and received multiple awards and grants. She has regularly published peer-reviewed articles and book chapters, as well as editing a theme issue on reproductive medicine for the *American Medical Association Journal of Ethics.*

Rasmus Rosenberg Larsen, Ph.D., is Visiting Assistant Professor at the University of Toronto, Mississauga, where he lectures in Philosophy and Forensic Science. He is particularly interested in the role psychiatric disorders play in the collection and assessment of forensic evidence. His research interests fall broadly within philosophy of science, with a current focus on psychopathology and value theory. Larsen is also associated with the Open Biomedical Ontologies (OBO) Foundry, where he is currently working on a project that involves data integration between affective science and psychiatric diagnostics.

Leslie Ann McNolty, D.P.S., M.A., is Program Associate with the Center for Practical Bioethics and teaches bioethics at Kansas City University of Medicine and Biosciences. She received B.A. degrees, with Honors, in Philosophy and Political Science with a Secondary Degree in Women's Studies from Kansas State University before completing her M.A. in Philosophy from Rice University and her Doctorate of Professional Studies in Bioethics from Albany Medical College. Her research focuses on feminist bioethics with a special focus on women's reproductive health, birthing ethics, and maternal mortality. She has published previously in the *American Journal of Bioethics* and *Hastings Center Report* and presented her research at the American Society for Bioethics and Humanities Annual Meeting, among other venues.

Leah M. Omilion-Hodges, Ph.D., is Associate Professor in the School of Communication at Western Michigan University. Her research focuses on leadership and health communication within the larger context of organizational communication, allowing her to fuse her academic and industry experience. More recently, she has parlayed her leadership and group work within the palliative-care setting, working with national samples of practitioners to explore the nuances of this medical specialty. Her research has been featured on OncToday.com in addition to venues such as *Communication Yearbook*, the *International Journal of Business Communication*, the *Leadership Quarterly*, and *Health Communication*.

David Peña-Guzmán, Ph.D., is an Assistant Professor of Humanities and Liberal Studies at San Francisco State University. His research is at the intersection of the history and philosophy of science, animal studies, feminist philosophy, bioethics, and social theory. His work has appeared in journals such as *Foucault Studies*, *The Journal of French and Francophone Philosophy*, *Animal Sentience*, and *Hypatia*. Before joining SFSU, Dr. Peña-Guzmán was a postdoc at The Centre for Evolutionary Ecology and Ethical Conservation (CEEEC) in Ontario, Canada, and at the Johns Hopkins Berman Institute of Bioethics in Baltimore, MD.

Michael S. Pritchard, Ph.D., is Emeritus Professor of Philosophy at Western Michigan University, where he taught from 1968 to 2016. He served as director or co-director of WMU's Center for the Study of Ethics during 1985–2016 and as chair of WMU's Department of Philosophy for 15 years. In addition to his many published articles on ethical issues, his books include: *Teaching Ethics Across the Curriculum: Pedagogical Challenges*, co-editor (Springer 2018); *Engineering Ethics: Concepts and Cases*, 6th ed., co-author (Cengage 2018); *Obstacles to Ethical Decision-Making*, co-author (Cambridge University Press 2013); *Professional Integrity: Thinking Ethically* (University Press of Kansas 2007); and *Medical Responsibility: Paternalism, Informed Consent, and Euthanasia*, co-editor (Humana Press 1979).

Robert W. Rebar, M.D., is Professor and Founding Chair Emeritus of Obstetrics and Gynecology (OB/GYN) at the Western Michigan University Homer Stryker M.D. School of Medicine. Rebar has also taught at the University of California, San Diego, and Northwestern University, as well as served as Associate Executive Director of the American Society for Reproductive Medicine. He is a member of numerous professional societies, has served on the editorial boards of several journals and is currently an Associate Editor for *Journal Watch Women's Health* and *OB/GYN Clinical Alert*. Robert has contributed to many books, has authored more than 250 articles on menopause, fertility, and reproductive endocrinology, and has been the PI or co-PI for various grants from the National Institutes of Health.

Samuel Reis-Dennis, Ph.D., is Assistant Professor at Albany Medical College in the Department of Bioethics Education and Research. He received his B.A. in Philosophy from Cornell University, and his M.A. and Ph.D. in Philosophy from the University of North Carolina, Chapel Hill. From 2017 to 2019, he was a Hecht-Levi Postdoctoral Fellow in the Berman Institute of Bioethics at Johns Hopkins University. His research in ethics and moral psychology focuses on response to wrongdoing, and the connections between emotional attitudes and responsible agency. His work has appeared in philosophy and bioethics journals, including *The Australasian Journal of Philosophy*, *Philosophical Studies*, *The Journal of Medical Ethics*, and *The Hastings Center Report*.

Joel Michael Reynolds, Ph.D., is Assistant Professor of Philosophy at the University of Massachusetts, Lowell and the Rice Family Fellow in Bioethics and the Humanities at The Hastings Center. His research focuses on analyzing and improving biomedical practice and theory with respect to people with disabilities. He is the author or co-author of more than 20 peer-reviewed journal articles and book chapters appearing in outlets including the *American Journal of Bioethics*, *Hastings Center Report*, *Kennedy Institute of Ethics Journal*, and *AMA Journal of Ethics*. He is the author of *Ethics after Ableism: Disability, Pain, and the History of Morality* (University of Minnesota Press, forthcoming) and co-editor of *The Disability Bioethics Reader* (Routledge, forthcoming).

Robin Rockhold, Ph.D., F.A.P.E., is Professor and Deputy Chief Academic Officer at the University of Mississippi Medical Center, Jackson, Mississippi. He oversees the Office of Interprofessional Simulation, Training, Assessment, Research, and Safety. He is an active lecturer in the Schools of Medicine, Dentistry and Graduate Studies in the Health Sciences, with areas of concentration in cardiovascular agents, opioid analgesics, and drugs of abuse. An award-winning educator, Rockhold is a Fellow of the Academy of Pharmacology Educators, American Society of Pharmacology and Experimental Therapeutics.

Devora Shapiro, Ph.D., is Associate Professor of Philosophy at Southern Oregon University. She specializes in philosophy of science, feminist epistemology, and philosophy of medicine. Her previous work has centered on the articulation of non-propositional accounts of experiential knowledge, as well as critiques of the political and epistemic value of "objectivity." Her current work focuses on applying intersectional theory within the context of medical diagnosis and pharmaceutical trials, as well as in the philosophy of epidemiology.

Jordan Joseph Wadden, M.A., is a Ph.D. candidate in the Department of Philosophy at the University of British Columbia. His primary research areas are in bioethics and the philosophy of medicine, with a focus on issues of access to health care, exchanges between health-care providers and patients, and biotechnology. His recent work includes: a project on disability and human flourishing within the context of medical aid in dying at the Centre for Inclusion and Citizenship at UBC's Vancouver campus, and the development of a course for UBC Extended Learning where he taught health-care policy and ethics to Vancouver community members.

Index

Printed in the United States
by Baker & Taylor Publisher Services